Essentials
of
Clinical Nutrition

Essentials
of
Clinical Nutrition

ELAINE B. FELDMAN, M.D.
Professor of Medicine and Physiology and Endocrinology
Chief, Section of Nutrition
Medical College of Georgia
Augusta, Georgia

ESSENTIALS OF MEDICAL EDUCATION SERIES

DAVID T. LOWENTHAL, M.D., Ph.D. / Editor-in-Chief
Professor of Geriatric Medicine and Adult Development
Professor of Medicine and Pharmacology
Mt. Sinai School of Medicine
New York, New York

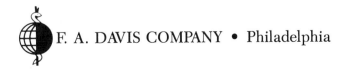 F. A. DAVIS COMPANY • Philadelphia

Printed in the United States of America

NOTE: As new scientific information becomes available through basic and clinical research, recommended treatments and drug therapies undergo changes. The author(s) and publisher have done everything possible to make this book accurate, up-to-date, and in accord with accepted standards at the time of publication. However, the reader is advised always to check product information (package inserts) for changes and new information regarding dose and contraindications before administering any drug. Caution is especially urged when using new or infrequently ordered drugs.

LIBRARY OF CONGRESS
Library of Congress Cataloging-in-Publication Data

Feldman, Elaine B., 1926-
    Essentials of clinical nutrition / Elaine B. Feldman.
       p.   cm. — (Essentials of medical education series)
    Includes bibliographies and index.
    ISBN 0-8036-3431-5
    1. Diet therapy.   2. Nutrition.   3. Nutrition disorders.
  I. Title.   II. Series.
    [DNLM: 1. Diet Therapy.   2. Nutrition.   3. Nutrition Disorders.
  orders.
    QU 145 F3125e]
    RM216.F42 1988
    613.2—dc19
    DNLM/DLC   88-3709
    for Library of Congress   CIP

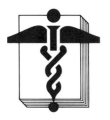

Preface

Clinical nutrition has achieved respectability and recognition as a discipline in medicine. While some current medical curricula may not include specific basic or clinical science courses in nutrition, the knowledge base in nutrition is necessary in order to understand the etiology, prevention, and treatment of disease. Nutrition support is a part of life support and is as vital as breathing or cardiac or renal function. Nutritional assessment and provision of an appropriate nutritional prescription are basic components of patient evaluation and care.

Whether nutrition is taught as a separate preclinical or clinical course, or nutritional principles are presented as part of other courses, a certain minimum body of nutritional knowledge, or competence, is necessary for the physician. These "essentials" are covered in this book. References to some more detailed texts and sources of information are provided.

The Chapters are organized under Sections encompassing basic principles of required nutrients and aspects of their molecular function, regulation, and food sources; nutritional assessment; the diet and nutrient intake; food hazards and fads; nutrition throughout the life cycle; modalities for nutritional support using therapeutic diets, enteral and parenteral nutrition; disorders of undernutrition and overnutrition; and nutritional aspects of diseases, nutrition-related organ failures, and trauma and critical care.

The brief case studies that illustrate the clinical entities all summarize patients cared for in recent years at the Medical College of Georgia. Recognition of these problems will continue to be relevant in clinical medicine. Most important is the need to think "nutritionally" with regard to primary patient care bringing to the bedside a basic, learned, intuitive and applied awareness. Appropriate concern for nutritional status must be taken for granted and implicit in health promotion, disease prevention, and patient care.

The material in this book should be useful not only to medical students, residents, and physicians, but also to other health practitioners, especially dentists and nurses. This text also should prove informative for students in undergraduate and graduate nutrition training or in dietetics.

In addition to the sources listed in the References (p. 561), the reader is referred to a variety of sources for additional and updated nutrition information: journals including the American Journal of Clinical Nutrition, Nutrition Reviews, the Journal of Nutrition, the Annual Review of Nutrition, the Journal of the American College of Nutrition; publications of the American Cancer Society, the American Diabetes Association, the American Heart Association (especially for materials for patient education); and government publications including reports of the Food and Nutrition Board, the Food and Drug Administration, the National Institutes of Health, and the Department of Agriculture.

The educator is referred to the *Guide to clinical nutrition teaching materials* (see References) that will be updated by the American Society for Clinical Nutrition every few years.

The author assumes full responsibility for the opinions expressed and the selections, omissions, and interpretations of the nutrition literature.

ELAINE B. FELDMAN, M.D.

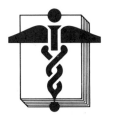

Acknowledgments

This book would not have been possible without the encouragement and assistance of my colleagues at the Medical College of Georgia: Drs. Terrence Kuske, Natalie McLeod, Diane Smith, and R. J. Teague; Mrs. Jane Greene and Mrs. Sandra Leonard; and the many medical students, residents, and fellows who previewed portions of the book. Many of my nutrition colleagues kindly read chapters and provided constructive criticism—thanks (and no responsibility for errors) go to Drs. Steve Heymsfield, Dick Rivlin, Dan Rudman, Rob Russell, and Noel Solomons. Other colleagues at MCG provided "in-house" review, including Drs. Tom Huff, Henry Middleton, Max Stachura, and Nancy Stead.

My career in nutrition began in the laboratory and clinic of Dr. David Adlersberg at Mount Sinai Hospital in New York and was fostered by Dr. Anne C. Carter at the State University of New York Downstate Medical Center. Dr. A. J. Bollet recruited me to the Medical College of Georgia where Dr. Kuske and I expanded nutrition teaching, service, and research in medicine. Dr. Paul Webster, Dean Fairfield Goodale, and President William Moretz provided further resources. Their interest and foresight established nutrition as a significant discipline at MCG.

The completion of this book was enabled by the hard work of industrious office assistant Ms. Frances Saddler and my skilled and efficient secretaries Mrs. Barbara Trill, Myra Cox, Ms. Theresa Hodge, and Rita Youngblood. Thanks also to Dr. Sylvia Fields, Linda Weinerman, and Bernice Wissler at F. A. Davis for their patience, understanding, and helpful editing.

Finally, no work such as this, over 4 years in preparation and development, could have been accomplished without the constant support, encouragement, and affection of my husband, Dr. Daniel Feldman, who made the ultimate sacrifice of making available to me *his* microcomputer word processor (complete with instructions, supervision, and graphics).

ELAINE B. FELDMAN, M.D.

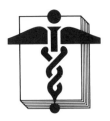

Contributors

DRUCY BOROWITZ, M.D.
Instructor of Pediatrics
University of Washington
Director, Failure to Thrive Clinic
Children's Hospital Medical Center
Seattle, Washington

JANE M. GREENE, M.S., R.D., L.D.
Research Scientist
Medical College of Georgia
Augusta, Georgia

SANDRA B. LEONARD, M.S., R.D., L.D.
Assistant Research Scientist
Medical College of Georgia
Augusta, Georgia

RALPH V. McKINNEY, Jr., D.D.S., Ph.D.
Professor and Chairman, Oral Pathology
Professor, Oral Biology
Medical College of Georgia
Augusta, Georgia

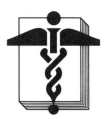

Contents

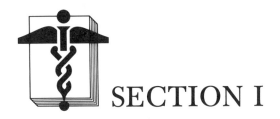 SECTION I

Basic Principles of Nutrition

Tell me what you eat, and I will tell you what you are.

Anthelme Brillat-Savarin, 1755–1826, *La Physiologie du Gout*, "Fundamental Truths" (tr. by R.E. Anderson as *Gastronomy as a Fine Art*).

In this section we deal primarily with the approximately 40 nutrients (water, energy, essential amino acids, essential fatty acids, vitamins, and minerals) considered essential for the maintenance of health; also we examine the procedure for evaluating a patient's nutritional status, ways of optimizing the diet, and the potential hazards posed by certain foods and by fads and myths.

In Chapter 1—**Essential Nutrients: Macronutrients and Energy**—we discuss the normal composition of the human body, including the variations in distribution of its components. In addition, the body's requirements for water, protein, amino acids, carbohydrates, and fat are explained. The chapter concludes with a general analysis of how the composition of body weight lost during a weight loss diet differs depending on the dietary regimen used.

Chapter 2—**Essential Nutrients: Vitamins and Minerals**—delineates the four fat-soluble and nine water-soluble vitamins and discusses their requirements in the daily diet, their sources and availability, and their metabolism. The chapter then covers the 15 essential minerals, including their sources and normal metabolism.

Chapter 3—**Nutritional Assessment**—first defines what nutritional assessment is, and then deals with its components: the medical and diet history, the physical examination, and the appropriate clinical laboratory tests. A discussion of how to apply the information thus gleaned concludes the chapter.

In Chapter 4—**Optimizing the Diet**—nutrients meeting daily requirements are translated into foods, consumed as meals, that compose the usual American diet. Among the subjects covered are sources of nutrient data, dietary guidelines, the four food groups, food composition and labeling, vegetarian diets, and diet for athletic activity.

In Chapter 5—**Food Additives, Toxins, and Hazards**—we present a straightforward look at the hazards that various foods can present, including the risks posed by food additives, environmental contaminants, food toxins, food allergies and intolerance, and food accidents.

Chapter 6—**Fads, Myths, and Quackery**—discusses the many myths relating to foods, and the fads and quackery that stem from some of these myths. In particular, we look at specific food fallacies and the corresponding facts, vitamin myths, unreliable nutritional services and practices, natural and organic foods, nutritional supplements, and fad diets.

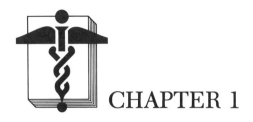

CHAPTER 1

Essential Nutrients: Macronutrients and Energy

BODY COMPOSITION

"You are what you eat," or more correctly, "what you eat **becomes** you." Regardless of its caloric content or balance of nutrients and molecules, the food we eat is digested, absorbed, transported, and metabolized to form and sustain our bodies.

Although the composition of the body can be specified in terms of the amount and distribution of nutrients, this composition is not static, but varies with gender and age. For example, the amount of body fat is proportionately higher in women (25 percent) than in men (12 percent), and the proportion increases in adults of both sexes with age (Fig. 1–1). At the same time, the lean body mass (the fat-free portion) decreases with age at a rate of approximately 3 kg every 10 years. These changes can be modified by food intake or exercise or both, since excess calories regardless of source—fat, carbohydrate, or protein—are stored in the body as fat. All these body proportions can be quantified through various means.

Total body weight is composed of water (one half to three fourths of total), fat, protein, carbohydrate, and minerals or ash (Table 1–1 and Fig. 1–2). Their proportions can be determined by measuring the body density by

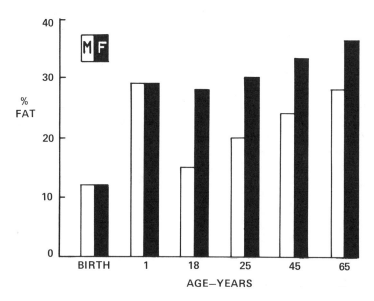

Figure 1–1. Body fat content throughout life. The proportion of fat in the body increases from birth to puberty, with a peak at age 1 year. Thereafter, fat content rises more in females. (Data derived in part from Friis-Hansen, B.: Hydrometry of growth and aging. In Brozek, J. (ed.): Human Body Composition. Pergamon Press, Oxford, 1965, p. 197.)

Table 1-1. APPROXIMATE PERCENTAGES OF WATER, FAT,
PROTEIN, ASH, AND CARBOHYDRATE IN THE BODY

Component	Percentage	Comment
Water	50–75%	Total body water can be measured with stable isotopes.
Fat (density 0.9)	15% (12% males, 25% females, in 18-yr-olds)	Half of the fat is located in the subcutaneous fat depots. This compartment represents calorie stores and can be estimated by skinfold thickness measurements (see Chapter 3) or by measurements of total body impedance or electrical conductivity. Fat tissue contains less than 10% water.
Protein	15%	The protein is divided primarily among muscle, assessed by arm muscle measurements and by creatinine excretion (see Chapter 3); skeleton; viscera, assessed by serum protein levels; and skin and extracellular components (see Table 1-2).
Ash	6%	
Carbohydrate	0.5%	

underwater weighing. The average adult body has a density of 1.06 g per cc. Because of their greater proportion of body fat, women's bodies have a lower average density (1.04 g per cc) than men's bodies (1.07 g per cc). Because muscle is denser than fat, the larger the lean body mass of an individual, the greater the body density.

Body mass can be further divided into the **extracellular** portion and the **cellular** or **cell mass** portion. These are approximately equal in size. The cellular part of the body consists of 60 percent muscle, 20 percent internal organs and blood cells, and 20 percent connective tissue. Body **structural (or somatic) protein,** of which **collagen** is the most abundant type, is found in muscle, bone, the internal organs, and skin, while **transport (visceral) proteins** are found in blood.

The minimal carbohydrate stores in the body are found primarily in muscle, liver, and blood. In muscle, carbohydrate is stored as **glycogen,** which is only available for use by that muscle. In contrast, carbohydrate stored in the liver (glycogen) is released to the circulation as free glucose and is available to all cells. The amount of stored carbohydrate will fill only about one-half day's energy needs. Thus, the body stores energy mostly in the form of fat, not carbohydrate. Because it can be stored with minimal water, fat is more energy dense and thus is a more efficient energy store.

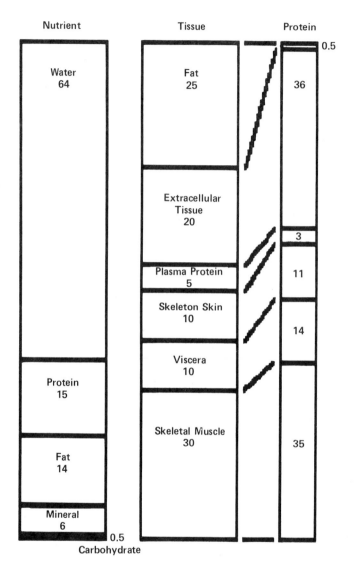

Figure 1–2. The major subdivisions of body composition. The height of the bar = 100 percent. The size of each divisin is proportional to its contribution to body weight. The relative proportion of total body protein contained in the tissue compartment also is indicated. Values are approximate.

FLUID AND ENERGY REQUIREMENTS

Fluid

Carbohydrate, fat, protein, and 1 to 4 liters of water enter the body each day in the form of ingested food and liquid to provide fuel for metabolic functions and nutrients essential for cellular growth and repair. The general requirement for water is about 1 ml per kcal ingested. In addition, approximately 8 liters of liquid are secreted daily into the gastrointestinal tract as a result of digestion.

- saliva (1 liter)
- gastric acid (2 liters)
- pancreatic and biliary juice (2 liters)
- intestinal juice (3 liters)

Most of this liquid is absorbed as it passes through the entire length of the digestive tract. Active sodium transport is the principal driving force for the absorption of water from the lumina of the small and large intestines. This sodium transport is followed by passive transport of chloride along its electrochemical gradient, and water follows sodium and chloride passively down the osmotic gradient created.

Energy Requirements

Energy expenditure is proportional to body size (see Table 3–3) and increases progressively from the basal to the resting state, and with increasing levels of activity and stress. The **basal metabolic rate** is the minimal rate of energy usage necessary to sustain life processes. This basal energy expenditure is measured in an awake person at complete rest in bed who has not eaten in 12 hours, such as one who has awakened from a night's sleep. Approximate energy expenditures for subjects at the various levels follow:

- **Resting** – 10 percent increase over basal (any conscious activity at all, including that within 3 hours of eating)
  Note: To accomplish usual activities while on complete bed rest, a patient will expend about 20 percent over basal.
- **Sedentary** – 30 percent over basal
- **Moderately active** – 50 percent over basal
- **Laboring** (heavy labor) – 100 percent over basal (work equivalent to walking 30 miles per day)
- **Fever** – 13 percent over basal per °C increase above normal
- **Major trauma, sepsis, and burns** (hypermetabolic states) – 35, 50, and 100 percent over resting, respectively (see Chapter 25)

Table 1–2. CALCULATION OF "IDEAL" BODY WEIGHT
(IBW) AND CALORIC REQUIREMENTS

1. **Calculate IBW**

	Men	Women
IBW at 60 inches of height, lb	106	100
Add per inches height >60, lb	6	5

   Example: Male, 67 inches height: 106 + (7 × 6) = 148 lb*

2. **Calculate basal calories required per day**
   Basal calories = IBW (lb) × 10
   Example: 148 × 10 = 1480 kcal

or

Harris-Benedict Equation

♂66.47 + 13.75 Wt (kg) + 5 Ht (cm) − 6.76 Age (yr)
♀655 + 9.46 Wt (kg) + 1.86 Ht (cm) − 4.68 Age (yr)

3. **Add for activity**

	Sedentary (Medical Student)	Moderate (Salesman)	Strenuous (Lumberjack)
% Basal calories	30	50	100

   Example: Moderate = 1480 + (0.5 × 1480) = 2220 kcal

---

*These calculations assume average, or medium, body frame. Add or subtract 10% for large or small frame, respectively. A simple method to assess body frame is to measure the wrist circumference by wrapping the thumb and middle finger of one hand around the other wrist. If the fingers meet, the frame is medium; if the fingers do not meet, the frame is large; if the fingers overlap, the frame is small (see Chapter 3).

(Adapted from Feldman, E.B., Greene, J.M., Kirchhofer, A.K.: Nutrition. In Taylor, R.B. (ed): Health Promotion: Principles and Clinical Applications. Appleton-Century-Crofts, New York, 1982, p. 162.)

Ideal Body Weight and Estimate of Energy Expenditure

For adults, the basal energy requirement can be estimated by multiplying the ideal body weight by 10 if the weight is in pounds or by 22 if it is in kilograms. As seen in Table 1–2, a gross estimate of "ideal" or desirable body weight for men and women can be determined relating body weight to height. In addition, the energy requirements for each sex can be estimated from the Harris-Benedict equation (Table 1–2), and from many other suggested formulas. Unfortunately, these calculations may be in error by as much as 1000 kcal.

Energy Expenditure and Respiratory Quotient

The amount of energy expended can be quantitated by measuring the heat produced by the body. This is **direct calorimetry**. Alternatively, **indirect calorimetry** may be used. In indirect calorimetry the patient breathes room air and the expired air is analyzed for O_2 and CO_2. The calculation requires knowledge of the volume of air breathed per unit time. Caloric expenditure is calculated from oxygen consumption and carbon monoxide production using the modified Weir equation:

$$kcal = 3.9 \times liter\ O_2\ used + 1.1 \times liter\ CO_2\ produced$$

The **respiratory quotient** (RQ) is the ratio of carbon dioxide production to oxygen consumption. RQ measurements represent the sum of metabolic processes in different organs and provide an estimate of the type of fuel being burned (fat and carbohydrate primarily—sometimes protein). If carbohydrate were being burned by the body as its main fuel, the RQ would be 1.0. If fat were dominant, the RQ would approach 0.7. For a typical American diet, the measured RQ is around 0.85, which indicates that a mixture of fat and carbohydrate is being used as the nonprotein source.

A typical American diet in 1980 (Table 1–3) contained 40 percent of its calories as fat, which supplies 9 kcal per g. Sixty percent of these calories came from animal sources, 40 percent from vegetable sources. Approximately half the calories in the diet were from carbohydrates, which yield 4 kcal per g. Of these, over half were from simple carbohydrates and the remainder from complex. Protein made up the remaining 10 percent of the calories in the diet. On the average, protein produces about 4 to 5 kcal per g. Seventy percent of the protein in the American diet was from animal sources and the rest from plants. (See Chapter 4 for recent changes in food consumption in the United States.)

Table 1-3. AMERICAN FOOD CONSUMPTION*

	% kcal	g	g
Carbohydrate	46	408	192 complex
			216 simple
Fat	42	169	98 animal
			71 vegetable
Protein	12	104	71 animal
			33 vegetable
Calories	3580		

*U.S. food supply per capita per day, 1980, U.S.D.A.

PROTEIN

Requirements

The **recommended dietary allowance (RDA)** represents a level of intake for most essential nutrients based on the amount that should meet the needs of at least 97.5 percent of the healthy population. Protein allowances are set at 0.8 g per kg of body weight per day; however, the usual high protein intake in the United States provides 1 to 2 g per kg body weight per day.

Essential or Indispensable Amino Acids

In addition to the requirement for protein in general, adults need as part of the daily diet eight amino acids that the body cannot make (Table 1-4). These are a source of nitrogen for the biosynthesis of other major protein constituents of the body such as enzymes, hormones, and antibodies. They include the five large **neutral branched chain** and **aromatic amino acids:** leucine, isoleucine, valine (branched chain, BCAA); phenylalanine and tryptophan (aromatic, AAA); the **dibasic** amino acid, lysine; sulfur-containing methionine; and threonine. Histidine, tyrosine (which can be made from phenylalanine), and cystine (which can be made from methionine) are required in the diet of infants. Arginine, glycine, alanine, and proline may be necessary for optimum protein status. These amino acids can be synthesized by humans, but not in sufficient quantities to provide optimal health and growth for infants or some sick children and adults. Recent studies indicate that the healthy adult may require higher levels of the essential amino acids than earlier recommendations.

Metabolism of the amino acids may be via the Krebs cycle for **gluconeogenesis** (isoleucine, valine, phenylalanine, tryptophan, lysine, methionine, threonine, histidine, arginine). The ketogenic amino acids (leucine, iso-

Table 1-4. ESSENTIAL AMINO ACIDS AND DAILY
REQUIREMENTS (ADULTS)

	Required g/day
Leucine	1.1
Isoleucine	0.7
Valine	0.9
Phenylalanine	1.1
Tryptophan	0.5
Lysine	0.8
Methionine	1.1
Threonine	0.5

Table 1-5. FOODS AS SOURCES OF ESSENTIAL
AMINO ACIDS

Food Source	% Total N, From Essential Amino Acids	Biologic Value of Protein
Eggs, milk	35	93
Meat, fish, beans, peas	30–34	76
Lentils, cornmeal, white potato, rice	25–29	67
Barley, wheat flour, peanuts	20–24	40

leucine, phenylalanine, lysine) are so called because they generate acetyl-CoA. The large neutral amino acids compete with each other for transport.

Other amino acids used in protein synthesis can be made in the body from various precursors and are therefore termed **nonessential** or dispensable in the diet. These amino acids (i.e., glutamic acid, aspartic acid, serine, glutamine, asparagine) cannot be converted to the essential amino acids.

The proportion of essential amino acids required to be present in the dietary proteins as a source of nitrogen for cellular functions varies from at least 20 percent to maintain health in adults to 36 to 43 percent to maintain health as well as to sustain growth in infants and children. The necessary proportions of individual essential amino acids must be provided in the same meal. The adult who is repleting body protein requires about the same proportion of essential amino acids as the infant (40 percent).

Eggs and milk provide the highest proportion of essential amino acids, followed by meat, fish, legumes, and finally vegetables, grains, and nuts (Table 1-5). Their biologic value varies similarly. The ideal amino acid pattern, such as that in egg albumin, provides an optimum proportion of the essential amino acids for protein synthesis (Table 1-6). In cereals, the proportion of lysine is low and methionine is high, whereas in legumes lysine is high and methionine low. Eating a combination of proteins from different sources,

Table 1-6. IDEAL AMINO ACID PATTERN

	%
Leucine	7.0
Isoleucine	4.0
Valine	5.0
Phenylalanine (+ Tyrosine)	6.0
Tryptophan (limiting in corn)	1.0
Lysine (limiting in wheat)	5.5
Methionine (+ Cystine)	3.5
Threonine	4.0

including solely plants, can provide a diet that contains adequate amounts of all essential amino acids (Table 1–6). Therefore, to improve the protein quality of strict vegetarian diets, foods with **complementary** proteins should be eaten, such as combining tortillas (grain low in lysine, high in methionine) with beans (legume high in lysine, low in methionine) (see Chapter 4). Since lacto-ovovegetarians consume milk and eggs, they should achieve an adequate intake of essential amino acids.

Amino Acid Metabolism

Muscle is the main site of catabolism of the branched chain amino acids (BCAA). Insulin acts on the muscle to promote the entry of BCAA; protein synthesis in muscle increases, and protein breakdown decreases. With impairment in insulin activity, the utilization of BCAA by muscle decreases. The availability of the BCAA for protein synthesis by other tissues (i.e., liver, brain) is related inversely to their utilization by muscle. The transport system of large neutral amino acids across cell membranes involves both the BCAA and the **aromatic amino acids** (AAA), which compete for binding sites. As these amino acids may serve as precursors for neurotransmitters, alterations in the availability of BCAA and changes in the ratio of BCAA to AAA in the blood may have important effects on brain function and play a role in hepatic encephalopathy (see further on and Chapter 22).

The plasma amino acid pool is available for clinical sampling and characterization (Table 1–7). Plasma amino acids can be quantified after chromatographic separation and colorimetric and fluorometric visualization of derivatives. Despite some limitations in extrapolating plasma values to intracellular amino acid metabolism, the plasma amino acid profile provides important insight into disorders and deficiencies of amino acid metabolism and nutriture. For example, inborn errors in urea cycle enzymes can be diagnosed by the plasma amino acid pattern. Organ failure leads to widespread metabolic disorders that may be accompanied by changes in levels of multiple plasma amino acids reflecting loss of several enzyme pathways. Because of the liver's important role in amino acid metabolism, liver failure leads to marked changes in the amino acid profile. In cirrhosis there is an elevation of the amino acids degraded exclusively by the liver [i.e., the sulfur containing (methionine) and AAA] and a decrease in the amino acids that are predominantly metabolized extrahepatically (i.e., the BCAA) (see Chapter 22).

Dietary factors play a complex role in determining the plasma amino acid profile. Generally, when the dietary intake of an amino acid is low, plasma levels are low, and begin to rise when tissue levels approach adequacy owing to provision of the amino acid. Plasma levels of amino acids plateau at excessive intakes, indicating degradation of excess dietary amino acids. When the relative amounts of essential amino acids in the diet are altered so that one amino acid is severely limiting, there is a decrease in that amino acid in

Table 1-7. PLASMA AMINO ACID PATTERN

Amino Acid	Normal, μM Range	Normal, μM Mean
Fluoro-phenylalanine	—	—
Aspartic acid	8–42	25
Glutamic acid	25–87	56
Asparagine	29–65	47
Serine	70–168	119
Glutamine	404–688	546
Histidine	76–144	110
Glycine	137–385	261
Threonine	117–261	189
Alanine	241–523	382
Taurine	30–94	62
Arginine	41–121	81
Tyrosine	27–99	63
Methionine	19–51	35
Valine	152–328	240
Tryptophan	27–75	51
Phenylalanine	49–85	67
Isoleucine	38–118	78
Leucine	85–209	147
Ornithine	60–116	88
Lysine	103–263	183

plasma. Often there is an accompanying increase in nonessential amino acids that cannot be utilized for protein synthesis because of the relative deficiency of the limiting amino acid. In kwashiorkor, a syndrome of protein deficiency in children, there is a decline in the plasma levels of all the essential amino acids (plus tyrosine and arginine) regardless of the limiting amino acid in the protein food, resulting in the so-called kwashiorkor pattern. Most of the nonessential amino acids are not decreased and some may be abnormally high (see Chapter 13). Dietary factors other than amino acids also affect the plasma amino acid profile. Dietary glucose suppresses circulating BCAA levels preferentially, stimulating insulin release and insulin-mediated transport of the BCAA into muscle.

Digestion and Absorption

The small intestine normally absorbs all of the ingested protein after it has been digested into small peptides and amino acids, which are then actively transported into the portal blood. Gastric pepsin action yields large peptones, and pancreatic peptidases rapidly hydrolyze these products of digestion into dipeptides and tripeptides. The final digestion of amino acids occurs in the microvilli of the intestinal brush border by dipeptidases. Dipeptides and tripeptides are absorbed by active mechanisms that are more rapid than absorption of amino acids. Peptide absorption is independent of sodium.

Amino acids are absorbed with specificity from the intestinal lumen. Only naturally occurring L–amino acids are actively transported, with the exception of D-methionine. Amino acid transport is coupled with sodium transport, exactly analogous to coupled sodium and monosaccharide transport.

There are at least four different amino acid transport mechanisms for classes of basic, neutral, acidic, and imino acids as well as specific transport for some individual amino acids (methionine/phenylalanine). A sodium-independent mechanism for amino acid transport also exists. Basic amino acids are absorbed more easily than neutral amino acids. Glutamic and aspartic acids are transaminated to alanine during absorption.

Absorption of small peptides and amino acid normally is nearly complete at the end of the jejunum. It is important to be aware of the variety of inborn errors of amino acid transport in the intestine and the renal tubule.

Nitrogen Balance

A healthy adult should have a daily nitrogen intake that at least equals the amount of nitrogen that is lost in order to maintain nitrogen equilibrium or positive balance. Nitrogen balance can be used to evaluate whether the subject is in an anabolic (nitrogen retention) or catabolic (nitrogen loss) state (Table 1–8). Nitrogen balance measures the difference between intake (I) and output (O), where the intake is the protein content of the diet and the output is the nitrogenous end products, excreted mainly in urine and feces (unabsorbed protein), with a fairly constant amount (less than 2 g daily) through skin, breath, nasal secretion, hair, menses, and semen. Skin losses of nitrogen represent about 10 percent of the value of the fecal nitrogen excretion.

Table 1–8. NITROGEN BALANCE

N Intake (I) —	N Output (O) =	Balance (I−O)
Diet (Protein ÷ 6.25)	Urine	Positive (I > O)
	Urea Nitrogen	Equilibrium (I = O)
	Nonurea Nitrogen	Negative (I < O)
	Feces	
	Skin	
	Miscellaneous	

Nitrogen output in healthy individuals on usual diets totals between 8 and 15 g per day. Nitrogen in urine is excreted primarily as urea nitrogen (UUN, 6 g) and also as nonurea nitrogen (NUN, 1.5 g), with their usual ratio 4:1 (Table 1–9). Urea nitrogen is the primary reflection of body protein metabolism. Excretion of 1 g of urea in urine requires about 50 ml water. The nonurea nitrogen components include ammonia, creatinine, and uric acid. Creatinine excretion is proportional to the lean body mass, namely muscle, with 1 mg creatinine in urine equivalent to 18 g of muscle. (See Chapter 3 for the creatinine/height index in nutritional assessment.)

An easy way to estimate nitrogen balance in clinical situations is to use the formula:

$$\frac{\text{Protein intake}}{6.25} \; - \; [(1.25 \times \text{UUN}) + 2 \text{ to } 3]$$

For this calculation, we need to measure protein intake (average nitrogen content 16 percent) and urinary urea nitrogen excretion. Nitrogen balance is positive when intake exceeds output. Nitrogen is retained by the body, protein is synthesized, and excess protein calories are used to synthesize fat for storage. There are no protein stores as such in the body; excess input can be used for anabolism (repletion) or as fuel. Nitrogen balance is negative when intake is less than output; the result is nitrogen loss. Body protein breaks down to yield an energy substrate to provide calories and maintain gluconeogenesis.

Urinary nitrogen components vary with the protein and calorie intake (Table 1–9). With fasting, the proportion of urinary nitrogen excreted as urea declines, whereas that excreted as ammonia (and glutamine) increases. With prolonged starvation, total nitrogen excretion falls markedly. With a low protein but adequate caloric intake, urea falls still further and the proportion of urinary nitrogen excreted as creatinine rises; total urinary nitrogen decreases markedly. During high protein intake, the total nitrogen increases significantly, with the proportion as urea also increased.

Table 1–9. URINARY NITROGEN COMPONENTS

	Dietary Regimen				
Compound	Usual	Fasting 4–5 Days	Starvation Prolonged	Low Protein kcal Adequate	High Protein
Total N_2, g/24 hr	8–15	9	4	4	17
Urea, %	80+	75	11	62	88
Ammonia, %	5	12	54	11	3
Creatinine, %	14	4	35	17	4
Uric acid, %		2		2	1

Protein-Nitrogen Relations

Although protein on average contains 16 percent nitrogen, the proportion of nitrogen in food proteins varies from 15.7 percent nitrogen in milk proteins to 19 percent nitrogen in protein from nuts. To convert nitrogen to protein, multiply by 6.25. The lean body mass (muscle, viscera) is about 21 percent protein (the balance is water), which calculates to about 3 percent nitrogen. We can thus calculate that 1 g nitrogen is equivalent to approximately 30 g lean body mass:

1	×	6.25	÷	0.21	≈	30
(g nitrogen)		(conversion factor N to protein)		(protein content)		(g lean body mass)

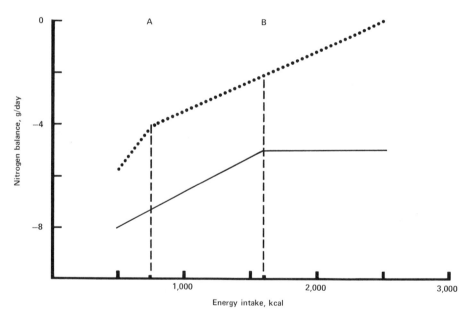

Figure 1-3. An increase in energy intake from 800 (*A*) to 1600 kcal (*B*) results in improved nitrogen balance at low (*solid line*) and adequate (*dotted line*) levels of protein intake. At the low protein intake increments in energy intake beyond 1600 kcal (*B*) are not effective in improving nitrogen balance. (Adapted from Munro, H.N. and Allison, J. (eds): Mammalian Protein Metabolism. Academic Press, New York, 1965, p. 420.)

Protein-Energy Relations

Nitrogen balance is related both to the energy intake and to the protein content of the diet. When the diet is deficient in protein, nitrogen equilibrium is **not** achieved, regardless of the energy intake. When no protein is provided, the individual remains in negative nitrogen balance even if the energy intake increases from about 700 to 2500 kcal (Fig. 1–3). Similarly, at a low energy intake (17 to 50 percent of requirements), despite increasing protein intake from the equivalent of 4 to 9 g of nitrogen per day, the person remains in negative nitrogen balance (Fig. 1–4). At 3000 kcal intake of a mixed carbohydrate and fat diet, the person achieves nitrogen balance at an intake of about 8 g of nitrogen daily. The protein level required to achieve nitrogen balance is related inversely to the calorie level; thus nitrogen balance is achieved at a lower protein intake if the energy intake is higher (e.g., more than 50 percent of requirements). In healthy, eating individuals the optimal calorie-to-nitrogen ratio approximates 300:1.

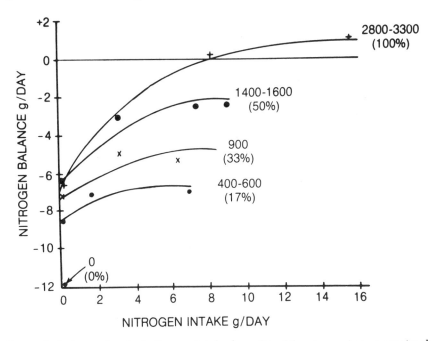

Figure 1–4. At any level of nitrogen intake from 0 to 15 g, increasing energy intake from 500 to 3000 kcal (indicated to the right of the isobar) improves nitrogen balance. At any level of energy intake, increasing nitrogen intake improves nitrogen balance, but only when energy intake exceeds 50 percent of daily expenditure (number in parentheses below range of energy intake) does nitrogen balance become positive. (From Greene, H.L., Holliday, M.A., and Munro, H.M.: Clinical Nutrition Update: Amino Acids. American Medical Association, Chicago, 1977, p. 49, with permission.)

CARBOHYDRATES

Nutrient Interconversions

Carbohydrates are a cheap and available dietary source of energy, derived primarily from plant sources. Excess carbohydrate calories are stored as triglycerides, which are synthesized in the liver and adipose tissue.

Total breakdown of glucose yields acetate, which can be used to synthesize fatty acids. Glucose can be used to synthesize the nonessential amino acids, while amino acid breakdown products can serve as precursors for glucose synthesis (gluconeogenesis). Long chain fatty acids are not converted directly to synthesize glucose (see Fig. 13–1). Fatty acid oxidation first yields acetate, which then can be used for synthesis.

Types of Carbohydrates in Foods

Complex polysaccharides (see Table 1–3) include mainly dextrins and starches, which are digestible forms of complex polysaccharides. Nondigestible fiber and partially digestible fiber account for 3 percent and 2 percent, respectively, of the dietary carbohydrate intake.

Simple or refined carbohydrates account for most of the dietary carbohydrate, with the disaccharide sucrose providing 60 percent of refined carbohydrate calories, and lactose, glucose, and fructose providing the remainder. The refined carbohydrates are essentially "empty calories," that is, without

Table 1-10. DIETARY SOURCES OF FIBER

Nondigestible (Not Absorbed)	
Structural Component of Plant Cell Wall	
Cellulose	Unpeeled apples and pears, stalks, grains, all bran, fresh carrots, brazil nuts
Lignin	Fruits (pears), all bran, toasted whole wheat bread, fried or browned potatoes
Partially Digestible	
Noncellulose	
Hemicellulose	Onions, legumes, all bran, beets, eggplant, radishes
Pectin	Fruits (skins), potatoes, cabbage
Algal (polysaccharides)	Seaweed
Gums, mucilages	Guar, beans, oatmeal, sesame seeds

any associated minerals or vitamins. Sucrose has been associated with a variety of diseases, but to date the only certain relationship is with dental caries. Refined sugars are usually eliminated from the diet in controlling body weight in obese subjects (see Chapter 16). Commercial use of corn syrup added for sweetening food products is increasing, as fructose (found in corn syrup) is sweeter per unit weight than sucrose (found in cane sugar, beet sugar).

Dietary **fiber** can be classified into nonabsorbed, nondigestible structural components of plant cell walls (cellulose, lignin) and partially digestible noncellulose fibers, which include hemicellulose, pectin, algal mucilages, and gums. Some dietary sources of fiber are provided in Table 1–10. Dietary fiber may shorten transit time and have a favorable effect in lowering blood sugar and lipids. In addition, foods containing high fiber provide satiety and may therefore be of value in the control of obesity. (See also Chapters 1, 18, and 19.)

Digestion and Absorption

Dietary carbohydrates are digested in the duodenum by the enzymes pancreatic amylase and some intestinal amylase. The products of digestion are primarily the disaccharides (maltose and isomaltose), maltotriose, some α-dextrins, and small amounts of the monosaccharides (glucose, galactose, and fructose). Only monosaccharides can be absorbed across the intestinal mucosa into the portal blood, as the intestinal mucosa is relatively impermeable to the disaccharides. Disaccharides are digested into monosaccharides and absorbed simultaneously at the brush border or microvilli of the intestinal mucosal columnar epithelial cells. The disaccharidases (maltase, lactase, and sucrase) and α-dextrinase are located in the brush border. Digestion by the brush border enzymes yields glucose, galactose, and fructose, which are transported across the intestinal mucosa into the general circulation.

Glucose presents about 80 percent of the total monosaccharide load to be transported, with about three fourths of that glucose derived from digested starch and the remaining derived from digested sucrose (19 percent) and lactose (6 percent). The major portion of glucose is transported by an energy-requiring process of active transport. Glucose transport and sodium transport are coupled. Absorption of glucose occurs mainly in the upper third of the intestine. Galactose represents about 5 percent of total monosaccharide absorbed and is also absorbed primarily by active transport. Fructose absorption (the remaining 15 percent of total monosaccharide absorbed) does not involve metabolic energy even though a specific carrier system is involved in a passive facilitated transport process. Carbohydrates are thereby normally absorbed in the duodenum and the proximal half of the jejunum.

FATS

Food Sources

Animal product sources of fat in the typical American diet include meats (34 percent), dairy products (12 percent), and animal fat per se (8 percent). The rest of the dietary fat comes predominantly from vegetable fats and oils, with a small proportion from legumes and cereals. More than 40 percent of dietary fat is ingested as visible fat. Thus, the first step in trying to reduce the fat intake, if advisable, is to eliminate visible fat and fatty meats in the diet.

The visible fat in the diet is provided as either monounsaturated or polyunsaturated liquid oils, primarily of vegetable origin. Fish oils, of animal origin, are also highly polyunsaturated. The other sources of visible fat (shortening, margarine, butter, lard, and tallow) are solid fats composed of saturated fatty acids and may be of vegetable (palm or coconut oils) or animal origin.

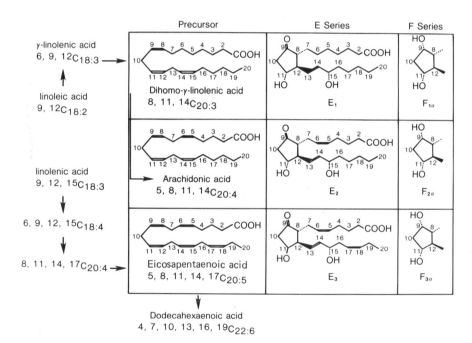

Figure 1–5. Prostaglandins of the E and F series, subseries $_{1,2,3}$, and their fatty acid precursors. The sequence of fatty acids derived from linoleic acid are the n-6 or omega-6 series, whereas those derived from linolenic acid are the n-3 or omega-3 series.

Essential Fatty Acids

The only dietary fat that is definitely proven essential in humans is the fatty acid linoleic acid, ingested primarily from liquid vegetable oils. It is converted to arachidonic acid in the body. The families of polyunsaturated fatty acids are precursors for the various prostaglandins (Fig. 1–5) and other biologically important eicosanoids which among others play a role in platelet aggregation, coronary artery dilation and constriction, and blood pressure regulation. Some of these fatty acids with unique biologic function are obtained from fish oils. The characteristic fatty acid composition of fats and oils in the American diet is provided in Chapter 19 (see Fig. 19–10).

Digestion and Absorption

Digestion of fats occurs in the intestine primarily by pancreatic lipase. Fat is absorbed more slowly than carbohydrate, reaching a peak in blood at about 3 hours, in contrast to a glucose load which peaks within one-half hour after ingestion. Long chain fatty acids and monoglycerides are solubilized in mixed micelles with conjugated bile acids. These are absorbed in the small intestine and then re-esterified to triglycerides, which combine with specific

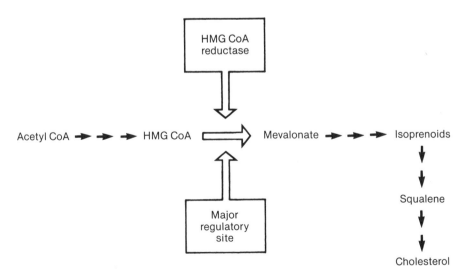

Figure 1–6. Simplified schema of cholesterol synthesis from acetate. The rate limiting step is the conversion of β-hydroxy beta methylglutaryl CoA (HMG CoA) to mevalonic acid, catalyzed by HMG CoA reductase.

proteins, cholesterol, and phospholipids to form lipoprotein particles called chylomicrons. These particles are released into the lymphatic circulation and delivered into the blood. (See Chapter 19 for a discussion of lipoprotein metabolism.) Shorter chain fatty acids (C_{12} and lower) are absorbed directly into the portal circulation. This simpler, faster pathway makes the so-called medium chain fats (MCT) useful in patients with fat malabsorption syndromes (see Chapter 21). About 95 percent of the fat ingested is absorbed.

Cholesterol

The typical American diet contains 300 to 450 mg of cholesterol (180 to 190 mg per 1000 kcal), about half of which is absorbed. In contrast to other fats, cholesterol comes only from animal sources and is synthesized from acetate most importantly in the liver and also in other tissues (Fig. 1–6). Cholesterol is not used for energy production but rather occurs as an essential part of membranes and serves as a precursor for steroid hormone and bile acid synthesis. Cholesterol is an integral component of cell membranes and can be synthesized in all animal cells. Bile acids secreted from the liver in the bile must be present in the intestinal lumen in order for cholesterol to be absorbed. Unabsorbed cholesterol derived from the diet and sterol and bile acid metabolites produced by intestinal flora are excreted in feces (see Chapters 19, 21, and 24).

Table 1–11. COMPOSITION OF WEIGHT LOSS
ON VARIOUS LOW CALORIE DIETS (10 DAYS)

	Treatment		
	800 kcal Mixed (Balanced)*	800 kcal Ketogenic†	0 kcal
Body weight loss, g/day	278	467	761
Composition weight loss, g/day			
Protein	10	18	50
Fat	165	165	243
Water	103	284	468
Fat:Protein	16:1	10:1	5:1
Nitrogen loss, g/day	1.6	2.9	8.1
Ketones, mg/day	—	3.0	9.0

*Mixed (balanced)—30% fat, 45% carbohydrate
†Ketogenic—70% fat, 5% carbohydrate

Table 1-12. COMPOSITION OF WEIGHT DIFFERENCE
ON INCREASE TO 1200 kcal MIXED DIET

	Previous Diet: 800 kcal Mixed (Balanced)	800 kcal Ketogenic or 0 kcal
Body weight difference, g/day	−163	+145
Composition weight difference, g/day		
Protein	−6	+2
Fat	−122	−128
Water	−40	+271
Fat:Protein	19:1	∞

WEIGHT LOSS DIETS

There is one unifying principle for all successful weight loss diets: In order to deplete body fat, the number of calories ingested must be smaller than the number used in daily activity. However, the complexities of metabolism cause the amount and composition of weight loss to vary with the form in which the energy is provided, as well as with the energy balance. Table 1-11 shows the weight loss that will occur with two 800 calorie diets containing different composition of nutrients. More weight is lost with the ketogenic low carbohydrate, high fat diet. However, much of this loss is water and the rest is due to an undesirable loss of body protein. Such changes are even more severe if a no-calorie or starvation diet is used.

Changing individuals from these three dietary plans to one containing 1200 kcal of a mixed (balanced) composition of fat and carbohydrate results in continued weight loss only for those previously on the 800 kcal mixed (balanced) diet (Table 1-12). This weight loss consists of body fat, water, and a small amount of protein. For those previously on the starvation or ketogenic diet, fat continues to be lost but weight is gained, primarily due to an increase in body water.

SUMMARY

This chapter has served as a general introduction to the study of nutrients in relation to body composition, energy, and weight. Succeeding chapters in this section will explore the essential nutrients in greater depth, while the topic of weight loss diets, an area of much American popular interest, will be considered more intensely in Chapter 6 on quackery and Chapter 16 on obesity.

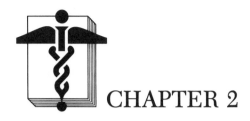

CHAPTER 2

Essential Nutrients:
Vitamins and Minerals

Fluoride
Chromium
Selenium
Molybdenum

CLASSIFICATION AND REQUIREMENTS

Vitamins are organic compounds that are essential to life but are not synthesized by the body in the adequate small amounts required. Because of this, they must be obtained from the diet.

Classification

The 13 vitamins people require are grouped as fat-soluble (A, D, E, and K) and water-soluble [C, thiamin (B_1), riboflavin (B_2), niacin (B_3), pyridoxal (B_6), B_{12}, folic acid, pantothenic acid, and biotin] (Figs. 2–1 and 2–2). Because the fat-soluble vitamins are stored, their ingestion in high doses can lead to toxicity. Also because of storage, it takes a long time to deplete the body of these vitamins even without any dietary source. On the other hand, the water-soluble vitamins are generally contained only in minute amounts within the body. With the exception of vitamin B_{12}, which is stored in the liver, body stores are limited. For example, only 30 mg of thiamin and 1 to 2 g of vitamin C are found in the body. Since there is little storage, body tissues are rapidly depleted of these vitamins if there is no dietary source. Conversely, when excessive amounts of the water-soluble vitamins are ingested, they are lost in the urine, either in their original form or as metabolites, and are less likely to be toxic.

Requirements and Supplementation

Because they are required in the diet in quantities of less than 100 mg per day, vitamins are termed micronutrients. The daily requirement of a vitamin is defined as the amount needed to avoid deficiency symptoms. On the other hand, the recommended dietary allowance (RDA) is set at two standard deviations above the daily needs (Table 2–1). The RDA attempts to determine the average daily amounts that the population of healthy adults should consume for good health. The RDA as given throughout this chapter as well as in Table

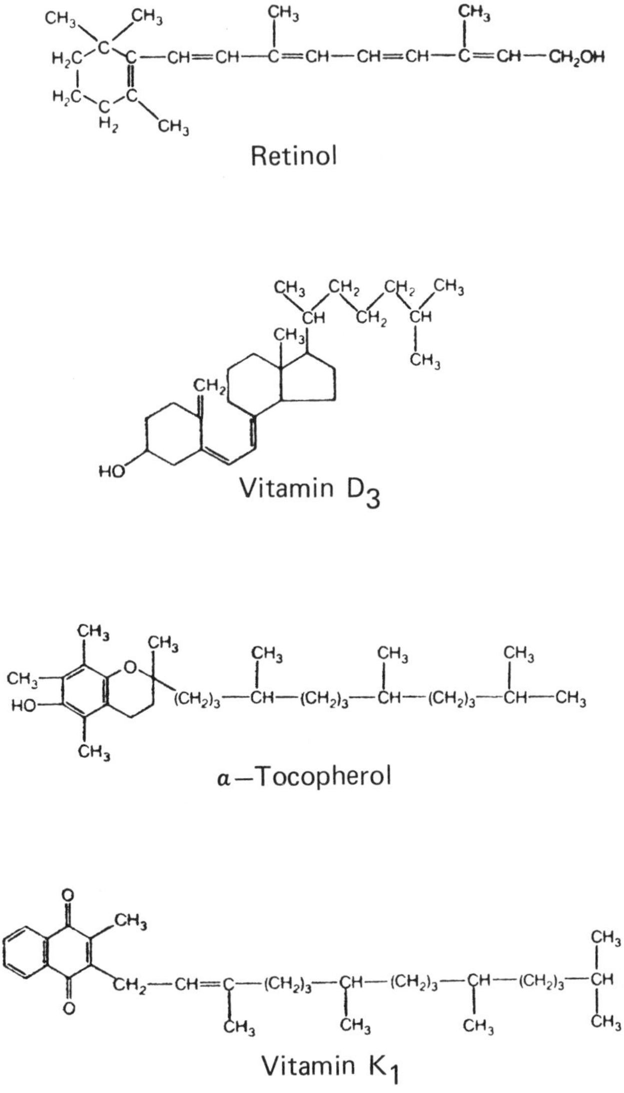

Retinol

Vitamin D₃

α—Tocopherol

Vitamin K₁

Figure 2–1. Chemical formulas of fat-soluble vitamins.

2–1 should be adequate to supply the known nutritional needs of 97.5 percent of the healthy population. Note that vitamin requirements vary with age and gender and are increased during pregnancy and lactation. For more information on the special needs of pregnant and lactating women, children, and the elderly, see Chapters 7, 8, and 9.

This chapter describes the function, dietary allowance, and food sources

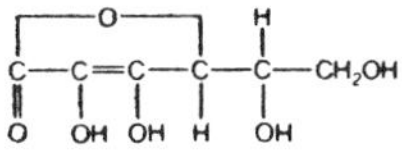

Ascorbic acid

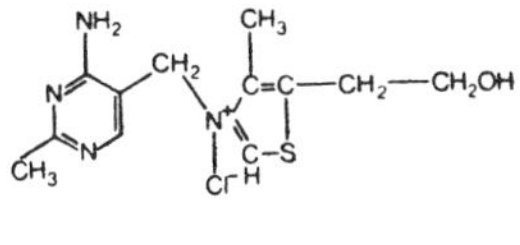

Thiamine chloride

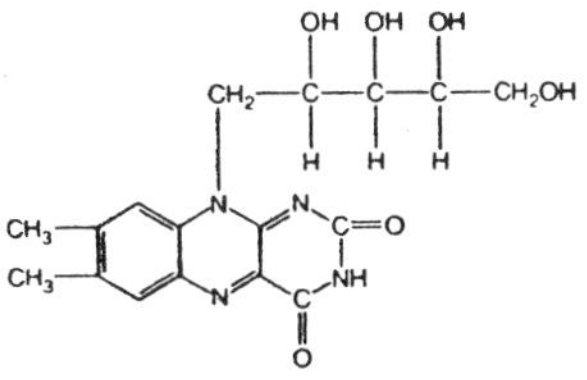

Riboflavin

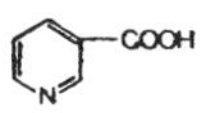

Niacin

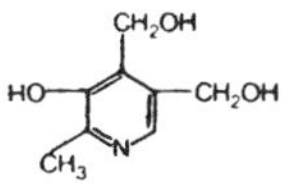

Pyridoxol

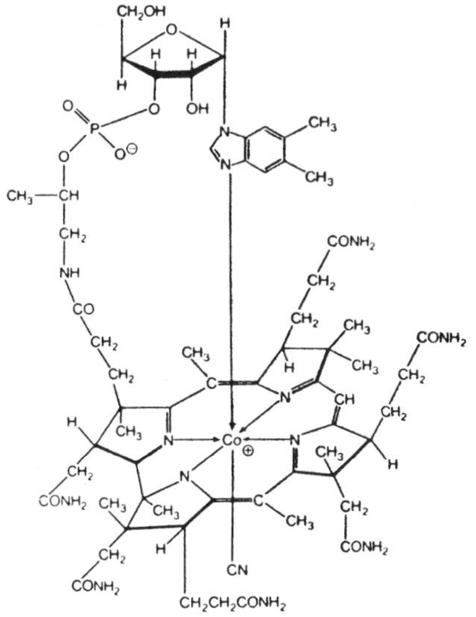

Cobalamin

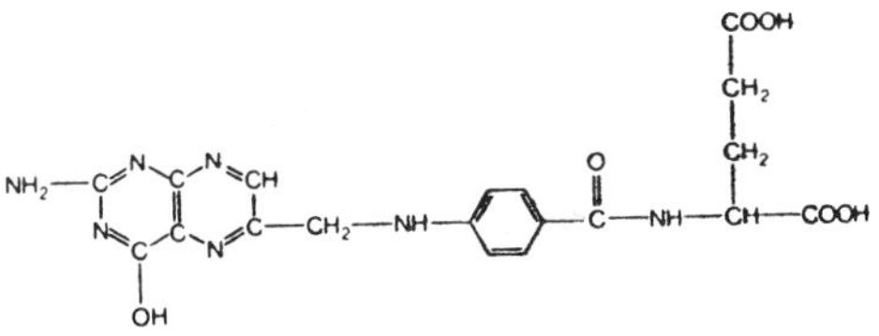

Pteroylglutamic acid (PGA)

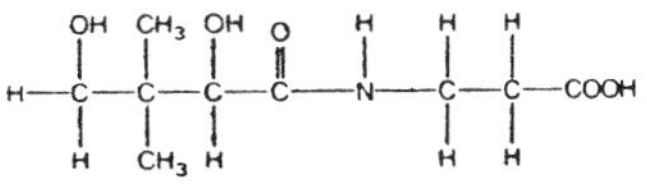

Pantothenic acid

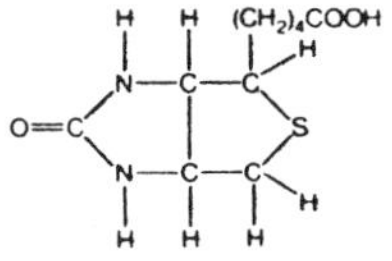

Biotin

Figure 2–2. Chemical formulas of water-soluble vitamins.

Table 2-1. RECOMMENDED DIETARY ALLOWANCES
(RDA) OF VITAMINS FOR HEALTHY ADULTS
IN THE UNITED STATES

Vitamin	Males	All	Females
A (retinol equivalents), μg	1000		800
D (cholecalciferol), μg		7.5, 5.0*	
E (α-tocopherol equivalents), mg	10		8
K, μg†		70–140	
C (ascorbic acid), mg		60	
B$_1$ (thiamin), mg	1.5, 1.4*		1.1, 1.0*
B$_2$ (riboflavin), mg	1.7, 1.4*		1.3, 1.2*
B$_3$ (niacin equivalents), mg	19, 16*		14, 13*
B$_6$ (pyridoxine), mg	2.2		2.0
B$_{12}$ (cobalamins), μg		3.0	
Folacin, μg		400	
Pantothenic acid, mg†		4–7	
Biotin, μg†		100–200	

*The first number is for younger adults, the second for older adults.
†Estimated safe and adequate daily dietary intake.

for each vitamin. Vitamin deficiency symptoms and syndromes, as well as vitamin toxicities, may be found in Chapter 14.

Vitamins can be provided as natural parts of the diet or added to foods as enrichment or fortification. White flour and its products contain added B vitamins and the mineral iron. Many fruit juices and soft drinks have added vitamin C. Vitamin D is added to milk and vitamin A to margarine.

Vitamin supplements can be provided as multivitamin tablets or capsules that contain approximately the RDA for almost all the vitamins. Such multivitamin supplements are indicated for adults if the balanced diet contains less than 1300 calories or if the diet is restricted in certain kinds of foods, as are extremely low fat diets. There are no differences in the effects of vitamins derived from food sources or as synthetic preparations. However, the bioavailability may differ.

Therapeutic Administration

Multivitamins also may be provided at therapeutic levels in the form of high potency vitamins. These also are over-the-counter (nonprescription) preparations. The content of individual vitamins allowed per tablet or capsule in these preparations is limited for folate (less than 1 mg) and vitamins A (not more than 7.5 mg retinol or 25,000 IU) and D (not more than 30 μg or 1200 IU) in order to avoid toxicity or exacerbation of other nutrient deficiencies.

Prescription of vitamins at the therapeutic level, which may be 2 to 10 times the RDA, is usually indicated for patients with deficiency diseases, for those who have undergone significant weight loss, and for those with alcoholism, hypermetabolism, limited dietary intake, malabsorption, or excessive vitamin loss.

Requirements in Disease and Deficiency States

There also are special requirements for some vitamins in patients with specific disorders. For example, patients with end-stage renal disease undergoing dialysis have increased needs above the RDA for folate and vitamins B_6 and C. The vitamin requirements of patients receiving chronic hemodialysis may be met by prescribing folic acid 1 mg, pyridoxine 10 to 25 mg, ascorbic acid 100 mg, plus thiamin, riboflavin, vitamin B_{12}, and pantothenic acid at levels equal to or less than the RDA. The patient with renal failure can develop high levels of vitamin A and a bone disease that is responsive especially to 1,25-dihydroxy vitamin D.

Individual vitamins in dosages 10 or more times the RDA level may be required in the management of inborn errors of metabolism. Examples include

- **thiamin**–maple syrup urine disease or Leigh's syndrome
- **nicotinic acid**–Hartnup's disease
- **pyridoxine**–homocystinuria or cystathionuria

Biotin is used in the treatment of propionic acidemia and multiple carboxylase deficiency. Doses as high as 40 mg per day may control biotin-dependent inborn errors. The coenzyme combines with the apoenzyme within the cell; very large amounts of coenzyme may serve to improve the function of a limited amount of apoenzyme in this and other inborn errors of metabolism.

Folic acid and vitamin B_{12} in high doses are also used in the treatment of some inborn errors of metabolism.

Those alcoholic patients who develop Wernicke-Korsakoff's encephalopathy may be predisposed by a specific inherited defect in brain transketolase, with thiamin a limiting factor in this syndrome as well (see Chapter 14).

Intravenous Administration

The requirements listed earlier refer to vitamins ingested as tablets or liquid, or given by the enteral route, where absorption is variable. When vitamins are given by the intravenous route, the requirements may be increased or decreased. An example of an appropriate multivitamin formulation for intravenous administration to adults is given in Table 2–2. This mixture provides 12 essential vitamins and does not contain vitamin K. Most of

Table 2–2. INTRAVENOUS MULTIPLE
VITAMIN PREPARATION

Vitamin	Daily Supply
A (retinol equivalents), μg	1000.0
D (ergocalciferol), μg	5.0
E (tocopherols), mg	10.0
C (ascorbic acid), mg	100.0
B$_1$ (thiamin), mg	3.0
B$_2$ (riboflavin), mg	3.6
Niacin, mg	40.0
B$_6$ (pyridoxine), mg	4.0
B$_{12}$ (cobalamin), μg	5.0
Folic acid, μg	400.0
Dexpanthenol, mg	15.0
Biotin, mg	0.06

the vitamins are provided at about twice the RDA, a few at the RDA (vitamins A and E, and folate), and some at a lesser level.

FAT-SOLUBLE VITAMINS

Vitamin A

Function

Vitamin A was identified in 1913. Its structure, a 20-carbon polyene, relates it to the provitamin beta carotene, which provides about half the vitamin A in the American diet. Carotene is converted to vitamin A alcohol (retinol) in the intestine. Restinaldehyde, a derivative of retinol, is an essential component of the visual pigment rhodopsin. The chemical alterations of vitamin A in response to light (Fig. 2–3) are essential for adaptation to dim light and for rod excitation. Some of the carotene product is retinoic acid, which supports cells growth but does not have the vision or reproduction effects of vitamin A. Vitamin A also stabilizes lysosomal membranes, plays a role in gene expression, and, by aiding glycoprotein synthesis, is important for mucus-secreting epithelial tissues. Vitamin A and carotene have been implicated in the prevention of cancer, and derivatives (retinoids) are used in the treatment of acne and psoriasis.

Requirements and Sources

Although the precise daily requirement for vitamin A is uncertain, the RDA is set at 800 μg for women and 1000 μg for men. The vitamin A activity

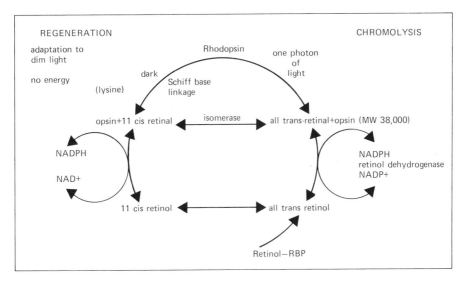

Figure 2–3. The steps in the chemical reactions of retinol in the eye involved in vision. Light activates the vitamin A–containing photopigment rhodopsin to yield retinaldehyde and opsin. These biochemical and conformational reactions are reversed during dark adaptation.

in food is expressed commonly as international units (IU). One IU is equal to 0.3 μg retinol (0.344 μg of retinyl acetate) or 0.6 μg of beta carotene. The RDA is given in retinol equivalents (RE):

	One Retinol Equivalent	
	Retinol	*β-Carotene*
μg	1.0	6.0
IU	3.3	10.0

These discrepancies arise because the absorption of carotene is less efficient than that of retinyl esters in the diet. Vitamin A is found only in animal foods; the vitamin A precursors (beta carotene, carotenoids) are of vegetable origin (Table 2–3). To ensure adequate intake in the general population, dairy products and margarine are supplemented with retinyl esters.

Metabolism

Intake of both vitamin A and carotene is reflected only in part by their serum levels. Retinol is transported in blood bound to a retinol binding protein (RBP), which in turn is bound to prealbumin. Vitamin A is stored in the liver, which can replenish and maintain serum levels. Vitamin A is usually ingested as the retinyl ester, which is hydrolyzed by pancreatic and brush border enzymes prior to absorption (Fig. 2–4). Absorbed retinol is then re-

Table 2-3. DIETARY SOURCES OF VITAMINS

Retinol (A)	Liver, fish liver oils, butter, carrots, spinach, cantaloupe, sweet potatoes
Cholecalciferol (D)	Fortified milk, fish liver oils, fish, egg yolk
Tocopherol (E)	Vegetable oils, margarine, meat, peas, nuts
Phylloquinone (K)	Green tea, turnip greens, broccoli
Ascorbic acid (C)	Citrus fruits, melon, strawberries, green pepper, broccoli, brussel sprouts, turnip greens
Thiamin (B$_1$)*	Enriched or whole grain cereal products, pastas, peas, nuts, beans, pork
Riboflavin (B$_2$)	Liver, milk, yogurt, cottage cheese, eggs, leafy vegetables
Niacin (B$_3$)	Liver, peanuts, chicken, salmon, tuna
Pyridoxine (B$_6$)	Liver, meat, fish, poultry, peanuts
Cyanocobalamin (B$_{12}$)	Liver, meat, eggs, shellfish
Folacin*	Liver, leafy vegetables, oranges, peanuts
Pantothenic acid*	Liver, eggs, wheat, peanuts
Biotin*	Liver and other organ meats, egg yolk

*Brewer's yeast is a good source.

esterified to retinyl ester and incorporated into chylomicrons. Ingested beta carotene may be converted in the intestine to two retinols or absorbed intact. The liver also can convert carotene to retinol. Both forms of the vitamin are absorbed primarily into the lymphatics. Retinyl esters are stored in the liver or may be converted to retinol for transport to other tissues bound to RBP. Some hepatic retinol is converted to retinoic acid via the intermediate retinaldehyde. Retinoic acid is conjugated to glucuronide and excreted in the bile.

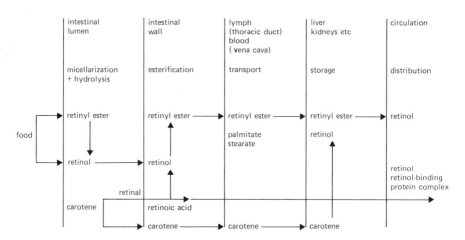

Figure 2-4. The absorption and transport of retinol.

Retinol is released into the blood from the liver bound to RBP, while a small amount of retinol circulates bound to prealbumin. Prealbumin binds RBP (and retinol) in a complex of molecular weight 80,000, which is not normally filtered by the kidney. RBP is a small molecule (molecular weight 21,000) that is partially filtered by the kidney. Receptors for RBP are present in virtually all tissues.

Vitamin D

Function

Vitamin D, purified in 1931, is now considered a hormone that regulates calcium and phosphate metabolism by mobilizing calcium from bone in the presence of parathyroid hormone, promotes intestinal absorption of both calcium and phosphate, and influences bone mineralization. Renal reabsorption of calcium also is increased by vitamin D. Cholecalciferol (vitamin D_3) is formed by the action of sunlight on 7-dehydrocholesterol in the skin. It is then hydroxylated in liver and kidney to yield the active biologic form of the vitamin (1,25-dihydroxy vitamin D_3).

Requirements and Sources

The RDA of vitamin D is given in μg, with 0.025 μg equal to 1 IU. The RDA for vitamin D has been set at 5 μg for adults and 10 μg for children, with 2.5 μg considered adequate to prevent rickets, the major vitamin D–deficiency disease. The dietary intake of vitamin D is important in persons with limited exposure to sunlight, whose endogenous production from 7-dehydrocholesterol may be inadequate. Natural food sources of vitamin D are listed in Table 2–3.

Metabolism

Dietary vitamin D is absorbed after micellar solubilization. It is incorporated into very low density lipoproteins or chylomicrons and delivered to the liver. The liver adds a 25-hydroxyl group, whereas in the kidney, hydroxyl groups are added either at the 1 or the 24 position. These hydroxylated vitamin D metabolites are stored in adipose tissue. 25-hydroxy and 1,25-dihydroxy vitamin D_3 are excreted in bile and undergo an enterohepatic circulation.

Vitamin E

Function

The specific functions of vitamin E (tocopherols), discovered in 1923, are as yet unknown. However, it may play a role in biologic oxidations protecting intracellular membranes from damage due to lipid peroxidation.

Requirements and Sources

The RDA for vitamin E (see Table 2–1) is set at 7 to 13 mg of alpha-tocopherol equivalents (10 to 20 IU). Requirements for vitamin E vary inversely depending on the intake of selenium and sulfur amino acids. In addition, the requirement for vitamin E is increased in proportion to the intake of polyunsaturated fatty acids, with 1 mg of vitamin needed for each 0.6 g of polyunsaturated fatty acid ingested. The sources of the fatty acids, vegetable oils (see Table 2–3), may contain the appropriate amounts of vitamin E, with the daily intake averaging about 7 mg.

Metabolism

Vitamin E is absorbed passively, transported with lipoproteins, and deposited in adipose tissue, which represents its major storage pool.

Vitamin K

Function

Vitamin K was isolated in 1939 and is necessary for the hepatic synthesis of several blood-clotting factors: factors II (prothrombin), VII, IX, and X. It also is necessary for the synthesis of osteocalcin, a calcium-binding protein in bone.

Requirements and Sources

Vitamin K exists in two natural forms: vitamin K_1 (phylloquinones) found in plants and vitamin K_2 (menaquinones) found in bacteria and animals through the intestinal flora. It also exists in one synthetic form, vitamin K_3 (menadione). Half of the vitamin K requirement in humans is met by vitamin K synthesized by the intestinal flora. These are capable of synthesizing approximately 2 μg of the vitamin per kilogram of body weight. Because of this, the dietary requirement for vitamin K is difficult to determine. However, a range has been recommended by assuming that only half the intestinal bacterial production is absorbed. The remainder must be supplied by the diet. Thus, the safe and adequate intake is set at 70 μg. Green leafy vegetables are good dietary sources of vitamin K (see Table 2–3).

Metabolism

Vitamin K is absorbed passively in the small intestine following micellar solubilization. It enters into the lymph and is then metabolized in the liver. There are no large tissue stores of this vitamin. Vitamin K is not a component of oral or intravenous multivitamin preparations and, if required, must be prescribed separately.

WATER-SOLUBLE VITAMINS

Vitamin C

Function

Vitamin C (ascorbic acid) was identified as a vitamin in 1928 and synthesized in 1933. The deficiency disease, scurvy, is ancient. The efficacy of citrus fruits in the prevention of scurvy was known as far back as the 16th century.

Ascorbic acid can be synthesized in the liver, from glucuronic acid, by most species of animals. Among the exceptions are primates (including humans), guinea pigs, some birds (red-vented bulbul), and some fish (catfish). The chemical functions of vitamin C have not been well defined. However, it is known to be involved as a cofactor in proline hydroxylation, collagen formation, metabolism of tyrosine, synthesis of the adrenal hormones and the neurotransmitters serotinin and norepinephrine, conversion of folic acid to folinic acid, and stimulation of phagocytosis by leukocytes. It also functions in hydrogen ion transfers, regulates the intracellular redox potential of some enzyme systems, and acts as an antioxidant (reducing agent) for vitamins A and E. Another function of vitamin C is to enhance the absorption of non-heme iron when the two nutrients are ingested together. This can produce as much as a fourfold increase in iron absorption.

Requirements and Sources

A dietary allowance of 60 mg ascorbic acid per day is recommended, with absorption approximately 80 to 90 percent complete. Scurvy can be prevented by an intake of only 10 mg daily. Complete tissue saturation with vitamin C is achieved at a daily intake of 200 mg, with the body pool of ascorbic acid about 1500 mg. Ascorbic acid is present in especially high concentrations in green vegetables and citrus fruits (see Table 2–3) but is heat labile and easily destroyed by oxidation or exposure to iron or copper. About 50 percent of the ascorbic acid content of foods is lost in processing and cooking.

Metabolism

Ascorbic acid is catabolized to oxalate and under normal conditions accounts for 20 to 30 percent of urinary oxalate.

Thiamin (Vitamin B₁)

Function

Thiamin, or vitamin B_1, was synthesized in 1936 and is essential for reactions in carbohydrate metabolism, such as the transketolase reaction in the pentose phosphate cycle and in the pyruvate dehydrogenase reaction. After conversion to the pyrophosphate, thiamin functions as a coenzyme in the oxidative decarboxylation of α-ketoacids to aldehydes (Fig. 2–5). Thiamin also is involved in nucleotide synthesis, in the generation of NADPH for fatty acid synthesis, and in steroid hydroxylation. Thiamin deficiency can result in beriberi.

Requirements and Sources

The RDA for thiamin varies from 1 to 1.8 mg per day, depending on the caloric intake (0.5 mg per 1000 kcal per day). Its requirement is proportional to energy intake when calories are derived primarily from carbohydrates. Thus, the thiamin requirement is estimated at 0.35 mg per 1000 kcal per day, but 0.4 mg or more per 1000 kcal per day may be required by the elderly. When calorie intake is significantly reduced, as in "starvation" diets, a minimal intake of thiamin is still recommended. Although thiamin is abundant in all foods, excellent sources of thiamin include enriched bread and rice, meat, and peas (see Table 2–3). Unfortunately, much of the thiamin is lost in cooking.

Metabolism

Thiamin is rapidly absorbed from the upper small intestine by active and passive transport mechanisms. Absorption is greater than 80 percent. About 1 mg per day of thiamin can be metabolized to pyrimidine metabolites, which are excreted. At higher intakes, unmetabolized thiamin is excreted in the urine. Only about 30 to 40 mg of thiamin is retained in the body.

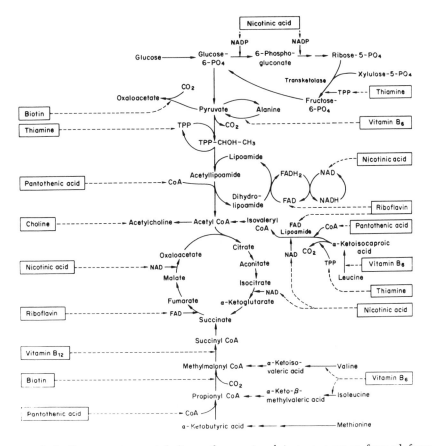

Figure 2–5. Some major metabolic pathways involving coenzymes formed from water-soluble vitamins. (From Gilman, A.G., et al.: Goodman and Gilman's The Pharmacological Basis of Therapeutics, ed. 7. Macmillan, New York, 1985, Fig. 66–1, p. 1552, with permission.)

Riboflavin (Vitamin B₂)

Function

Vitamin B_2, or riboflavin, was synthesized in 1935. The vitamin functions primarily as the reactive portion of the prosthetic group of flavoproteins concerned with biologic oxidations. Flavoproteins are involved in hydrogen transport, tricarboxylic acid and fatty acid dehydrogenation, electron transport, and oxidase action (see Fig. 2–5). Because of the diversity of reactions utilizing riboflavin, the required intake is dependent on protein and energy needs and overall metabolic activity.

Requirements and Sources

The RDA for riboflavin ranges from 1.1 to 1.8 mg per day, with allowances computed as 0.6 mg per 1000 kcal. The requirement to prevent deficiency is probably at a level of 0.4 to 0.5 mg per 1000 kcal. Riboflavin is found especially in leafy vegetables, with milk and eggs among the other usual dietary sources (see Table 2–3). Riboflavin is free in milk but is conjugated with protein in other foods. It is sensitive to ultraviolet light, and approximately 15 to 20 percent is lost in cooking water. The average diet contains about 2.7 mg of riboflavin per day, an amount that exceeds the RDA.

Metabolism

Riboflavin is absorbed rapidly in the proximal small intestine by a specific saturable transport process and is phosphorylated by a flavokinase. The phosphorylated flavin mononucleotide is hydrolyzed prior to absorption as riboflavin. Riboflavin is not metabolized, so that excretion in the urine correlates well with recent dietary intake. Riboflavin circulates in blood 75 percent bound to protein. The average concentration in blood is 32 μg per liter.

Niacin

Function

Niacin, also known as nicotinic acid or 3-pyridinecarboxylic acid, was recognized as a vitamin in 1937. The niacin deficiency disease pellagra has been known since the early 1700s. Niacin is a component of the important respiratory coenzymes NAD and NADP. These participate in oxidation/reduction reactions in glycolysis, fat synthesis, and tissue respiration (see Fig. 2–5).

Requirements and Sources

The RDA for niacin ranges from 12 to 18 mg per day based on an intake of 6.5 mg per 1000 kcal, while the actual requirement is presumed to range between 8.8 and 12.3 mg per day. Nicotinic acid is present in most nonfat foods, with meat, fish, and grains particularly rich sources (see Table 2–3). The average diet provides about half the niacin intake as nicotinic acid and the other half as tryptophan, some of which can be converted to niacin in a reaction requiring vitamin B_6. The rate of tryptophan conversion produces an equivalent activity of one-sixtieth the activity of niacin.

Metabolism

Nicotinic acid is one of the most stable vitamins. In some cereals, especially corn, niacin is bound and unabsorbable. Nicotinic acid occurs naturally in the body as nicotinamide.

Pyridoxine (Vitamin B$_6$)

Function

Vitamin B$_6$, synthesized in 1936, includes pyridoxine, pyridoxal, and pyridoxamine. These function as coenzymes for the transaminases, decarboxylases, and deaminases of amino acid metabolism (see Fig. 2–5).

Requirements and Sources

The RDA for vitamin B$_6$ is estimated by using a ratio of 0.02 mg per g protein ingested. Thus, the RDA varies from about 1 to 3 mg per day depending on the protein intake. The daily requirement varies from about 0.75 to 2.2 mg per day. Since the vitamin in some form is present in low concentration in all plant and animal tissues, dietary deficiency is uncommon. Foods high in vitamin B$_6$ content are listed in Table 2–3.

Metabolism

Vitamin B$_6$ is rapidly absorbed in the upper intestine. It is in the form of pyridoxal phosphate that most enzymes utilize the coenzyme (see Fig. 2–5). Vitamin B$_6$ is excreted as pyridoxal, pyridoxamine, and the metabolite 4-pyridoxic acid.

Folate

Function

Folic acid (pteroylglutamic acid) was synthesized in 1945. Folacin, or folate, is the generic term for compounds resembling folic acid and having similar biochemical activity. The principal function for folate-containing coenzymes is the transport of one-carbon fragments. Folate is essential for synthesis of nucleic acid bases, purines, and thymidylate, and for the metabolism of serine and homocysteine, particularly true in rapidly growing tissues. Folate coenzymes methylate biogenic amines and are required for the initiation of protein synthesis in bacteria.

Requirements and Sources

The relative availability of folate varies in different foods. In addition, some forms are readily destroyed by heat so that only 25 to 50 percent of dietary folate may be available. Folate requirements are difficult to determine because of:

- variation in structure and function of pteroylglutamic acid (PGA) vitamers
- variation in absorption, which does not correlate with retention
- variations in bioavailability from foods
- varying enterohepatic recirculation
- assessment of requirement using PGA, which is less readily utilized and retained than natural methylated or reduced folates found in food

The adult RDA for folate is set at 400 μg per day. However, the daily requirement may be only half that amount. The folacins in food occur largely as polyglutamates. The pentaglutamate predominates, and forms with four or six residues also are common. Most folacins in food are methylated (60 to 95 percent of dietary folacin) or reduced (10-formyl PGA—14 to 40 percent). Unsubstituted reduced PGAs are unstable. Because of this, cooking losses can be as high as 80 to 90 percent. Foods with folacins of high bioavailability include bananas, lima beans, liver, and yeast. Folacins are also present in green leafy vegetables and organ meats (see Table 2–3). The usual diet contains an average of about 700 μg folacin per day.

Metabolism

Polyglutamates must be deconjugated to the monoglutamate for absorption. The folate conjugase is found in salivary, gastric, pancreatic, and jejunal secretions, with intestinal mucosa, liver, pancreas, kidney, and placenta also having enzyme activity. Reduced folates are better absorbed than oxidized forms. PGA in tablets is not as well utilized as food folates which are reduced further by a specific enzyme, dehydrofolate reductase, to tetrahydrofolic acid (THFA) and are absorbed efficiently. The THFA is converted in the liver to 5'-methyl THFA, which enters plasma, is stored, or is re-excreted in bile. The enterohepatic circulation of THFA is about 100 μg per day, which is equivalent to the amount utilized daily.

Cobalamin (Vitamin B_{12})

Function

Vitamin B_{12}, isolated in 1948, is a group of cobalt-containing compounds (cobalamins) that play an important role as coenzymes in methylation to form methionine and in the metabolism of amino acids and odd chain fatty acids. In addition to its well-known hematopoietic action, vitamin B_{12} is required to provide reduced glutathione for glyceraldehyde-3-phosphate dehydrogenase and carbohydrate metabolism and for the action of methylmalonyl CoA isomerase (propionyl to succinyl) in lipid metabolism and the maintenance of myelin (see Fig. 2–5). Vitamin B_{12} is also linked to nucleic acid metabolism and folate metabolism by regenerating tetrahydrofolate from methyl folate. The vitamin is not absorbed in the absence of the highly specific binding protein, **intrinsic factor**, which is secreted in the stomach. Vitamin B_{12} is recycled in the enterohepatic circulation and has a long biologic half-life.

Requirements and Sources

The total body content of cobalamins is approximately 2.5 mg, primarily in the liver. The RDA of 3 μg per day is sufficient to meet daily losses from the liver and maintain body pool size. The average diet provides 5 to 15 μg per day. Cobalamin content of food is highest in liver, oysters, and clams (see Table 2–3). Because vitamin B_{12} is found only in foods of animal sources, deficiency can occur in vegetarians who ingest absolutely no animal products (vegans). Vitamin B_{12} deficiency may also occur in patients with malabsorption syndromes.

Metabolism

Serum vitamin B_{12} usually correlates with body stores, since cobalamin concentration in red cells is not higher than serum. Because serum vitamin B_{12} levels may be decreased up to 30 percent in patients with folate deficiency, these levels do not always reflect the vitamin status. In general, however, a serum vitamin B_{12} level of less than 120 pg per ml is associated with low body stores.

Cobalamin is tightly bound to food protein and its absorption requires digestion by gastric proteases to liberate free cobalamin. After digestion, the free vitamin is bound to an R protein (nonintrinsic factor-binding protein) in the stomach. In the upper small intestine, pancreatic enzymes hydrolyze R protein, thus liberating free cobalamin. Intrinsic factor then binds cobalamin, and this complex is picked up by a specific ileal mucosal receptor and taken up by the cell. The free cobalamin is then released into the plasma. In the circulation, cobalamin is bound primarily to transcobalamins I and III, with only 10 to 20 percent bound to transcobalamin II, a protein that delivers cobalamin to tissues. In the liver, cobalamin is bound again to an R protein and secreted in bile, while in the intestine, the R protein–cobalamin complex is digested and absorbed to undergo an enterohepatic circulation.

Biotin

Biotin was synthesized in 1943 and plays an important role in the synthesis of fatty acids and in gluconeogenesis as a component of enzymes transporting carboxyl units and fixing carbon dioxide (see Fig. 2–5). The RDA for biotin is 100 to 200 μg per day. It is found in abundance in liver, other organ meats, and egg yolk. The intestinal microflora makes a significant contribution to the body pool.

Pantothenic Acid

Pantothenic acid, isolated in 1939, is a component of coenzyme A and is important for acyl group activation reactions (see Fig. 2–5). These reactions release energy and are important in gluconeogenesis, synthesis and degradation of fatty acids, and synthesis of sterols, steroid hormones, porphyrin, acetylcholine, and so forth. The RDA for pantothenic acid is 4 to 7 mg daily. It is found in liver, eggs, wheat, and nuts.

MINERALS

Fifteen minerals are required in the daily diet (Table 2–4, and Fig. 2–6). Six minerals are required in relatively **large** amounts and are present in large quantities in the body:

- calcium (Ca)
- phosphorus (P)
- magnesium (Mg)
- sodium (Na)
- potassium (K)
- chloride (Cl)

Nine essential minerals are **micronutrients** and are termed trace elements or trace minerals:

- iron (Fe)
- zinc (Zn)
- iodine (I)
- copper (Cu)
- manganese (Mn)
- fluoride (F)
- chromium (Cr)
- selenium (Se)
- molybdenum (Mo)

Table 2–4. RECOMMENDED DIETARY ALLOWANCES (RDA)
OF MINERALS FOR HEALTHY ADULTS IN THE U.S.

Mineral	Males	All	Females
Calcium, mg		800	
Phosphorus, mg		800	
Magnesium, mg	350		300
Sodium, mg*		1100–3300	
Potassium, mg*		1875–5625	
Chloride, mg*		1700–5100	
Iron, mg	10		18, 10†
Zinc, mg		15	
Iodine, mg		0.15	
Copper, mg*		2–3	
Manganese, mg*		2.5–5.0	
Fluoride, mg*		1.5–4.0	
Chromium, mg*		0.05–0.2	
Selenium, mg*		0.05–0.2	
Molybdenum, mg*		0.15–0.5	

*Estimated safe and adequate daily dietary intake.
†First figure is for younger age group; second figure is for older age group.

Table 2–5. DIETARY SOURCES OF MINERALS

Calcium	Milk, cheese, sardines (with bone), tortillas, almonds, broccoli, and other green vegetables
Phosphorus	Milk, bologna, liver, hamburger, cheese
Magnesium	Milk, meats, seafood, cereal, peanuts, bananas, dark green leafy vegetables
Sodium	Table salt, cheese, milk, shellfish, condiments
Potassium	Meat, milk, fruits (bananas) and fruit juices, beans
Chloride	Table salt
Iron	Meat (calves' liver), poultry, fish, beans, raisins
Zinc	Red meat, shellfish (oysters), eggs
Iodine	Seafood (haddock, cod, lobster), iodized salt, dairy products, bread
Copper	Liver, oysters, crustaceans, nuts
Manganese	Nuts, grains, vegetables, fruits, tea
Fluoride	Fish (sardines), tea
Chromium	Brewer's yeast, black pepper, spices, meat, cheese, eggs, whole grains
Selenium	Seafood, organ meats, muscle meats, whole grains
Molybdenum	Meat, grains, legumes

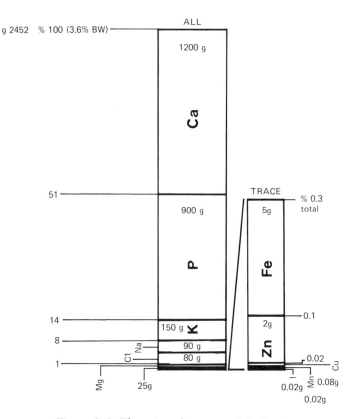

Figure 2-6. The mineral content of the body.

Sulfur and cobalt are also considered essential but have no specific recommended allowances. Dietary sources of the major minerals are provided in Table 2–5.

The bulk of the total mineral content of the body is in the skeleton, since bone is the major site of deposition of calcium, phosphorus, magnesium, fluoride, and zinc. However, bone is not considered a storage site for zinc, as it cannot be recovered readily for nutritional use. Lesser amounts of minerals are constituents of essential proteins such as thyroxin or hemoglobin, exist as free ions, or are loosely bound to other proteins. Minerals are major activators of cellular enzyme systems and are important for the control of pH of body fluids and the osmotic balance between the cell and extracellular fluids.

The body content of minerals is regulated by the intake from food, water, or other sources in the environment. Additional control mechanisms include intestinal absorption and kidney, skin, lungs, and gastrointestinal tract. The maintenance of balance of these inorganic elements in the body requires

Table 2–6. ELECTROLYTE CONTENT OF SWEAT AND
GASTROINTESTINAL FLUIDS (mEq/L)

Source	Na	K	Cl	HCO$_3$	H
Saliva	60	20	16	50	—
Gastric content, mean	59	10	89		90
range	30–90	4.3–12.0	53–155	0–1	
Bile, mean	145	5	100		—
range	134–156	3.9–6.3	83–110	35–50	—
Pancreatic juice, mean	142	4.6	77	≈70	—
Upper small bowel, mean	105	5.1	99	≈10	—
range	72–128	3.5–6.8	69–127		—
Ileum, mean	117	5.0	106		—
range	91–140	3.0–7.5	82–125	15–20	—
Diarrheal fluid	50	35	40	45	—
Sweat	50	5	50	—	—

Adapted from Randall HT: Fluid, electrolyte and acid-base balance. Surg Clin North Am 56:1040, 1976.

their presence in the diet not only in adequate amounts but also in appropriate **balance** with one another. For example,

- excess potassium increases sodium loss
- excess calcium results in decreased absorption or increased excretion of zinc
- excess ratio of calcium to phosphorus impairs mineralization of bone
- excess magnesium increases calcium excretion in the presence of phosphate deficiency
- the presence of molybdenum, sulfate, and copper modify the requirements for one another

Ordinarily, these interactions are not major influences in healthy people receiving a well-balanced diet.

Blood levels of minerals usually do not correlate with body stores. Electrolytes are present in most body secretions (Table 2–6) and can become depleted when losses are excessive. Laboratory tests of mineral status, deficiency states, and some toxicities are discussed in Chapters 14 and 15.

Calcium

Function

Calcium, the major cation of bone, is necessary for bone mineralization as well as skeletal growth and maintenance. Ninety-nine percent of the body calcium is located in teeth and bones. Approximately 1.2 kg of calcium is present in the skeleton of a young adult male as calcium phosphate (hydroxy-apatite). The calcium outside the bone (less than 110 g) has a vital role in controlling neuromuscular transmission, blood clotting, myocardial and skeletal muscle function, and the integrity of intracellular substances and membranes. In addition, calcium plays a role in many secretory processes.

Requirements and Sources

There is disagreement over whether the current RDA for calcium in adults, 800 mg per day, is too low and should be increased to at least 1 g. Median calcium intake in women is estimated at about 700 mg per day in late adolescence, declining to less than 500 mg per day with advanced age. Milk and cheese contribute about 60 percent of the calcium intake in the United States (see Table 2–5).

Availability and Metabolism

Vitamin D is required for absorption of calcium, which is a very inefficient process (less than 30 percent). Calcium must be absorbed in the ionized form (Ca^{++}) and is most readily absorbed in the duodenum, where there is a high affinity active transport system. The active form of vitamin D, 1,25-dihydroxy vitamin D_3, increases calcium absorption. Vitamin D levels are regulated by parathormone, which is secreted in response to a decrease in the level of plasma calcium.

Calcium in plant foods is less bioavailable than that from animal sources. Oxalic acid (found in green vegetables) and phytic acid (found in abundance in unleavened wheat bread) combine with calcium to form insoluble salts. These compounds do not impair net calcium uptake or delivery significantly if total intake is adequate.

Human beings may tolerate a calcium-to-phosphorus ratio between 2:1 and 1:2. The ideal calcium-to-phosphorus ratio has not been established, but the average ratio in the United States is 1:1.5. Excessive intake of phosphorus may lead to increased bone resorption and increased calcium loss in feces, presumably as a result of secondary hyperparathyroidism.

The relationship of dietary protein intake to calcium excretion is unclear. High dietary intakes of protein or low intakes of phosphate, or both, increase calcium excretion and bone resorption.

Aging is accompanied by a reduction of calcium absorption and decrease in gastric acidification. All of these factors suggest that the dietary intake of calcium should be ample throughout life to avoid significant loss of calcium from bone.

Bone Mineralization

Osteopenia denotes a reduction in bone mass that may result in spontaneous fracture. Whether the primary mechanism of bone loss in osteopenic patients is decreased bone formation or increased resorption has not been resolved. There is considerable controversy concerning the role of calcium intake in the prevention of osteoporosis, or decreased bone density. An adequate calcium intake is necessary for normal skeletal growth. Skeletal calcium accumulates with growth, with the maximum occurring at the time of the adolescent growth spurt, and calcium intake affects the peak bone mass achieved. Middle-aged and elderly individuals may require additional dietary calcium to maintain positive calcium balance because of decreased absorption. Osteoporosis is estimated to affect at least 10 percent of Americans over age 50, particularly postmenopausal women, and is a factor in the high incidence of spontaneous fractures in that age group. Bone loss with osteoporosis coincides with reduction in physical activity in later years (see Chapter 9).

Phosphorus

Function

Phosphorus is a major component of all cells. Combined with calcium, it contributes to the skeleton and as an important anion is involved in a variety of chemical reactions within the cell. Since phosphorus is present in nearly all foods, a dietary deficiency is unlikely. However, in parenteral feeding, serum phosphorus will be depleted rapidly unless appropriate amounts are provided, since it is utilized in glucose metabolism. The level of phosphorus in the body is regulated primarily by obligatory urinary excretion. With a decrease in kidney function, phosphorus will be retained. Phosphorus excess in renal disease may require treatment by the administration of nonabsorbable antacids.

Requirements and Sources

Because of its natural abundance in all the major food sources, especially milk, phosphorus intake can be two to five times higher than calcium intake in American diets. The phosphorus RDA is similar to that of calcium. Approximately 1 g of phosphorus is needed for each 17 g of nitrogen retained.

Metabolism

Phosphorus is absorbed well (60 to 70 percent) by the intestine in inorganic and organic forms. It is reabsorbed readily (80 to 90 percent) by renal tubules.

Magnesium

Function

Ninety percent of the body magnesium is found in bone and muscle. Next to potassium, it is the predominant intracellular cation. Total body stores are about 25 g (see Fig. 2–6).

Magnesium is an essential part of many enzyme systems responsible for the transfer of energy. The enzymes include those that hydrolyze and transfer phosphate groups (phosphokinases). Magnesium is also involved in adenosine triphosphate (ATP)–dependent reactions including oxidative phosphorylation and oxidative decarboxylation. It is required for the conversion of ATP to cyclic adenosine monophosphate by adenylate cyclase. Magnesium also activates amino acids and influences ribosome aggregation, messenger RNA binding, and synthesis and degradation of DNA. Magnesium plays an important role in neuromuscular transmission and activity and is important in maintaining nerve and muscle electric potentials. Low cellular magnesium may be involved in the pathogenesis of hypertension and atherosclerosis.

Requirements and Sources

Although we need magnesium in relatively large amounts (several hundred mg per day), ordinarily little attention is paid to dietary adequacy because magnesium occurs widely in foods, especially cereals and vegetables. Intake averages about 120 mg per 1000 kcal.

Metabolism

About 30 to 40 percent of dietary magnesium is absorbed by active transport, mainly in the ileum. Absorption varies inversely with dietary intake and can range from 70 percent to 20 percent. There is secretion of magnesium in bile and in pancreatic and intestinal juices. This is followed by reabsorption and reutilization.

Sodium

Function

Sodium, the principal cation of extracellular fluid, is involved with maintenance of osmotic equilibrium and extracellular fluid volume. Sodium homeostasis is regulated primarily through the kidney.

Requirements and Sources

Most of the dietary sodium is added to foods as sodium chloride (table salt). Other dietary sources include meat and dairy products and processed foods with sodium added in a variety of compounds. Minimum sodium needs of healthy adults can be met by an intake of 90 to 180 mg daily unless there is increased sweating or prolonged vomiting. The estimated safe intake of sodium is generally exceeded twofold to threefold in the usual Western diet, which contains greater than 2 to 7 g daily. Reduction of sodium intake has been recommended because of a possible relationship to high blood pressure. In hot climates with increased sodium losses in sweat, dietary sodium restriction may produce sodium deficiency manifested by muscle cramps. When more than 3 liters of water are required daily to replace sweat fluid losses, extra sodium chloride should be provided.

Metabolism

Sodium absorption is very efficient. Sodium is absorbed in the jejunum by bulk flow coupled with sugars and amino acids. The ileum and colon absorb sodium by active transport. Renal tubular reabsorption conserves sodium. Total sodium in adults ranges from 48 to 60 mEq per kg, or 90 g (see Fig. 2–6) in the whole body, with 25 percent in the skeleton.

Potassium

Function

This electrolyte is widely distributed in foods and is absorbed readily. Potassium is the principal cation in the intracellular fluid, which contains approximately 98 percent of the body potassium. Along with sodium and calcium, potassium maintains normal transmembrane electrical potential and controls membrane depolarization.

Variations in the sodium-to-potassium ratio in the diet may affect blood pressure; a high sodium-to-potassium ratio tends to elevate blood pressure.

Requirements and Sources

The recommended daily potassium intake has been estimated at 2.5 g, with the usual dietary intake averaging 4 g per day. Body potassium averages 54 mEq per kg body weight. Although dietary deficiency of potassium in healthy adults is rare, hypokalemia can be caused by prolonged diarrhea (including that induced by laxative abuse), renal disease, diuretics, and diabetic ketoacidosis. Patients for whom diuretic therapy is prescribed may meet potassium needs by consuming high potassium foods such as citrus fruits, tomatoes, potatoes, and bananas.

Metabolism

Body stores of potassium are regulated by renal excretion and conserved by renal tubular reabsorption. Potassium is also secreted into the colon (see Table 2–6).

Chloride

Function

Chloride, found in the secretions of the gastrointestinal tract—especially gastric juice (see Table 2–6)—is an important anion functioning primarily to regulate osmotic pressure. It is a coenzyme for amylase, a component of hydrochloric acid in the stomach, and part of the buffer system that maintains acid-base balance. Metabolic alkalosis may result from large chloride losses from vomiting. By passing readily from erythrocyte into plasma, chloride enhances the ability of the blood to transport CO_2. Chloride also aids in the conservation of potassium.

Requirements and Sources

Approximately 7 g chloride are ingested daily, primarily in the form of table salt.

Metabolism

Chloride is actively absorbed in the ileum and colon in exchange for actively secreted bicarbonate and is also absorbed passively accompanying sodium.

TRACE MINERALS

Iron

Function

Iron is an integral part of hemoglobin, myoglobin, the cytochrome system, peroxidase, and catalase. Iron-binding proteins are of crucial importance in resistance to infection. The 3 to 5 g of iron in the average adult are essential for cellular respiration and oxygen transport. The distribution of iron in the body is about 60 to 75 percent in the red blood cells as hemoglobin, 5 percent as myoglobin, less than 0.5 percent as heme-containing enzymes, about 10 percent as nonheme enzymes, and less than 0.1 percent circulating bound to transferrin. Ferritin and hemosiderin storage in liver, spleen, and bone marrow accounts for about 20 to 30 percent of iron stores. Iron deposits are roughly divided into one-third liver parenchyma, one-third skeletal muscle, and one-third reticuloendothelial system (liver, spleen, and bone marrow). Iron stores are controlled primarily by the rate of intestinal absorption.

High tissue iron concentrations are toxic, possibly because of free radical formation. In the inherited disease hemochromatosis, iron transport and intestinal uptake are excessive. In addition, chronic toxicity may occur with the use of iron cooking pots or with frequent transfusions.

Requirements and Sources

Iron requirements are determined by fixed losses primarily from feces (unabsorbed dietary iron), and also from skin, blood, and urine. There are additional menstrual losses in women. Because of this, the RDA for males and postmenopausal females is less than that for premenopausal females (see Table 2–4). Iron intake averages 15 mg on a 1500 kcal diet.

It is advisable for infant formulas to contain iron, and iron supplementation is advised for breast-fed infants, especially those of low birth weight, and for adolescent girls and young women. Pregnant or lactating women should double or triple their iron intake. It is difficult for some women to achieve the RDA (18 mg) by eating iron-rich foods such as meat, poultry, fish, and beans (see Table 2–5), so supplementation may be necessary.

Metabolism

Only about 10 percent of dietary iron is absorbed. The iron found in meats (heme iron) is better utilized than that found in egg yolk, vegetables, whole grains, or fortified bread. Nonheme iron is absorbed by active transport in the duodenum and proximal jejunum, while heme iron is absorbed over the entire length of the small intestine. The mean absorption of the total iron content of heme iron averages 23 percent and is little influenced by intraluminal factors in the intestine. Heme iron ordinarily accounts for only 1 to 3 mg iron per day. Absorption is inhibited by phosphate, phytate, dietary fiber, tannin, and possibly antacids. Ascorbic acid enhances absorption of iron in a linear fashion, by reducing ferric to ferrous iron. The presence of meat enhances the absorption of nonheme iron, while the most potent known inhibitor of iron absorption in a meal is tea—one cup in a meal reduces absorption by a factor of 4.

Iron transport depends on iron stores. The iron-depleted individual absorbs more than one who is iron-replete up to a maximum of about 5 mg daily. The nonheme iron absorption varies from about 3 percent in a meal with little meat (less than 30 g) or ascorbic acid (less than 25 mg), to 5 percent in a meal of medium availability (25 to 75 mg ascorbic acid, 30 to 90 g meat), to about 8 percent or more when greater than 90 g of meat or greater than 75 mg of ascorbic acid are present.

Iron is absorbed as a divalent cation in the duodenum, and absorption is stimulated and regulated by negative iron balance and red cell production. In iron-excess states, absorbed ferrous ions are oxidized to ferric ions and trapped in the intestinal mucosa as ferritin granules. This blocks further iron absorption. Iron can then be lost by desquamation of intestinal cells. Iron is transported in plasma bound to transferrin, which normally is not fully saturated.

Zinc

Function

Zinc is a constituent of several enzymes involved in nucleic acid synthesis and degradation. A body pool of biologically available zinc is small (about 2 g) and turns over rapidly. Most of the body zinc is in bone. Copper and nonheme iron share absorptive pathways with zinc and may compete for absorption. Calcium and phosphate reduce the utilization of dietary zinc.

Zinc is an essential component of more than 80 zinc metalloenzymes participating in all major metabolic pathways. These metalloenzymes include carbonic anhydrase, carboxypeptidases, aminopeptidases, alkaline phosphatase, thymidine kinase, and alcohol, retinol, malate, lactate, glutamate, and glyceraldehyde-3-phosphate dehydrogenases. Zinc is also essential for the synthesis of DNA, RNA, and protein. Zinc stabilizes cell membranes and ribosomes during protein synthesis, is required for DNA and RNA polymerase activity, and is essential for spermatogenesis and ova formation. Other functions of zinc include possible roles in taste and in the synthesis of collagen. Mobilization of vitamin A from the liver requires zinc, and insulin stored in the pancreas contains zinc. Cell-mediated immunity is decreased in zinc deficiency, and such a deficiency may play a role in the impaired immunocompetence seen in protein-energy malnutrition.

Requirements and Sources

The RDA for zinc is 15 mg per day. However, the average intakes are barely adequate and range from 6 to 15 mg per day. Zinc intake correlates with protein intake. Atlantic oysters are the richest dietary source of zinc. Zinc in whole grain products may be unavailable because of the presence of phytate and fiber.

Metabolism

Zinc absorption ranges from 10 to 40 percent. The exact absorption site in the small intestine is unknown. Absorption of zinc seems to be controlled by the zinc status of the individual. Metallothioneins, low molecular weight cytoplasmic proteins, have a high affinity for binding zinc and may participate in the homeostatic regulation of zinc metabolism and absorption, providing zinc at times of deprivation. Zinc losses can be exacerbated by liver or gastrointestinal disease, or following burns or trauma.

Plasma zinc is bound tightly to α_2-macroglobulins (30 to 40 percent), or loosely to albumin and amino acids (60 to 70 percent). About 80 percent of circulating zinc is in red blood cells, with 60 percent in hemoglobin and 20 percent in carbonic anhydrase. Zinc is lost mainly into the feces, and also through sweat and menses.

Iodine

Function

Iodine is an integral part of the thyroid hormones thyroxine (T4) and triiodothyronine (T3). The only known functions of iodine are associated with its presence in these hormones. Iodine is taken up by the thyroid as iodide, oxidized to elemental iodine, and incorporated into iodotyrosine. This then forms the hormone T4, which is activated in the tissues to T3. The iodine content of the body is 15 to 20 mg, with 60 to 80 percent found in the thyroid gland.

Requirements and Sources

Lack of dietary iodine causes endemic goiter. However, goiter was abolished as a major medical problem in the United States by the addition of iodine to table salt. The present dietary intake in the United States is estimated at 200 to 700 µg per day, which is considerably higher than the RDA of 150 µg per day. An intake of 2 g of iodized salt ensures an adequate intake of iodine. Additional food items providing iodine in the American diet are milk products from cattle given iodine supplementation, bread supplemented with iodized salt, shellfish, and saltwater fish. Absorption is inhibited by antithyroid substances (goitrogens) found in rutabagas, turnips, cabbage, and other members of the *Brassica* genus.

Metabolism

Dietary iodine is converted to iodide in the gastrointestinal tract and is nearly completely absorbed. About 30 percent is taken up by the thyroid gland (60 μg per day) with the remaining iodine excreted in the urine (more than 50 μg per day).

Copper

Function

Copper is contained in a number of copper metalloenzymes involved in oxidation-reduction reactions. These include cytochrome oxidase, which reduces molecular oxygen to water and produces ATP; lysyl oxidase, required in crosslinking collagen and elastin; tyrosinase, required for the formation of melanin; superoxide dismutase, which protects cells from damage by superoxide radicals; uricase; and histaminase. Ceruloplasmin transports copper and also functions in the oxidation of ferrous to ferric iron. The highest concentration of copper in the body is in the liver.

Requirements and Sources

The copper content of foods (see Table 2–5) is influenced by the copper content of the soil as well as environmental contamination. Copper also may be present in the water supply. The average daily intake in the United States (1 to 2 mg per day) is below the recommended level of 2 to 3 mg per day.

Metabolism

Copper is absorbed actively complexed to L–amino acids or by passive diffusion. Ascorbic acid decreases absorption. Copper is transported from the gastric and intestinal mucosa into the portal vein complexed with albumin. Copper is stored in the liver and incorporated into ceruloplasmin or other copper enzymes, or is excreted in the bile. Metallothionein binds copper tightly and may play a role in accepting albumin-bound copper from plasma into liver, binding about 80 percent of hepatic copper.

Copper content of the body is about 80 to 160 mg, with one third in the liver. Ceruloplasmin transports 90 to 95 percent of the circulating copper to peripheral tissues, and albumin binds the remainder. There is no significant enterohepatic circulation of copper secreted into bile because of its low reabsorption (about 30 percent).

Manganese

Function

Manganese, a divalent cation, activates many enzymes but, in part, may be substituted for by magnesium. Manganese is required for the synthesis of mucopolysaccharides in cartilage by activation of the galactotransferases and polymerases important in their synthesis. Manganese is also a component of the metalloenzymes pyruvate carboxylase and mitochondrial superoxide dismutase. Many metal enzyme complexes (hydrolases, kinases, and dicarboxylases) contain manganese, which also is required for clotting factors.

Manganese toxicity occurs in miners inhaling ore dust. The neurologic symptoms resemble those of Parkinson's or Wilson's disease.

Requirements and Sources

The recommended intake for manganese is set at 2.5 to 5 mg per day. The average intake is 2.5 mg per day, and dietary intakes up to 10 mg are probably safe. The body contains about 12 to 20 mg of manganese. Manganese is abundant in plant products such as nuts, grains, fruits and vegetables, and tea (see Table 2–5). It is present only in small concentrations in animal products.

Metabolism

Manganese absorption by the small bowel is less than 20 percent and varies inversely with dietary iron, calcium, and phosphorus. Loss is mainly through the bile, with urinary excretion being negligible.

Fluoride

Function

Fluoride protects teeth from dental caries by its incorporation into the crystalline structure of hydroxyapatite. This has resulted in the recommendation of fluoridation of water.

Requirements and Sources

Fluoride is present in soil, water, plants, and animals. The fluoride in food is of minor importance compared with water to which fluoride is added at about 1 ppm. The recommended safe and adequate intake ranges from 1.5 to 5 mg per day for adults, for the prevention of dental caries. With fluoridation, food intake provides an average of 2.6 mg (from food preparation) and water intake provides 1 to 1.5 mg. Without fluoridation of water, intake averages 0.9 mg from food and 0.1 to 1.6 mg from water.

Fluoride deficiency during infancy and childhood results in increased susceptibility to dental caries. Fluoride toxicity from dietary ingestion is rare. At higher levels of fluoride intake in growing children, the tooth enamel may become mottled or stained. Higher levels deform teeth and bones or erode tooth enamel. This mottling will not occur in adults given fluoride, which may be used as therapy to strengthen bone in osteopenia.

Metabolism

About 80 to 90 percent of the fluoride ingested is absorbed mainly by passive diffusion in the stomach. Approximately half of the fluoride ingested is retained in teeth and bones. Fluoride is excreted primarily in the urine, with small amounts lost in sweat and feces.

Chromium

Function

Chromium is essential as a component of glucose tolerance factor, a cofactor for insulin. Chromium may also play a role in lipid metabolism, lowering serum cholesterol levels. The body contains 5 to 10 mg.

Requirements and Sources

The safe and adequate intake has been set at 30 to 200 μg per day, with the average intake estimated at 60 μg. At present, the best source of chromium is brewer's yeast.

Metabolism

Chromium in foods is present as trivalent chromium or in the organic complex of the glucose tolerance factor. Absorption is very inefficient—only 0.5 to 3 percent. Chromium circulates bound to transferrin and as glucose tolerance factor. When chromium is administered, the excess is excreted mainly by the kidney. Ingestion of chromium produces little toxicity.

Selenium

Function

Selenium is a component of the enzyme gluthathione peroxidase, which is present in high concentrations in red blood cells and in liver. This enzyme catalyzes the reduction of hydrogen peroxide to water and of fatty acid hydroperoxides to hydroxy acids. This protects cell membranes from peroxidation. Selenium also plays a role in electron transfer functions. It overlaps in function with vitamin E, another important antioxidant.

Requirements and Sources

In most biologic material, selenium is found largely in the protein fraction. Selenium in serum is mostly bound to protein. Selenium deficiency may accompany protein-energy malnutrition. Because geographic areas vary in the soil content of selenium, the selenium content of plants varies. This variation is then passed up the food chain to animals and humans. Selenium in wheat may vary threefold depending on where the grain was grown. In some low selenium areas of the world, such as Keshan Province in China, selenium deficiency is associated with a fatal cardiomyopathy of children. Environmental selenium levels are also low in the South Island of New Zealand and in Finland. The west coast and southeastern coastal plain of the United States are low selenium areas, and blood levels of healthy subjects in those regions are below the average for the United States. The recommended safe and adequate intake ranges from 50 to 200 μg per day.

Since the days of Marco Polo, selenium toxicity has been known in horses grazing in soils with excessive selenium content—so-called blind staggers. Human selenium toxicity, or selenosis, has occurred in coal-mining areas in seleniferous soil in China and in persons ingesting excessive supplements. It is estimated that intake in excess of 1.5 mg daily is toxic. Symptoms include loss of hair and nails.

Metabolism

Selenomethionine is better absorbed than inorganic selenium. Elemental selenium and inorganic salts are relatively poorly absorbed. Intestinal absorption of selenium in food is about 80 percent, occurring mostly in the duodenum. Principal control of homeostasis is by urinary excretion in the kidney.

Molybdenum

Function and Metabolism

Molybdenum is an integral part of xanthine oxidase and aldehyde oxidase. It may inhibit formation of dental caries. Its absorption is from 40 to 100 percent efficient, and the major route of excretion (up to half the daily intake) is through the urine.

Requirements and Sources

The safe and adequate daily dietary intake of molybdenum is estimated at from 150 to 500 μg. Molybdenum is found in meat, grains, and vegetables, with the amount in plants varying according to soil content. Intake ranges from 0.5 to 2 mg daily.

CHAPTER 3

Nutritional Assessment

Every patient evaluation should include nutritional assessment in order to ascertain the patient's nutritional status—normal, malnourished, or at risk of developing some form of malnutrition. From such evaluation an effective nutritional prescription, or plan, is developed. A plan appropriate for a particular individual may require obtaining additional information beyond routine assessment, as well as determining whether some modification of the patient's usual diet is needed.

The standard tools of the physician may be supplemented by some special ones when making a nutritional assessment (Table 3–1). The history places special emphasis on certain elements of the medical and social background. An initial diet history is taken by the admitting health professional,

Table 3-1. INITIAL NUTRITIONAL ASSESSMENT

Compartment	Examination/Test
	I. History
	Medical
	Social
	Dietary
	II. Physical examination including anthropometrics
	Height (Ht)
	Weight (Wt)
Fat	Triceps skinfold thickness (TSF)
Skeletal muscle	Mid-arm circumference (MAC) → Mid-arm muscle circumference (MAMC)
	III. Laboratory data
Visceral protein	CBC (complete blood count) with differential and indices (total lymphocyte count)
	SMA-6 and SMA-12 (including cholesterol/triglycerides)
	Magnesium (Mg)
Visceral protein	Transferrin (prealbumin, retinol-binding protein)
	PT/PTT (prothrombin time/partial thromboplastin time)
	If indicated:
	Serum and RBC
	Folic acid
	Vitamin B_{12}
	Plasma
	Zinc (Zn)
	Copper (Cu)
	Assays of other vitamins and minerals, amino acids
	Urine study
Skeletal muscle	24-hour urine nitrogen and creatinine for calculation of nitrogen (N) balance* and creatinine-height index†
Visceral protein	IV. Skin testing for determination of cell-mediated immunity

* Nitrogen balance = $N_{in} - (N_{out} + 3)$
† Creatinine-height index = 24-hour urine creatinine, divided by expected 24-hour creatinine excretion of a healthy adult of the same gender and height × 100.

but more extensive evaluation may require the attention of the dietitian. The physical examination should note specific signs of nutritional deficiencies, protein-energy malnutrition, or obesity. In addition, anthropometric measurements are made from height, weight, skinfold thickness (to evaluate fat stores), and mid-arm muscle circumference (an indicator of somatic protein stores).

    Laboratory tests include routine clinical tests that offer clues to nutritional status as well as more specific tests of circulating transport proteins, of indicators of nitrogen balance and body composition, of the cellular immune status and immune response, and of specific levels or functional action of electrolytes, trace minerals, lipids, essential fatty acids, and vitamins. Tests of intestinal absorption may be indicated. The clinical relevance of the anthropometric and biochemical measurements that assist in recognizing malnutrition is not yet firmly established; however, some of these may predict complications, morbidity, or mortality.

Other factors weighed in the nutrition prescription include age, gender, level of activity, and degree of stress. In cases of undernutrition, extent of depletion is determined and the appropriate route of nutritional support considered. For example, the nutritionally depleted patient may require repletion, and the catabolic patient needs to have appropriate adjustments made. It should be kept in mind that overeating can also represent a form of malnutrition, so limits in caloric intake also need to be considered.

ROLE OF NUTRITIONAL ASSESSMENT

When assessing the individual patient, the clinician must determine whether the patient is malnourished and whether the conditions causing malnutrition are likely to persist. Rather than wait for malnutrition to appear, the physician should take prophylactic action by predicting the course and nature of the illness and its probable impact on the need, intake, and utilization of nutrients.

A "five day rule" has been recommended that charges the clinician to prepare within this period an estimate of the patient's metabolic and nutritional status and to project whether the patient will be able to eat within 1 week. An example of initial assessments and appropriate plans is shown here.

Patient's Status	Nutritional Plan
Anatomic or physiologic loss of gastrointestinal function has occurred and will continue	Implement nutritional support
Clinically malnourished on initial evaluation	May need to initiate nutritional support immediately
Normal	Preserve body cell mass
Cachectic	Restore body cell mass

The primary goal should be to prevent malnutrition rather than to attempt to replete patients after the fact.

HISTORY

Significant information from several areas may be elicited during the health assessment interview. Thus, the history can be divided into medical, social, and dietary data.

Medical History

When obtaining the medical history, among the pertinent questions to ask are

- What is the patient's usual weight?
- Has there been any recent change in weight?
- If so, how much? Over what period of time?

Possible causes of any malnutrition must be explored, and these normally fall into one or more categories, including abnormal intake, inadequate absorption, decreased utilization, increased losses, and excessive destruction and increased requirements.

Abnormal Intake

Changes in smell and taste, depression, alcoholism, dental problems, or other conditions may influence appetite. Dietary intake may be inadequate because of poverty, special diet prescriptions, food idiosyncrasies, or food fads such as those described in Chapter 6. It is important to ask about possible soreness of the tongue, or a history of ingesting such non-nutrients as clay, starch, or ice (pica).

Inadequate Absorption

Absorption may be affected by some medications (antacids, laxatives, oral contraceptives, and anticonvulsants), parasites, surgical resection of portions of the gastrointestinal tract, or malabsorption syndromes.

Decreased Utilization and Increased Losses

Nutrient utilization may be impaired by the use of anticonvulsants, oral contraceptives, antimetabolites, or isoniazid, or by inborn errors of metabolism, while nutrient losses are increased with alcohol abuse, blood loss, diarrhea, vomiting, draining wounds, burns, proteinuria, dialysis, fistulas, or ostomies.

Excessive Destruction and Increased Requirements

Nutrient requirements are increased with fever, sepsis, and hypermetabolic states such as hyperthyroidism, multiple trauma, and burns, in part because of excessive destruction. The patient should be asked about vitamin or mineral supplements that may have been taken in excessive amounts or that may tend to obscure underlying deficiency diseases.

Additional Risk Factors

Multiple nutrient deficiencies may be associated with chronic disease or recent major surgery. A history of excessive alcohol intake may be difficult to elicit, but it is prudent to consider all alcoholic patients to be at risk of nutritional deficiency. Chapter 17 contains more information on problems of patients who abuse alcohol.

Social History

The psychosocial evaluation should generate information concerning the patient's income and living conditions.

- Does the patient live alone?
- Does he or she have access to shopping?
- Are facilities adequate for storage and cooking of food?
- Who prepares daily meals?
- Does the patient have a history of smoking?

Diet History

The diet history should yield a data base from which an accurate evaluation of the patient's nutrient intake may be obtained. The elements of such an inquiry must be covered by the physician in every patient evaluation, although more extensive assessments are best done by the professionally trained dietitian.

Meal patterns and food consumption must be determined. In the hospital, the dietitian can calculate the calories consumed from nurses' records of food intake. When the patient is not hospitalized, level of activity as well as social and cultural influences must be considered. Knowledge of this background will help the physician to avoid dietary prescriptions that the patient may be unwilling or unable to follow, and may also offer clues to possible deficiencies stemming from religious constraints or other dietary habits. Food allergies are important not only in the nutritional evaluation but also in the general health history because drugs and infusions may contain potential antigens such as egg.

The physician is unlikely to take the detailed dietary history, but should know what the dietitian can contribute to a full-scale evaluation. The consulting dietitian will aim to have an understanding of the patient's social situation, attitude regarding changes in food habits, and medical status, including those aspects of the physical examination relating to nutrition. If this information is not obtainable from the medical record or referral, the dietitian will make the appropriate inquiries.

When rapport with the patient has been established, the dietitian will ask questions concerning food intake. These will cover the content of meals, eating times, reasons for eating (or not eating), and food preferences. It is important to ensure that beverage consumption is also reported.

The following four basic methods for obtaining a food history may be used alone or in combination. None is without pitfalls, as the patient's memory and compliance with instructions are involved in each method. All of these methods may be adapted for computer analysis.

1. **24-Hour Recall.** This is probably the most frequently used method. The patient is asked to recall everything eaten during the previous 24 hours. This information may be obtained quickly and gives hints of eating habits and food preferences. There are significant sources of error, however: (1) the patient may not remember; (2) the previous day may have been atypical; (3) the patient may not be telling the truth for a variety of reasons; (4) the patient frequently tends to overestimate areas that are deficient and to underestimate those that are excessive.

2. **Food Frequency Questionnaire.** This tool can be used as a crosscheck of the 24-hour recall and to fill in the gaps left by that method. The dietitian solicits information on how many times a day, week, or month a particular food is eaten. The questioning may be selective so as to yield information about a specific deficiency or excess. In general, the patient is more likely to give honest answers in a frequency questionnaire than in a 24-hour recall, but answers are still only as good as the patient's memory.

3. **Typical Pattern.** This method is useful when the individual cannot remember the previous day's intake or states that the previous day was atypical, or when the interviewer suspects that the 24-hour recall is inaccurate. As this method is more general, the individual is more likely to give an accurate view of a typical day but is less likely to include significant details of intake he or she does not consider important.

4. **Diet Diary.** This is probably the most accurate method if done correctly, but it requires more time, understanding, and motivation on

the part of the patient. The individual is asked to write down everything he or she eats or drinks during a specified period of time—
usually 3 days (2 week days, 1 weekend day) or up to 7 days. The
method should be explained carefully to the patient, with special attention to recording the amounts eaten and the ingredients used in
preparation. The dietitian should then go over the diary with the
patient and ask questions where indicated to complete the history.

Whichever method(s) the dietitian chooses to use should provide information to aid in developing realistic goals for the patient. Information obtained may be used to assess excesses, deficiencies, imbalances, and adequa-
cies of the present diet, and to identify bizarre or unusual eating behaviors.
The dietitian also assesses the patient's understanding of previous dietary instructions and any need for change. Completion of an accurate history helps
the dietitian to establish a proper framework for future counseling at the
patient's level of understanding and to plan realistic increments of change.
(Chapter 10 details therapeutic uses of diet.) Details of the diet history can be
used to measure the intake of water, calories, protein, sugar, fiber, saturated
or unsaturated fat, and cholesterol, and to provide an index of vitamin/
mineral status.

PHYSICAL EXAMINATION AND ANTHROPOMETRICS

General Physical Examination

Many of the physical signs of malnutrition are apparent on observing
and examining the patient.

Hair	Luster, texture, depigmentation (flag sign), color (reddening), pluckability, areas of hair loss
Face	Skin color and texture, rash
Eyes	Color of conjunctiva, luster of cornea, blood vessel injection, corneal arcus, eyelid xanthelasma, eye muscle movements
Lips	Swelling, dryness, fissures
Tongue	Color, thickness, papillation
Teeth/Gums	Missing teeth, abnormal eruption, spots, cavities; turgor, color, bleeding, recession of gums; fit of dentures
Buccal mucosa	Ulceration, inflammation
Salivary glands	Enlargement
Neck	Thyroid gland

Skin	Texture, turgor, rash, edema, pigmentation or depigmentation, flakiness, bleeding, wrinkling
Nails	Shape, firmness, ridges
Muscle	Tone, tenderness, wasting
Bones and joints	Shape, enlargement, softening, tenderness, fracture deformities
Heart	Size, rhythm, blood pressure
Abdomen	Liver size
Neurologic examination	Mental status: orientation, memory, calculations
	Cranial nerves
	Motor performance, gait, ataxia
	Deep tendon reflexes
	Sensibility to light touch, position, vibration

The vital signs of blood pressure, temperature, pulse, and respirations may also provide an index of nutritional risk and altered nutritional requirements.

Anthropometric Measurements

Anthropometric measurements include height, weight, skinfold thickness at various sites, and mid-arm muscle circumference and are essential parts of the nutritional assessment. The simplest measurements—height and weight—should be considered as vital signs in all patients at the time of physical examination. Measurements of skinfolds and muscle circumference are compared with standards for healthy persons in the United States, classed by

Table 3–2. NUTRITIONAL ASSESSMENT, PERCENT OF STANDARD

	Male	Female
Triceps Skinfold, mm		
100%	12.5	16.5
50% *	6.0	8.0
20% †	2.5	3.0
Mid-Arm Muscle Circumference, cm		
100%	25.5	22.3
80% *	20.0	18.5
60% †	15.0	14.0

* Moderate depletion.
† Severe depletion.

Table 3-3. PERCENTILE FOR TRICEPS SKINFOLD THICKNESS*
OF ADULTS IN THE UNITED STATES

Age Group (yr) and Sex	Population Percentile						
	5	10	25	50	75	90	95
Men							
18–24	4.0	5.0	7.0	9.5	14.0	20.0	21.0
25–34	4.5	5.5	8.0	12.0	16.0	21.5	24.0
35–44	5.0	6.0	8.5	12.0	15.5	20.0	23.0
45–54	5.0	6.0	8.0	11.0	15.0	20.0	25.5
55–64	5.0	6.0	8.0	11.0	14.0	18.0	21.5
65–74	4.5	5.5	8.0	11.0	15.0	19.0	22.0
Women							
18–24	9.4	11.0	14.0	18.0	24.0	30.0	34.0
25–34	10.5	12.0	16.0	21.0	26.5	31.5	37.0
35–44	12.0	14.0	18.0	23.0	29.5	39.5	39.0
45–54	13.0	15.0	20.0	25.0	30.0	36.0	40.0
55–64	11.0	14.0	19.0	25.0	30.5	35.0	39.0
65–74	11.5	14.0	18.0	23.0	28.0	33.0	36.0

*In millimeters.
Adapted from Bishop, C.W., Bowen, P.E., and Ritchey, S.J.: Norms for nutritional assessment of American adults by upper arm anthropometry. Am J Clin Nutr 34:2530, 1981. (Data from Health and Nutrition Examination Survey, 1971–1974.)

sex, age, and in some instances, race. Each value is usually compared with a norm defined as a fixed percentage of the standard or ideal value (Table 3–2), or with percentile values of the measurement obtained from the normal distribution of measurements in healthy individuals (Tables 3–3 and 3–4).

Height

In older children and adults, height is measured with the patient standing erect, if possible, commonly using a horizontal arm that moves vertically on a calibrated scale. The individual must stand straight, with shoes removed, heels on the ground, and the horizontal arm resting lightly on the crown of the head. A better method, not available in most hospitals, is to use a measuring scale fixed to a wall (anthropometer). If the patient is unable to stand, the length of the body may be ascertained with a tape measure.

Weight

Weight should be measured on balance beam scales that are calibrated and checked frequently. Patients who are keeping track of their weight should

Table 3-4. PERCENTILES FOR MID-ARM MUSCLE
CIRCUMFERENCE* OF ADULTS IN THE UNITED STATES

Age Group (yr) and Sex	Population Percentile						
	5	10	25	50	75	90	95
Men							
18–24	235	244	258	272	289	308	323
25–34	242	253	265	280	300	317	329
35–44	250	256	271	287	303	321	330
45–54	240	249	265	281	298	315	326
55–64	228	244	262	279	296	310	318
65–74	225	237	253	269	285	299	307
Women							
18–24	177	185	194	206	221	236	249
25–34	183	189	200	214	229	249	266
35–44	185	192	206	220	240	261	274
45–54	188	195	207	222	243	266	278
55–64	186	195	208	226	244	263	281
65–74	186	195	208	225	244	265	281

*In millimeters.
Adapted from Bishop, C.W., Bowne, P.E., and Ritchey, S.J.: Norms for nutritional assessment of American adults by upper arm anthropometry. Am J Clin Nutr 34:2530, 1981. (Data from Health and Nutrition Examination Survey, 1971–1974.)

consistently be weighed on the same scale. Patients at home are advised to weigh themselves unclothed in the morning after arising and urinating, but before eating or drinking. In the clinic, only light clothing should be worn, with pockets emptied and shoes off; in the hospital the patient should be weighed each time in approximately the same weight of clothing, without slippers. There are devices to measure weight while sitting, as well as scales designed for the bedridden patient.

A commonly used gauge of impaired nutrition is a loss of more than 10 to 15 percent of body weight. The presence or absence of edema should also be noted, as it suggests that water and salt are being retained or lost, with a proportionate effect on body weight. As shown in Chapter 1, ideal body weight (IBW) can be determined when the patient's height is known. This figure is used to calculate calorie and protein requirements. The percentage IBW generally indicates the degree of nutritional depletion, although protein malnutrition may exist in the obese person in the presence of excessive fat stores. Calculation of the IBW by the simple formula in Chapter 1 is easy, available, and relatively accurate in comparison to using reference tables for height and weight to calculate relative weight as a percentage of "desirable," or "ideal," average weight.

Table 3-5. FRAME SIZE*

Height (inches)	W	E Male	E Female
<62	$5^1/_2$–$5^3/_4$	$2^1/_2$–$2^7/_8$	$2^1/_4$–$2^1/_2$
62–65	6–$6^1/_4$	$2^5/_8$–$2^7/_8$	$2^3/_8$–$2^5/_8$
66–71	$6^1/_4$–$6^1/_2$	$2^3/_4$–3	$2^3/_8$–$2^5/_8$
>72		$2^3/_4$–$3^1/_8$	$2^1/_2$–$2^3/_4$

*Table lists *medium-framed* men and women. Measurements lower than those listed indicate a small frame. Higher measurements indicate a large frame.
W = Wrist circumference, inches.
E = Elbow width between epicondyles, inches.

Frame Size

Expected weight for height is adjusted for body frame size, which may be estimated by having the patient wrap the fingers of one hand around the opposite wrist. If the thumb and middle finger

overlap by 1 cm = small frame
touch = medium frame
cannot touch by 1 cm = large frame

Reference tables of wrist circumference are also available (Table 3-5). Wrist circumference is measured around the smallest part of the wrist, distal to the styloid process of radius and ulna. Body frame may also be determined by measurement of the distance between the lateral and medial epicondyles of the humerus with tape or calipers.

Body frame size can also be determined from a height–to–wrist circumference ratio developed by Grant at Duke University. The ratio (r) obtained by comparing height (cm, without shoes) to the wrist circumference (cm) indicates the following correspondence of frame sizes to r values:

	Women	Men
Small	>11	>10.4
Medium	10.1–11	9.6–10.4
Large	<10.1	<9.6

Body Mass Index (BMI)

Various indices of body mass have been developed to provide data relatively independent of frame size and height that provide an accurate measure of adiposity. These include

- weight-to-height ratio (W/H)
- Quetelet index (W/H^2)

- Khosla-Lowe index (W/H^3)
- Benn index (W/H^P)

The Quetelet index is the most widely accepted BMI and correlates with skinfold thickness and hydrostatic measurements of body fat. This BMI is discussed further in Chapter 16.

Skinfold Thickness

Skinfold thickness is a simple indicator of subcutaneous fat stores (which also can be assessed by soft tissue radiography and ultrasound). Calibrated calipers are required for skinfold measurements. They should exert a constant pressure of 10 g per mm^2, measure a range of at least 2 to 40 mm, have a contact of 20 to 40 mm^2, and be accurate to 0.1 mm.

Because it is readily accessible in both males and females, the tricep skinfold thickness (TSF) is the most commonly used measurement. Reproducible, valid measurements can only be obtained by use of a standardized procedure; standards for this measurement are based on the right arm, which should be bare. Using a tape measure, locate the midpoint of the upper arm, between the acromial process of the scapula and the olecranon process of the ulna. The arm should be bent while this point is located. Then, with the arm hanging relaxed at the patient's side, the skin is pinched and pulled away from the underlying muscle, and the calipers are applied 1 cm below the ridge of skin formed (Fig. 3–1). An average of three readings (taken to the

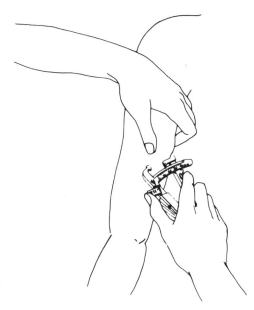

Figure 3–1. Technique for measuring triceps skinfold thickness.

Table 3-6. PERCENTILES FOR SUBSCAPULAR SKINFOLD
THICKNESS* OF ADULTS IN THE UNITED STATES

Age Group (yr) and Sex	Population Percentile						
	5	10	25	50	75	90	95
Men							
18–24	6.0	6.5	8.0	11.0	16.0	24.0	29.0
25–34	6.5	7.0	10.0	14.0	20.0	26.0	30.5
35–44	7.0	8.0	11.5	16.0	21.0	26.0	30.5
45–54	7.0	8.0	12.0	16.5	22.0	29.0	32.0
55–64	6.0	7.0	11.0	15.5	21.0	27.0	30.0
65–74	6.0	7.5	10.5	15.0	20.0	25.0	30.0
Women							
18–24	6.0	7.0	9.0	13.0	19.0	27.0	31.5
25–34	6.0	7.0	10.0	14.5	22.5	32.0	38.0
35–44	6.5	8.0	11.0	17.0	26.5	34.0	39.0
45–54	7.0	8.5	12.0	20.0	28.0	35.0	40.0
55–64	7.0	8.0	12.5	20.0	28.0	34.5	38.0
65–74	7.0	8.0	12.0	18.0	25.0	32.5	37.0

*In millimeters.
Adapted from Grant, J.P., Custer, P.B., and Thurlow, G.: Current techniques of nutritional assessment. Surg Clin North Am 61:443, 1981. (Data from Health and Nutrition Examination Survey, 1971–1974.)

nearest mm) is recorded. If it is not clear that the fat is being pinched firmly and cleanly away from the underlying muscle, have the patient contract and relax the arm muscles to ensure that no muscle is included in the pinch. Continue to pinch the arm while the caliper readings are being made. Skinfold thickness measurements are subject to observer error of ±1.5 mm.

Other skinfolds that may be measured in surveys or research protocols include the subscapular (below the shoulder blades), the suprailiac over the iliac crest (should be no thicker than the little finger of the patient), the thigh, the abdominal, the chest, or the axilla. The subscapular skinfold is measured with the patient sitting. The examiner pinches the skin and subcutaneous tissue at the tip of the right scapula, pulling the skinfold upward and medial. Caliper measurements are taken as with the TSF (Table 3–6).

The pattern of body fat distribution may influence health, so that excess fat deposition in the abdomen and upper body may be associated with risk of cardiovascular disease. The ratio of waist to hip circumference is calculated from measurements of girth with the subject standing. Waist circumference is measured at the level of the umbilicus and hip circumference at the level of the greater trochanters (widest point). A steel tape is used and is held firmly in the horizontal position. Two readings are taken and averaged. The significance of this ratio is discussed in Chapter 16.

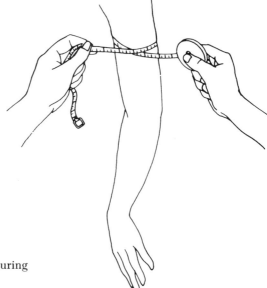

Figure 3-2. Technique for measuring mid-arm muscle circumference.

Mid-Arm Muscle Circumference

By comparing the triceps skinfold thickness (which measures fat stores) with the circumference of the mid upper arm, one can easily calculate the mid-arm muscle circumference (MAMC). The MAMC, a measurement of the lean tissue of the arm, is an indicator of muscle mass or somatic protein stores. To measure the arm circumference, allow the patient's right arm to hang relaxed at the side. A tape is held firmly around the upper arm at the midpoint, avoiding compression of the soft tissues. The circumference is recorded to the nearest 0.1 cm (Fig. 3-2).

MAMC is then calculated by the formula:

$$C_m = C_a - \pi S$$

where C_m = mid–arm muscle circumference (cm); C_a = mid–upper arm circumference (cm); and S = triceps skinfold thickness (cm).

Standards

Normal standards for comparing measurements from individual patients are not well defined, but Tables 3–3 and 3–4 list some standard TSF and MAMC percentile values. A patient's percentage of ideal caloric and somatic protein stores is indicated in Table 3–2. Serious depletion of caloric stores is more easily tolerated than similar depletion of protein stores. (See Chapter 13 for more information on protein-energy malnutrition.)

LABORATORY TESTS

Appropriate investigation includes certain routine laboratory tests (standard blood tests, liver function tests, and so on), as well as other, more specific measurements. These more specific tests can be roughly categorized as follows:

Skeletal muscle mass
    creatinine-height index (24-hour urinary creatinine excretion)
Nitrogen balance
Visceral proteins
    1. Plasma protein measurements (see Table 3–8)
    2. Acute phase reactants
Immune status
    1. Total lymphocyte count
    2. Skin test battery
Intestinal absorption
    1. Schilling test
    2. Fat absorption test
    3. Carotene levels
    4. Vitamin A absorption test
    5. D-xylose test

Blood Tests

The standard clinical blood tests SMA-6 and SMA-12 yield important measurements of blood urea nitrogen, glucose, electrolytes (sodium, potassium, and chloride), minerals (calcium and phosphorus), and renal and hepatic function useful in nutritional evaluation. Specifically, alkaline phosphatase may be an indicator of zinc status; serum glutamic-oxaloacetic transaminase, of pyridoxine status; and prothrombin time, of vitamin K activity. Blood levels of iron, transferrin, or total iron-binding capacity and of cholesterol and triglycerides may also be measured as part of the usual battery of blood tests. See Chapter 2, Chapter 14 (especially Tables 14–1 and 14–2), and Chapter 19 for standards.

Other blood tests of mineral or trace mineral status include those for magnesium and zinc (special tube required). Less readily available may be measurements of circulating copper and selenium.

Many hospital laboratories perform assays of serum or red blood cell folate or vitamin B_{12}. Measurements of levels of other vitamins (A, D metabolites, E, C, and B complex) can be obtained either by direct measurement of levels in blood or urine, or by measuring the activity of enzymes for which the vitamins are cofactors and determining the change in enzyme activity with the vitamin added in vitro (activity coefficient). Adequacy of fatty acid in-

Table 3-7. NUTRITION DATA FROM BLOOD TESTS

Lipids	Normal Range	
Free fatty acids, μEq/liter	300–700	
Plasma fatty acid composition, %		
Fatty Acid	**Normal Range**	**Mean**
16:0	23–36	27.6
16:1	1.6–4.0	3.0
18:0	8.5–22.4	14.2
18:1	14–45	30.8
18:2	8.1–16.2	13.2
20:3	0.8–2.0	1.5
20:4	1.3–6.5	4.5

Triene-to-tetraene ratio <0.3 is normal. An elevation of 20:3, which increases the ratio, is a sign of essential fatty acid deficiency.

take can be determined by the pattern of total fatty acids in plasma or in complex lipids (phospholipids, for example). Normal values for this test appear in Table 3-7.

Hemoglobin

Hemoglobin levels are useful in the assessment of nutritional status, since anemia may be an indication of prolonged protein starvation (normochromic normocytic) or may be vitamin-specific or mineral-related. Further discussion of nutritional anemias is found in Chapter 15. Clues to some specific nutrient deficiencies, liver disease, and alcoholism may also be found in indices of red cell size and hemoglobin content and concentration provided through measurement of the red blood cell count and hematocrit.

Total Lymphocyte Count

The total white blood cell count, when multiplied by the percentage of lymphocytes in the differential count, yields the total lymphocyte count (TLC). A TLC of less than 1500 per mm^3 may indicate depressed immune competence, which may result from protein malnutrition. A mild nutritional deficiency may be reflected in a TLC between 1200 and 1500 per mm^3; moderate deficiency, 800 to 1200; and severe deficiency, less than 800. It is important to remember, however, that the TLC is also affected by blood dyscrasias, infection, chemotherapy, and immunosuppressive therapy, and thus is not always useful in detecting malnutrition. In addition, anesthesia and surgery can depress the lymphocyte count for up to 48 hours.

Plasma Proteins

Visceral protein status is evaluated by measuring plasma proteins. Measurements of albumin, transferrin, thyroxin-binding prealbumin, and retinol-binding protein (RBP) are especially useful (Table 3-8). Low levels may indicate a decrease in hepatic protein synthesis owing to a limiting supply of substrate. The level of somatomedin-C may also be a sensitive marker of visceral protein status (range 0.34 to 2.2 units per ml).

Non-nutritional factors such as expanded extracellular fluid that reduces albumin, accelerated protein breakdown (as well as reduced synthesis), and liver and renal failure also influence the concentration of plasma proteins. In the absence of these confounding factors, the rate of change in levels of plasma proteins in response to change in nutritional status is in inverse proportion to their half-lives. Serum transthyretin (prealbumin) and RBP are thus more sensitive indicators of protein status than is serum albumin. Prealbumin is an early indicator of marginal protein intake, and may be depressed by infection, trauma, and short-term protein and calorie restriction. How-

Table 3-8. PLASMA PROTEINS

Protein	Normal Range	$T^{1/2}$, Days*	Levels Low In	Levels High In
Albumin	3.5–5.4 g/dl	18	Liver disease Pregnancy Overhydration Nephrotic syndrome	Dehydration
Transferrin	200–400 mg/dl	8	Chronic infection Chronic inflammation Liver disease Iron overload Nephrotic syndrome	Iron deficiency Pregnancy Renal insufficiency
Transthyretin (prealbumin)	23–43 mg/dl	2	Liver disease Inflammation Surgery Nephrotic syndrome	Renal insufficiency
Retinol-binding protein (RBP)	3–7 mg/dl	0.5	Liver disease Hyperthyroidism Zinc deficiency Nephrotic syndrome	Renal insufficiency

*$T^{1/2}$ = half-life.

ever, when measured twice weekly, prealbumin levels serve to monitor the effectiveness of treatment. RBP may be elevated in renal disease despite deficiencies in the visceral protein compartment. Tests for prealbumin and RBP can be done rapidly using commercially available radioimmunodiffusion kits (see Table 3–8 for normal values).

Transferrin is of intermediate sensitivity and may be calculated from the total iron-binding capacity (TIBC):

$$\text{Transferrin (mg/dl)} = \frac{\text{TIBC (mg/dl)}}{1.45}$$

However, transferrin values determined from TIBC do not correlate with and are substantially lower than those values obtained directly by radioimmunodiffusion, and transferrin may be elevated in patients with severe iron deficiency anemia.

Serum albumin and transferrin levels in acutely injured or postoperative patients may especially reflect the influence of non-nutritional factors and therefore not be predictive of outcome. In addition, because of albumin's long half-life, dependence on albumin levels alone to monitor visceral protein leads to delays in recognizing and treating deficits.

Acute Phase Reactants. Acute phase reactants have a role in host defense mechanisms (immune response, wound healing) and are stimulated by leukocyte endogenous mediator. These plasma proteins include α-1-glycoprotein, α-1-antitrypsin, C-reactive protein, α-2-macroglobulin, haptoglobin, ceruloplasmin, and fibrinogen.

Serum Carotene

Levels of serum carotene can reflect malnutrition or absence of carotene intake as well as nonabsorption in the intestine. Values above 50 μg per dl probably exclude intestinal malabsorption, as does a rise of 100 μg per dl of carotene following ingestion of 120 mg beta carotene (carotene tolerance test).

Vitamin A

A vitamin A absorption test, revealing impairment of intestinal absorption, can also be performed. The level of vitamin A in the blood is measured 4 to 8 hours after ingestion of 180,000 IU vitamin A in oil. More information on malabsorption is found in Chapter 21.

Urine Tests

Nitrogen Balance

As detailed in Chapter 1, nitrogen balance calculation requires knowledge of protein (nitrogen) intake and collection of at least one 24-hour urine for measurement of urea nitrogen. The same urine collection may be used to measure creatinine.

Creatinine-Height Index

Except in cases of very rapid loss of muscle, as in severe sepsis or trauma, creatinine production from creatine relates directly to skeletal muscle, with each milligram of creatinine equal to 17 to 18 g of muscle mass in women and 23 g in men. If renal function is normal in adults less than 55 years of age, 24-hour urinary creatinine excretion reflects lean body mass (skeletal muscle mass). Creatinine excretion can be expressed in terms of an expected value for body height—the creatinine-height index (CHI)—which is defined as the urinary excretion in 24 hours divided by the urinary excretion of a healthy person of the same gender and height and with ideal body weight. Accurate urine collections are required. This index correlates well with total body nitrogen and therefore reflects muscle bulk.

CHI values of 60 to 80 percent reflect moderate skeletal muscle depletion, and values of 40 to 50 percent indicate severe depletion. Although both measurements reflect skeletal muscle protein stores, arm muscle circumference and creatinine-height index do not correlate.

D-xylose Test

Some tests of intestinal absorption make use of urinary excretion. The D-xylose test of intestinal absorption, for example, requires measurement of urinary excretion 5 hours after oral ingestion of 25 g D-xylose. Twenty percent of the dose should appear in the urine, indicating adequate absorption into the blood and subsequent excretion.

Schilling Test

Absorption of cobalamin is measured by use of the Schilling test. An oral dose of radiocobalt-labeled cobalamin is administered, followed 2 hours later by an intramuscular flushing dose of unlabeled cobalamin. Urine is collected for 24 hours and radioactivity measured to yield excretion as a percentage of the oral dose. This test can be carried out with added intrinsic factor and two isotope labels of cobalt, one complexed with intrinsic factor. Thus, one can distinguish whether malabsorption, if revealed, is due specifically to lack of intrinsic factor.

Analysis of Stool Samples

Impairment of intestinal absorption may lead to nutrient deficiency. Fat absorption (which affects utilization of fat-soluble vitamins) may be evaluated by collection of a 72-hour stool sample from the patient, who should be ingesting at least 100 g of fat daily. The normal coefficient of fat absorption is 95 percent.

Skin Tests

Immune competence may be diminished due to a failure of protein synthesis. Along with calculation of the TLC, a battery of skin tests may be used to evaluate the patient's cell-mediated immunity. Skin test antigens should be those to which healthy persons in a particular geographic area commonly respond because of prior exposure. A positive response is defined as 5 mm or more of cutaneous induration at 24 to 48 hours following the test. The standard skin test battery includes four tests for sensitivity to Trichophyton, mumps, Candida, and one of the tuberculosis antigens. Streptokinase-streptodornase may be added for a fifth skin test. When five skin tests are employed, a normal response is two or more positive responses; one positive response indicates relative anergy; no positive response indicates anergy. The response may be graded on a scale of 1 to 4+, with induration progressively increasing at 5 mm increments.

Anergy may reflect immune deficiency or protein malnutrition or both. TLC may be monitored and the skin tests repeated and correlated with improvement in protein status. Provision of zinc may reverse negative skin test results, however, indicating that protein and energy malnutrition may not be the sole nutritional cause of anergy.

Non-nutritional factors that may depress cellular immunity include anesthesia, burns, corticosteroids, gastrointestinal hemorrhage, infections, liver disease, neoplasm, myocardial infarction, renal failure, sarcoidosis, shock, surgical operations, and trauma.

HOW TO APPLY THIS INFORMATION

The nutrition prescription prepared as a result of the complete nutritional evaluation will determine the method by which the patient can be fed: enteral (usual diet, with supplement, or tube fed) or parenteral (peripheral or central intravenous route). The level of calories, specific restrictions of any macronutrients because of the level of activity, and the presence of stress must be considered. The clinician must determine whether there is a need to replete; what level of protein to provide; whether there is pulmonary, cardiac, renal, or hepatic failure; and whether micronutrients should be provided at the usual level or at increased levels.

Is any portion of the assessment useful in predicting the outcome of a patient's illness? Certainly the incidence of abnormal nutritional indicators is high (occurring in 50 percent of hospitalized patients), and the patient's nutritional status commonly deteriorates during hospitalization. However, a single, ideal diagnostic test for nutritional risk is elusive. Our current armamentarium is nonspecific, and the patient's response to therapy may not necessarily correlate directly with appropriate changes in test values. Thus, multiple parameters must be determined and the interpretation must take into account the patient's entire medical status.

Certain facts are known, however. Mortality is increased in patients whose significant illness, injury, or surgery is accompanied by loss of 20 to 25 percent or more of their usual body weight. Patients with postoperative mortality or sustained complications had TSF values significantly lower than patients surviving without complications. Depressed visceral protein levels are predictive of increased postoperative morbidity and mortality in elective surgery. Anergy, regardless of cause, is associated with a poor prognosis in surgical patients.

Prognostic Nutritional Index

Mullin's group at the University of Pennsylvania has developed a prognostic nutritional index (PNI) that represents the risk of operative complications in a patient by the expression:

$$\text{PNI } (\%) = 158 - 16.6 \underset{\text{g/dl}}{(\text{Alb})} - 0.78 \underset{\text{mm}}{(\text{TSF})} -$$
$$0.20 \underset{\text{g/dl}}{(\text{transferrin})} - 5.8 (\text{skin test reactivity})$$

The skin test reactivity for any one of three antigens is graded 0 (nonreactive), 1 (less than 5 mm induration), or 2 (greater than or equal to 5 mm induration). A PNI less than 40 percent predicts a low risk of complications; the intermediate risk value is 40 to 49 percent, and the high risk value equals or exceeds 50 percent. Although valuable in assessing patients scheduled to undergo elective surgery, the PNI was not predictive of survival in critically ill patients following surgery or acute abdominal trauma.

Limitations and Significance

It should be recognized that the methods for performing nutritional assessment have certain limitations. They are less specific than may be desired, may have only minimal value in patient monitoring, and have only narrow predictive value. The application of nutritional assessment is also circumscribed by the lack of a clearly defined defect to treat or a goal to strive for. However, the methods are simple, promote awareness of nutritional deficits, indicate the potential for repletion, and thus have a significant role in patient care.

CHAPTER 4

Optimizing the Diet

The average American diet contains nearly 200 different food items. This chapter presents information concerning data on nutrient intake, determinants of food consumption, recommended normal dietary plans, tables of food composition, and nutritional labeling of foods. Some special dietary needs, such as those of athletes, and deviations from usual diet preferences, as in vegetarianism, also are discussed. The latter information is designed to assist the physician in the interpretation of patients' eating habits.

80

SOURCES OF NUTRIENT DATA

Information on the nutritional status of Americans comes from many sources, including
- agricultural data on food production and food imports/exports
- data on marketing, distribution, and storage of food
- cultural data pertaining to patterns of food consumption by groups, families, and individuals
- clinical nutrition surveys of deficiency signs
- anthropometric studies of physical development
- laboratory tests of nutrient levels
- vital statistics on morbidity and mortality
- epidemiologic information on the relation of diet to disease

Most of the information used is derived from dietary surveys, studies of food habits, anthropometric data, and clinical and laboratory nutrition surveys.

These data reveal that the American diet changed markedly over the past century, with two major differences from 1900 to 1976: (1) consumption of meat, poultry, fish, dairy products, sugar and other sweeteners, fats and oils, and processed fruits and vegetables increased; and (2) consumption of grain products, potatoes, sweet potatoes, fresh fruit, vegetables, and eggs decreased (Table 4–1).

In addition to monitoring per capita food consumption, the USDA estimates food intake from surveys such as the Ten State Nutrition Survey, the Health and Nutrition Examination Survey (HANES), and the Continuing Survey of Food Intakes by Individuals (CSFII). These surveys provide specific data on nutritional status and dietary practices.

Ten State Nutrition Survey

The Ten State Nutrition Survey was conducted from 1968 to 1970. It focused on low income groups in 10 states and evaluated 40,000 individuals.

Health and Nutrition Examination Survey

HANES was conducted in 1971. It consisted of four parts:
- a record of dietary intake based on 24-hour recall and food frequency questionnaires
- measurement of biochemical levels of various nutrients based on assays of blood and urine samples
- observation by a physician of clinical signs of nutrition deficiency
- anthropometric measurement

Table 4–1. CHANGES IN THE NUTRIENTS IN THE
U.S. DIET PER CAPITA CONSUMPTION

	Year			Change From 1977–1985 (percent)
	1900	1947	1976	
Fat, % kcal	32		42	−14
g/day	125	140	157	−6
Complex CHO, % kcal	37		21	
Sugar, lb/yr	89	110	119	−19
Refined sweeteners, % kcal	12		18	
CHO, g/day	492	403	376	+19
Protein, % kcal	19		19	—
g/day	102	95	101	—
Calories/day	3480	3230	3300	+6
Eggs, lb/yr	37	47	35	−26
Dairy products, qt/yr	177	236	222	
Butter, lb/yr	18	11	4	
Legumes, lb/yr	16	17	18	+41
Four/cereal, lb/yr	291	171	140	
Coffee/tea/cocoa, lb/yr	10	19	12	
Citrus fruits, fresh, lb/yr	17	52	29	
processed, lb/yr	0	14	47	
Other fruits, fresh, lb/yr	151	112	78	
processed, lb/yr	8	30	34	
Green/yellow vegetables, fresh	14	27	18	
processed	—	4	7	
Other vegetables, fresh	172	157	127	
processed	17	43	62	
Potatoes, white, fresh, lb/yr	182	111	54	
processed, lb/yr			22	
Potatoes, sweet, fresh	25	12	4	
processed			2	
Vitamin A, IU/day	7600.00	8800.00	8100.00	−6
Vitamin C, mg/day	104.00	114.00	118.00	+21
Vitamin B_1, mg/day	1.64	1.91	2.04	+15
Vitamin B_2, mg/day	1.86	2.30	2.46	+3
Vitamin B_3, mg/day	19.20	21.40	25.20	+9
Vitamin B_6, mg/day	2.26	1.99	2.26	+3
Vitamin B_{12}, µg/day	8.40	9.00	9.60	+24
Ca, g/day	0.82	1.00	0.93	+13
P, g/day	1.56	1.55	1.55	+6
Fe, mg/day	15.20	6.80	8.60	−1
Mg, mg/day	408.00	369.00	344.00	+6

Data derived from periodic nationwide food consumption surveys of individuals and apply to food intakes by adult men.

HANES data cover a sample of 28,943 persons ages 1 to 74, from 65 locations in the 48 contiguous states. Information on dietary intake, clinical and bio-chemical findings, anthropometric data, hemoglobin, serum iron, transferrin saturation, and serum cholesterol levels is available in publications from the National Center for Health Statistics. A follow-up survey, HANES 2, was carried out in 1974. HANES 3 is scheduled over 6 years, from 1988 to 1994. Estimates will be developed after 2 years and data will be made available by 1991.

Continuing Survey of Food Intakes by Individuals

The yearly Continuing Survey of Food Intakes by Individuals (CSFII) was conducted in 1985 and 1986 by the USDA, using a 1-day dietary recall collected by personal interview and 5 days of dietary data obtained by tele-phone at 2-month intervals over the year. The CSFII is a major component of the National Nutrition Monitoring System, a set of Federal activities intended to provide regular information on the nutritional status of the United States population.

The CSFII sampled households of women 19 to 50 years of age and their children 1 to 5 years of age. Data were collected for approximately 1500 women, 1100 men, and 500 children. Intakes by men in 1985 compared with 1977 (see Table 4–1) were lower in meat (principally beef), whole milk, and eggs. Intakes were higher in fish; low fat or skim milk; legumes, nuts, and seeds; and carbonated soft drinks (regular and low calorie). The percent of calories from fat decreased and from carbohydrate increased.

DETERMINANTS OF FOOD INTAKE

People choose foods—not nutrients—and their choices are determined by cultural, social, personal, and situational factors, including ethnicity and family tradition. Fads (discussed fully in Chapter 6) also affect food choices, while emotional associations with rewards or punishment may explain some selections.

In general, people will avoid foods that cause unpleasant symptoms and select those that are well tolerated. These factors especially influence sick people and postoperative patients. In addition, food choices may be restricted or influenced by poverty, lack of transportation, limited availability of foods in stores, poor food storage facilities, lack of cooking facilities or skills, or limited time for food preparation. Advertising and food labeling also may strongly influence choices.

In the United States, economic factors are more likely to limit the variety of food intake than directly to determine inadequate diet. Low income populations may be poorly educated and less likely to understand the food group classifications; their choices will be according to likes and dislikes, the influence of advertising, and the appearance of meal items.

DIETARY GUIDELINES

Several agencies have published guidelines to advise Americans on what constitutes a healthful diet.

Senate Committee Dietary Goals

In 1977 the Senate Select Committee on Nutrition and Human Needs issued *Dietary Goals for the United States*, based on concerns that overnutrition plays a role in the etiology of obesity, coronary heart disease, cancer, and stroke. The goals stipulated that Americans should consume less food, fat (especially saturated fat), cholesterol, refined sugar, and salt, and should increase consumption of fruits, vegetables, grain products, and unsaturated oils (Table 4–2). These goals suggest the following changes in food selection and preparation:

1. Increase consumption of fruits, vegetables, and whole grains.
2. Decrease consumption of red meats, and increase consumption of poultry and fish.

Table 4-2. DIETARY GOALS FOR THE UNITED STATES

1. Reduce overall fat consumption from approximately 40 percent to about 30 percent of energy intake.
2. Reduce saturated-fat consumption to account for about 10 percent of total energy intake and balance that with polyunsaturated and monosaturated fats, which should account for about 10 percent of energy intake each.
3. Reduce cholesterol consumption to about 300 mg per day.
4. Limit the intake of sodium by reducing the intake of salt (sodium chloride) to about 3 g per day (<2 g sodium).
5. Increase the consumption of complex carbohydrates and "naturally occurring" sugars from about 22 percent to about 45 percent of energy intake.
6. Reduce the consumption of refined and other processed sugars by about 40 percent to account for about 15 percent of total energy intake.
7. To avoid overweight, consume only as much energy (calories) as is expended; if overweight, decrease energy intake and increase energy expenditure.

From Report of the Select Committee on Nutrition and Human Needs, U.S. Senate: Eating in America: Dietary Goals for the United States, ed 2. MIT Press, Cambridge, MA, December, 1977, p. 12, with permission. [See also "Healthy People," the Surgeon General's report on health promotion and disease prevention, 1979. DHEW (PHS) Pub. No. 79-55071.]

3. Decrease consumption of foods high in fat, and partially substitute polyunsaturated fat for saturated fat.
4. Substitute nonfat milk for whole milk.
5. Decrease consumption of butterfat, eggs, and other high cholesterol sources.
6. Decrease consumption of refined sugars and foods high in sugar.
7. Decrease consumption of salt and foods high in salt.

Table 4–3 lists sample meals for a day, based on the 1977 goals.

**Table 4–3. SAMPLE MEALS FOR A DAY FOR A MAN
AGE 20–54 MEETING THE DIETARY GOALS**

Breakfast
    Cereal, 2 cups (with sugar*)
    Skim milk, 1 cup
    Toast, 3 slices
    Margarine*
    Juice, $1/2$ cup
    Coffee or tea, if desired
Lunch
    Macaroni salad, 1 cup
      (contains macaroni, $1/3$ egg, 2 tbs kidney beans, salad oil)
    Vegetable, $1/2$ cup
    Bread, 3 slices
    Margarine
    Milk, $1/2$ cup
Dinner
    Lean meat, poultry, or fish,† 5 oz
    Potato, $1/2$ cup
    Other vegetable or salad, $1/2$ cup
    Bread, 3 slices
    Margarine
    Cake
    Coffee or tea, if desired
Snack
    Biscuits, 3
    Juice, $1/2$ cup

*About 2 tbs of sugar or other sweets such as syrup, jams, and jellies and $3^1/2$ tbs of fats and oils per day may be added to foods during preparation or at the table.
†Meat and poultry (or fish) are served on alternate days.
From Peterkin, B.: The dietary goals and food on the table. Food Technol 32:34, 1978, with permission.

Nutrition Objectives for the Nation

Nutrition goals and objectives for the nation in relation to health promotion and disease prevention were first reported in the Surgeon General's Report on Health Promotion and Disease Prevention entitled *Healthy People,* published in 1979.

The specific nutrition objectives developed from that report were published in Public Health Reports, September-October, 1983. The nutrition goals and objectives are to be attained by 1990 and state that:

1. The proportion of pregnant women with iron deficiency anemia (as estimated by hemoglobin concentrations early in pregnancy) should be reduced to 3.5 percent.
2. Growth retardation of infants and children caused by inadequate diets should have been eliminated in the United States as a public health problem.
3. The prevalence of significant overweight (120 percent of "desired" weight) among the U.S. adult population should be decreased to 10 percent of men and 17 percent of women, without nutritional impairment.
4. Fifty percent of the overweight population should have adopted weight loss regimens, combining an appropriate balance of diet and physical activity.
5. The mean serum cholesterol level in the adult population 18–74 years of age should be at or below 200 mg per dl. The mean serum cholesterol level in children 1–14 years of age should be at or below 150 mg per dl.
6. The average daily sodium ingestion (as measured by excretion) by adults should be reduced at least to the 3 to 6 gram range.
7. The proportion of women who breast feed their healthy, full-term babies at hospital discharge should be increased to 75 percent and 50 percent at 3 months of age.
8. The proportion of the population which is able to correctly associate the principal dietary factors known or strongly suspected to be related to disease should exceed 75 percent for each of the following diseases: heart disease, high blood pressure, dental caries and cancer.
9. Seventy percent of adults should be able to identify the major foods which are low in fat content, low in sodium content, high in calories, high in sugars, good sources of fiber.
10. Ninety percent of adults should understand that to lose weight people must either consume foods that contain fewer calories or increase physical activity—or both.
11. The labels of all packaged foods should contain useful caloric and nutrient information to enable consumers to select diets that pro-

mote and protect good health. Similar information should be displayed where nonpackaged foods are obtained or purchased.

12. The proportion of employees and school cafeteria managers who are aware of, and actively promoting, USDA/DHHS dietary guidelines should be greater than 50 percent.

13. All states should include nutrition education as part of required comprehensive school health education at the elementary and secondary levels.

14. Virtually all routine health contacts with health professionals should include some element of nutrition education and nutrition counseling.

15. A comprehensive national nutrition status monitoring system should have the capability for detecting nutritional problems in special population groups, as well as for obtaining baseline data for decisions on national nutrition policies.

USDA/HEW Dietary Guidelines

In February 1980, the USDA and the Department of Health, Education and Welfare published *Dietary Guidelines* (updated in 1985). They recommend

1. Eat a variety of foods.
2. Maintain desirable weight.
3. Avoid too much fat, saturated fat, and cholesterol.
4. Eat foods with adequate starch and fiber.
5. Avoid too much sugar.
6. Avoid too much sodium.
7. If you drink alcoholic beverages, do so in moderation.

In Chapter 19, recent dietary recommendations from the American Heart Association and NIH for heart disease prevention are described in more detail.

Diet and Cancer

For guidelines aimed at cancer prevention, see **Diet to Prevent Cancer,** Chapter 24.

THE "BASIC FOUR" PLAN

In response to the need for simple, specific guidelines to enable an American household to plan and consume meals meeting the RDA, the United

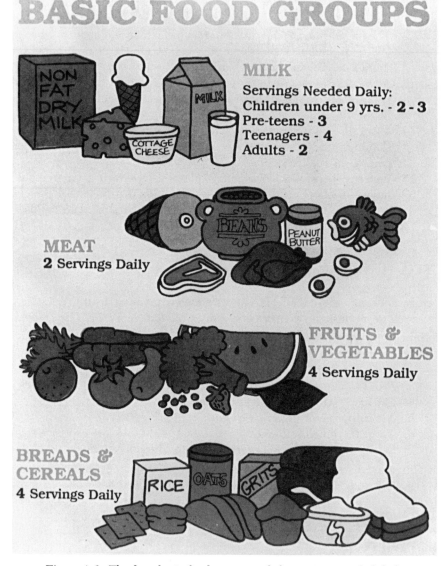

Figure 4–1. The four basic food groups and the servings needed daily.

States Department of Agriculture in 1956 established four major food groups—the "basic four" plan. The plan recommends a specific number of daily servings from each group: milk and milk products, meat and meat substitutes, fruits and vegetables, and breads and cereals. A well-balanced diet for an adult should include two or more servings daily from the milk and meat groups, and four or more servings from the fruit and vegetable and

Table 4–4. FOOD GROUPS AND SOME MAJOR NUTRIENTS

Food Group	Nutrient			Vitamins			Minerals	
	Protein	CHO	Fiber	A	B	C	Ca	Fe
Milk	X			X	Riboflavin		X	
Meat	X				X			X
Fruits and vegetables			X	X		X		X
Breads and cereals		X			X			X

bread and cereal groups (Fig. 4–1). The recommended number of milk servings increases for children and others with special needs.

As shown in Tables 4–4 and 4–5, each of the four groups provides different nutrients. Thus, individuals must select meals and snacks from each group in order to obtain all essential nutrients. In addition, it must be recognized that nutrients are not distributed evenly within each group. Thus, servings of fruits and vegetables, for example, should include one vitamin C–rich food daily and one vitamin A–rich food every other day (see Table 2–3).

While adhering to the basic four plan, there can be wide variation in total nutrient intake. For example, depending on the specific foods chosen, vitamin E intake may range from 10 to 100 mg, and calorie intake may range from 800 to 1800 calories (below the RDA for most adults). Isocaloric servings may have quite dissimilar nutrient content, and, conversely, sources of similar micronutrients may vary widely in calories. Thus, roughly the same calcium content (about 300 mg) is found in 1 cup of whole, low fat, or skim milk, chocolate milk, buttermilk, yogurt, pudding, or custard, or in varying amounts of nonfat milk powder, cheeses, and ice cream (Table 4–6). Similarly, cheeses, eggs, peanut butter, and beans can be substituted for meat, while bread and cereal equivalents include biscuits, crackers, and pasta (Table 4–7).

As can be seen from Table 4–5, eating only the recommended number of servings from each group may result in a diet deficient in calories, vitamins A and E, riboflavin, niacin, folacin, magnesium, iron, and zinc. Because the foods included provide a larger proportion of many nutrients than they do of calories, additional calories may be consumed by eating more servings of foods within the plan or by eating other, unlisted food.

Calorie-Dense Foods

Assuming that an adequate amount of fat occurs in foods or is added in food preparation and seasoning, the basic four plan makes no recommenda-

Table 4-5. NUTRIENT CONTENT OF THE FOUR FOOD GROUPS COMPARED WITH RDAS*

Food	Recommended Servings	Energy, kcal	Protein, g	Fat, g	Carbohydrate, g	Vitamin A, mg RE	Ascorbic acid, mg	Thiamin, mg	Niacin, mg	Calcium, mg	Iron, mg	Zinc, mg	Dietary fiber, g
RECOMMENDED DIETARY ALLOWANCES†													
Female (23–50 yr)		2000	44			800	60	1.0	13	800	18	15	
Male (23–50 yr)		2700	56			1000	60	1.4	18	800	10	15	
Milk Group	(2)												
2% low fat	2 cups	288	20	10	29	117	5	0.2	0.5	698	0.5	1.9	0
Meat Group	(3)‡												
Egg	1	70	6	5	0	156	0	0.1	0.1	24	1.1	0.5	0
Meat, fish, poultry	4 oz	285	31	18	0	26	0	0.3	7.3	14	3.1	5.4	0
Vegetable-Fruit Group	(5)‡												
Leafy green and deep yellow	1/4–1/3 cup	12	1	0	2	254	20	0	0.3	34	0.6	0.3	2.0
Other vegetables	1/4–1/3 cup	19	1	0	4	35	7	0	0.4	19	0.5	0.2	1.4
Potato	1 medium	113	3	0	26	0	24	0.1	2.0	11	0.8	0.3	3.5
Citrus fruit	1 serving	44	1	0	10	12	44	0.1	0.3	19	0.3	0.1	0.4
Other fruit	1 serving	92	1	0	22	50	5	0	0.4	10	0.6	0.2	1.5

Table 4-5. NUTRIENT CONTENT OF THE FOUR FOOD GROUPS COMPARED WITH RDAS* (Continued)

Food	Recommended Servings	Energy, kcal	Protein, g	Fat, g	Carbohydrate, g	Vitamin A, mg RE	Ascorbic acid, mg	Thiamin, mg	Niacin, mg	Calcium, mg	Iron, mg	Zinc, mg	Dietary fiber, g
Bread-Cereal Group	(4)												
Cereal, enriched or whole grain	¾ cup	135	4	1	29	0	0	0.1	1.3	13	1.1	0.5	3.8
Bread, enriched or whole grain	3 slices	205	7	2	39	0	0	0.2	2.0	68	1.9	0.8	6.4
Unlisted													
Fortified margarine	4 tsp	144	0	16	0	66**	0	0	0	4	0	0	0
Totals		1300	75	62	161	716**	105	1.9	14.6**	914	10.5**	10.2**	19

*Values represent the average nutrient content of a food group.
†From Recommended Dietary Allowances (see References).
‡Recommended 2 or more meat, 4 or more vegetable and fruit.
( ) Number of servings per day.
**Not meeting all RDAs.

Table 4–6. EQUIVALENT PROVIDERS OF CALCIUM IN THE DIET

Milk	1 cup
Yogurt	1 cup
Pudding	1 cup
Custard	1 cup
Nonfat, dry milk	1/3 cup
Cottage cheese	1 1/3 cup
Processed cheese	1 1/3 oz
Cheddar cheese	1 1/3 oz
Ice cream	1 1/2 cup

Table 4–7. FOOD GROUP SERVINGS

Meats	
Beef	
Lamb	
Pork	2 oz
Fish	
Poultry	
Cheddar cheese	2 oz
Cottage cheese	1/2 cup
Eggs	2
Peanut butter	2 tbs
Dried beans or peas, cooked	1 cup
Bread/Cereal (grains)	
Bread	1 slice
Muffin	1
Biscuit	1
Rolls	1/2
Cornbread	1 1/2 inch cube
Crackers	4–6
Cooked cereal, grits, pasta	1/2 cup
Breakfast cereal	3/4 cup
Tortilla	1
Fruits/Vegetables	1/2 cup or 1 medium piece

tions for fat consumption. In practice, however, more than enough fat is usually consumed in the American diet. Vegetable oils, lard, butter, margarine, and bacon are very high in calories with respect to the nutrients they contain (that is, they are "calorie dense").

Sweets and alcohol are also calorie-dense foods. Sugar, honey, syrup, jelly, candy, soft drinks, wine, beer, and hard liquor provide relatively "empty" calories. For this reason it is important to ensure that people include beverages, sweeteners, and snacks when reporting food consumption.

THE FOUR FOOD GROUPS

Milk and Milk Products

Milk is a good source of many nutrients. Cow's milk is a good source of protein, 80 percent of which is casein. The whey products resemble those in plasma and include lactalbumin and various immunoglobulins. Milk fat is for the most part easily digested. The carbohydrate in all milks is lactose, a sugar much less sweet than sucrose and not readily digested by some ethnic groups and sick people. Calcium is present in all milks in large quantities, chiefly combined with caseinogen, and is generally absorbed more readily than is calcium in other foods. Milk contains very little iron and is a useful, though not rich, source of vitamins. While its riboflavin and nicotinic acid may be valuable to people whose diets are poor, its ascorbic acid content is not high and is destroyed by pasteurization. Vitamin D, however, is generally added to milk.

Sour or curdled milk has all the protein, fat, calcium, and vitamins of the original milk. If yogurt is made from skim milk, the fat content decreases to 0.5 g per dl.

Cream contains all the fat and usually from one third to one half of the protein and lactose in milk. The fat content varies from 10 to 12 percent in "half-and-half" to 35 percent in whipping cream. The fat content of evaporated milk may vary, while condensed milk has added sugar. Skim milk contains the protein and calcium in the original milk and also contains the B vitamins. Dried skim milk may also be enriched with vitamins A and D.

Cheese

There are over 400 varieties of cheese, which is made from clotting of milk using rennet. The clot contains almost all the protein and fat in milk and many of the other nutrients. Ripening of cheese involves bacterial fermentation, giving the cheese its characteristic texture and flavor. Most cheeses contain 25 to 35 percent protein of high biologic value, with fat content usually varying from 16 to 40 percent. Cheeses are rich in calcium, vitamin A, and riboflavin.

Meat, Fish, Eggs, and Meat Substitutes

While meat is an excellent source of protein, protein of animal origin is not essential. As discussed in Chapter 1, proper combinations of vegetable proteins can supply all the essential amino acids. The perception that more land and energy are required for production of meat than for grain has led to a search for meat substitutes.

Meat

The digestibility of meat relates to the amount of muscle protein versus connective tissue, collagen, and fat. The collagen content may vary from 2.5 to 23.6 percent, while the proportion of fat in meat may vary from 5 to 50 percent. Tenderness is associated with marbling with fat, and is improved in beef that is appropriately stored. The flavor of meat derives in part from purines and amino acids.

The caloric value of meat depends primarily on the fat content. Lean meat contains about 20 percent protein and 5 to 10 percent fat; the protein is of high biologic value. Pork and chicken have a higher protein-to-fat ratio than beef and lamb.

Meats are usually rich in iron and zinc but contain little calcium. They are important sources of nicotinic acid and riboflavin. Muscle also provides moderate amounts of vitamin B_{12}, but very little vitamin A or ascorbic acid.

Fish

Fish is an important source of animal protein. Lean fish, such as cod, haddock, and sole, contains less than 1 percent fat, about 10 percent protein, is relatively low in calories, and is easily digested. Fatty fish, such as herring, salmon, and sardines, contains 8 to 15 percent fish oil, giving it double the calories of lean fish. Halibut, mackerel, and trout have intermediate fat content. Although the protein content of fish is less than that of meat, the protein is of high biologic value. Fish roe contains 20 to 30 percent protein, is rich in nucleic acid, and contains about 20 percent fat. Fish oils are rich sources of vitamins A and D, in addition to containing unique long chain, polyunsaturated omega-3 fatty acids (see Chapters 1 and 19). Iodine and fluoride are found in large quantities in marine fish, and small whole fish are high in calcium.

Shellfish. Shellfish have little fat and are low in calories. Protein content of oysters, mussels, and other molluscs is about 15 percent. These shellfish contain 5 percent glycogen and little fat. Oysters are the richest food source of zinc. See Chapter 5, however, for a discussion of allergic reactions to shellfish, toxins, and possible contamination.

Eggs

Naturally rich in essential nutrients, the average egg weighs about 2 ounces (60 g), contains 6 g protein, 6 g fat, and yields 80 calories. Egg proteins are mostly albumin, with the highest biologic value of all food proteins for human adults. The iron in egg is poorly absorbed, but the yolk is a fair source of vitamin A and contains significant amounts of B vitamins. There is about 250 mg of cholesterol in the average egg, with little or no ascorbic acid.

Meat Substitutes

(See section on **Vegetarian Diets**, p. 102.)

Textured Vegetable Protein. Derived from soybeans, textured vegetable protein is flavored to resemble meat. The natural ingredients contain no vitamin B_{12}. Vegetable proteins have less methionine than animal proteins and may be lower in iron, thiamin, and riboflavin than meat.

Legumes. Legumes are seeds of the family that includes peas, beans, and lentils. With a high protein content of about 20 g per 100 g dry weight, legumes qualify as meat substitutes. Although their low content of sulfur-containing amino acids reduces the biologic value of the protein, they are rich in lysine, in which many cereals are deficient. For this reason, a combination of legumes and cereal proteins may have a nutritive value as good as animal proteins, while also serving as an excellent source of fiber. Legumes also are a good source of B vitamins, except riboflavin, and there are no nutritive losses, as can occur in milling and cooking. Although legumes normally lack ascorbic acid, sprouted legumes will prevent scurvy.

Soybeans. Soybeans are very high in protein, with the whole dry grain containing 40 percent protein and up to 20 percent fat. Soya also provides B vitamins. See also Chapter 8 for soy-based infant formula products.

Peanuts and Other Legumes. Peanuts are seeds of a leguminous plant, and contain about 20 percent fat. Other legumes include lima beans, kidney beans, green beans, navy beans, baked beans, and broad beans. While their digestion and absorption is virtually complete, flatulence may be a byproduct.

Nuts. Although nuts are high in fat and protein content, they generally do not contribute significant nutrients to the diet.

Fruits and Vegetables

Fruits

With the widest variety of pleasing flavors, this class of foods can satisfy a sweet tooth without excessive calories. Nutritionally, however, ascorbic acid is the only essential nutrient in which fruits are rich. They are also sources of dietary fiber, and most contain small quantities of carotene and B vitamins. Most fruits have little or no protein or fat, and 5 to 20 percent carbohydrate. Ripe fruits provide fructose and glucose as the major sugars, often in equal proportions, but contain no starch. With much greater amounts of carbohydrates than most fruits, bananas serve as a useful energy source, but provide no protein. Some fruits, such as bananas and oranges, are high in potassium (see Chapter 2).

Vegetables

Although we all know what vegetables are, they are not easily described or classified. They may be leaves, roots, flowers, stalks, or gourds. Despite their differing botanic structure, however, vegetables' nutritive properties are similar. The chief nutritional value of vegetables is their contribution of carotene, ascorbic acid, and folate. In addition, they all contain dietary fiber. Although calcium and iron may be present in significant amounts, absorption is variable. Leafy vegetables may provide some B vitamins (riboflavin), but vegetables generally are poor sources of energy, protein, and amino acids.

Potatoes, a starchy root, are the inexpensive food most capable of supporting life as the sole diet. Starch supplies most of potatoes' calories. Although the protein content is low, it has relatively high biologic value. Potatoes are high in fiber and a good source of potassium. They are easily digested, well absorbed, and (contrary to myth) not especially fattening.

The quality and nutritional value of canned and frozen vegetables compare favorably with that of fresh produce; both contribute to the attractiveness of well-served meals. A single serving of fruit or vegetable usually is one-half cup, or one medium-size piece.

Breads and Cereals

The seeds of domesticated grasses, cereal grains remain the most important single food in many countries, including their consumption as bread and flour products. The principal cereals produced in North America are corn, wheat, barley, oats, and rye. Of these, only wheat and rye can be milled into flour.

Whole grain cereals are all similar in chemical constituents and nutritive value. They provide energy, good quality protein, and appreciable amounts of calcium and iron. Cereals contain no ascorbic acid and practically no vitamin A; yellow corn is the only cereal containing significant amounts of carotene. Except for corn, in which the nicotinic acid is not biologically available, whole grain cereals contain adequate amounts of B vitamins. However, milling and discarding of the outer portion of the seed diminishes the B vitamin content, especially from wheat and rice.

Wheat and Its Products

Wheat is usually ground into flour before being prepared as food. Wheat may contain from 10 to 20 g protein per 100 g, with lysine the limiting amino acid. In the average flour used to make white bread, protein provides about 13 percent of the energy. Bread has the nutritive properties of the flour from which it was baked, and all kinds are generally good sources of protein. Whole wheat flour does contain three times as much dietary fiber as white flour, but whole wheat is also high in phytate, which binds minerals (especially divalent cations), making them unavailable. Thus, although whole wheat flour contains appreciable amounts of calcium, iron, and zinc, absorption may be limited. In the United States each 100 g of white flour is enriched with up to 0.44 mg thiamin, 0.26 mg riboflavin, 3.5 mg nicotinamide, and 2.9 mg iron. In some states, calcium and vitamin D also may be added.

Pasta utilizes a portion of the wheat grain that is relatively poor in B vitamins, and so it too is frequently enriched.

Rice

With milling, rice undergoes changes similar to those in wheat, so that highly refined rice is almost devoid of vitamins. Parboiling fixes the vitamins so that they are not removed with milling, and is the simplest preventive measure against beriberi. Most rice contains 6.5 to 8.0 g protein per 100 g— less than other cereals—but it is of good quality.

Corn

The cereal structure of corn is similar to that of rice and wheat. The principal protein in corn (about half the total) is incomplete, lacking lysine and tryptophan. Yellow corn contains a mixture of carotenoids. Although the nicotinic acid in corn normally is bound, the preparation of Mexican tortillas makes it biologically available by heating the grains in lime water to soften them.

Other Grains

Oatmeal contains more protein (12 g per 100 g) and more oil (8.5 g per 100 g) than other common cereals. Barley produces the malt for brewers and is the basis of the best beers and types of whiskey. Bread made from rye flour is rich in B vitamins, and also contains fiber.

Breakfast Cereals

The chief nutritive value of breakfast cereals is derived from the addition of milk. Some cereals are fortified with B vitamins, iron, and, most recently, calcium.

OPTIMIZING MEALS AS SOURCES OF NUTRIENTS

Including smaller portions of a wider variety of foods can improve the nutritional quality of meals while maintaining or lowering the caloric content (Table 4–8). For example, 6 ounces of steak with a baked potato and a tomato contains fewer calories (480 kcal) than a protein-heavy meal of 10 ounces of steak and a tomato (655 kcal). Substituting a roll for a high-fat salad dressing will transform a 740 kcal chef's salad (very low in carbohydrate) to a more healthful 590 kcal sandwich, with room to have some fruit for dessert. Generally, reducing the intake of fatty and protein-heavy foods and increasing the proportion of starchy foods and fruit will provide more satisfying meals that offer both more micronutrients and more food. Often this change also causes a healthy increase in the dietary intake of fiber.

Simple changes in food preparation methods and seasonings (Table 4–9) can appreciably cut calorie content without altering intake of vitamins, minerals, or protein. Those who need to consume more calories can gain both calories and nutrients from healthful between-meal snacks such as milkshakes or peanut butter or other nut butter. Specific diets for weight reduction or weight gain are discussed in Chapter 16.

Determining Composition of Food

Tables of Food Composition

Food composition tables, providing average nutrient values based on quantitative analyses of many samples of each item, have been available for about 100 years. Most tables include data for five vitamins (vitamin A, thiamin, riboflavin, niacin, and ascorbic acid), calcium, iron, energy, protein, carbohydrate, and fat. The USDA periodically publishes updated food com-

Table 4–8. HOW TO OPTIMIZE THE DIET

	Common Choice		Wiser Choice	
	Menu	*Kcal*	*Menu*	*Kcal*
Breakfast	Orange juice, 1/2 cup		Orange juice, 1/2 cup	
	Black coffee		Skim milk, 1/2 cup	
	Fruit-flavored yogurt	320	Whole grain cereal, 1/2 cup	
			Toast, 2 slices	
			Butter/margarine, 1 tsp	325
Lunch	Tuna salad		Sliced turkey	
	Coleslaw, potato salad		Carrot sticks	
	Sliced tomato		Tomato	
	Crackers		Whole wheat bread	
	Mineral water	930	Cantaloupe, 1/2 melon	
			Milk, 1 cup	540
	or		*or*	
	Chef's salad and dressing	740	Ham, cheese, lettuce, tomato	
			Roll	590
	or		*or*	
	Meat patty		Meatballs	
	Cottage cheese		Grated cheese	
	Tomato		Tomato sauce	
	Lettuce		Spaghetti	445
	Pickle	465		
Dinner	Broiled chicken, 1/2		Broiled chicken leg	
	Tossed salad		Tossed salad	
	French dressing, 2 tbs		Dressing, 1 tbs	
	Green beans	410	Peas and onions, 1 cup	
			Roll	
			Grapes, small bunch	575
	or		*or*	
	Steak, 10 oz		Steak, 6 oz	
	Broiled tomato		Broiled tomato	
	Watercress	655	Watercress	
			Baked potato	480
Snack	0		Banana, popcorn (3 cups)	150
			or	
			11 Saltines	
			or	
			Fruit	
			or	
			Fruit juice and mineral water	

TABLE 4–9. SUGGESTIONS FOR INGESTING
FEWER CALORIES

Suggestion	Examples	Amount	Calorie Content
1. Use skim or low fat dairy products.	Skim milk	8 fl oz	90
	Whole milk	8 fl oz	160
2. Try seasonings or lemon juice instead of butter or margarine to bring out natural vegetable flavors.	Butter	1 tsp	35
	Margarine	1 tsp	35
	Lemon juice	1 tsp	1
3. Broil, bake, stew, or roast meat instead of frying. Use a rack to hold roast out of drippings. Skim excess fat from stew and soup.	Vegetable oil	1 tbs	125
	Lard	1 tbs	115
	Vegetable shortening	1 tbs	110
4. Poach or boil eggs rather than frying or scrambling.	Poached egg	1	80
	Boiled egg	1	80
	Scrambled egg	1	110
	Fried egg	1	110

position tables (e.g., Handbook No. 8, "Composition of Foods") in various sections. USDA Handbook No. 456 presents values for foods using household measures rather than the standard 100 g portions.

Labeling

Food Labeling. The Food and Drug Administration (FDA) has set standards for food labeling to provide information on the nutritional content of food products. Although primarily intended to protect consumers from deception, the requirements also permit consumers to gain useful nutritional information. Labels are required to include

- the name and address of the manufacturer
- the name of the product
- the quantity of the contents
- the ingredients listed in order of their predominance by weight for foods not defined by a standard of identity
- names of specific chemical preservatives used
- a statement that artificial flavoring or coloring has been used, although the specific flavor or color need not be named
- serving size (reasonable for an adult male engaged in light physical activity), if the number of servings is stated

Table 4–10. U.S. RECOMMENDED DAILY ALLOWANCES (AGE 4 YEARS AND OLDER)

Nutrient	Requirement
Protein	45–65 g*
Vitamin A	5000 IU
Vitamin D	400 IU
Vitamin E	30 IU
Vitamin C	60 mg
Thiamin	1.5 mg
Riboflavin	1.7 mg
Niacin	20 mg
Vitamin B_6	2.0 mg
Folic acid	400 μg
Vitamin B_{12}	3.0 μg
Pantothenic acid	10 mg
Biotin	0.3 mg
Calcium	1000 mg
Phosphorus	1000 mg
Magnesium	400 mg
Iron	18 mg
Zinc	15 mg
Iodine	150 μg
Copper	2.0 mg

*The U.S. RDA for protein is 45 g if the protein is "complete," that is, from an animal source. The U.S. RDA for protein becomes 65 g if the protein is "incomplete," that is, from a plant source. The U.S. RDA for foods with protein from both plant and animal sources should be in the 45 to 65 g range.

Nutrition Labeling. Nutrition labels are required for foods that are advertised for their nutritional properties (for example, low calorie, low fat) or food enriched or fortified with nutrients. Nutrition labels must follow a format established by the FDA, which includes

- calories per serving
- grams of protein, carbohydrate, and fat per serving
- content of protein, calcium, iron, vitamin A, vitamin C, thiamin, riboflavin, and niacin, listed in terms of percent of the U.S. RDA. (The U.S. RDA is the recommended *daily* allowance—not the recommended *dietary* allowance—and is based on the highest amount of each nutrient recommended for an adult by the National Academy of Science/National Research Council in 1968.) See Table 4–10 for the specific requirements for each nutrient.

Levels of other nutrients may be included, but this is not required. At present, listing the content of sodium, fat, cholesterol, simple sugars, and so forth, is voluntary, although federal legislation mandating labeling has been proposed. Serving sizes may vary. The labels of foods containing saccharin must contain a warning.

SPECIAL DIETARY NEEDS

Vegetarian Diets

Some people choose to adopt vegetarian diets, often out of philosophic or religious convictions. The Seventh Day Adventists, for example, encourage this practice. Vegetarianism can take several forms:

- abstinence only from red meat
- abstinence from red meat and poultry
- abstinence from flesh foods, but consumption of dairy products and eggs (lacto-ovovegetarian)
- consumption of dairy products but no eggs (lactovegetarian)
- consumption of eggs but no dairy products (ovovegetarian)
- abstinence from all foods of animal origin (strict or pure vegetarian; vegan)

Vegetarian regimens usually include less total fat, saturated fat, and cholesterol and more polyunsaturated fat and dietary fiber than the usual American diet. In a lacto-ovovegetarian, for example, the percent of calories from carbohydrate is higher (55 percent versus 45 percent) and from fat lower (32 percent versus 43 percent) than typical dietary intake.

The difficulty of meeting protein needs, and especially of consuming all the essential amino acids, increases in the more restricted forms of vegetarianism. The amino acids missing from grains and legumes, for instance, can be replaced by consuming them in the same meal as a complete protein: cereal with milk, macaroni with cheese, a peanut butter sandwich with milk. In this way, good quality dietary protein is consumed without meat.

Vegan Diets

Vegan diets are less likely to be nutritionally adequate, especially if there is undue reliance on a single plant food source. Infants and children are particularly likely to develop symptomatic clinical nutritional deficiencies, with retarded growth and development. Vegan diets require careful planning to ensure adequate supplies of lysine, tryptophan, and sulfur-containing amino acids (see Chapter 1 for a more complete explanation of the importance of these amino acids). The four groups of plant foods relied on are legumes, cereal grains, fruits and vegetables, and nuts and seeds. Cereal grains, for instance, are good sources of tryptophan and sulfur-containing amino acids but are low in lysine. By combining them in the same meal with another group that contains more lysine (such as legumes), their protein content can be more fully utilized (Table 4–11). Such complementary food combinations include wheat and beans; lentils and rice; or corn, beans, and rice.

Other nutrients that may be deficient in vegan diets are vitamin B_{12}, vitamin D (for children not exposed to sunlight), riboflavin, calcium (especially for children and women), and iron (for women of childbearing age). Generous servings of green leafy vegetables, dried beans, sesame seeds, onions, and soybean milk will supply riboflavin and calcium, while beans, seeds, nuts, green leafy vegetables, dried fruits, and grains will help to supply iron.

Table 4–11. FOOD SOURCES PROVIDING COMPLEMENTARY PLANT PROTEINS

Food	Amino Acids Deficient	Complementary Protein
Grains	Isoleucine and Lysine	Rice, corn, or wheat + legumes
		Wheat + peanut + milk
		Wheat + sesame + soybean
		Rice + sesame
		Rice + brewer's yeast
Legumes	Tryptophan and Methionine	Legumes + rice
		Beans + wheat
		Beans + corn
		Soybeans + rice + wheat
		Soybeans + corn + milk
		Soybeans + wheat + sesame
		Soybeans + peanuts + sesame
		Soybeans + peanuts + wheat + rice
Nuts and seeds	Isoleucine and Lysine	Peanuts + sesame + soybeans
		Sesame + beans
		Sesame + soybeans + wheat
		Peanuts + sunflower seeds
Vegetables	Isoleucine and Methionine	Broccoli ⎫
		Brussels sprouts ⎪ + sesame seeds,
		Cauliflower ⎬ Brazil nuts,
		Green peas ⎪ or mushrooms
		Lima beans ⎭
		Greens + millet or converted rice

The Athlete

The diet that will contribute to the best performance by the athlete (whether recreational or world-class competitor) is similar to that which is best for the nonathlete: a nutritionally balanced diet supplying appropriate quantities of water, energy, protein, fat, carbohydrate, vitamins, and minerals. If the recommended dietary allowances are followed, all necessary nutrients for a physical conditioning program should be received. Commercially promoted food supplements and drugs offer nothing to the healthy, well-nourished athlete and should be rejected.

Protein

There is no difference in physical performance of individuals with protein intake ranging from 50 to 160 g per day. A high-protein diet is associated with increased fat and may deprive the athlete of needed carbohydrate; other hazards include ketosis, dehydration, and gout. The protein that is consumed, however, should be of high quality, such as that found in meat, fish, cheese, eggs, and milk. Care should be taken to consume vegetable protein along with either animal protein or a complementary vegetable protein.

Carbohydrate

The increased calories for training should be supplied by increased portions of all foods found in a good diet. However, it may be that these needs should be met chiefly by extra portions of foods from the bread-cereal and fruit-vegetable groups, resulting in a diet somewhat higher in calories derived from carbohydrate and lower in calories derived from protein than the usual American diet. A high carbohydrate diet leads to increased glycogen storage and subsequent greater endurance during prolonged exercise.

Glycogen Loading

Some athletes may wish to use a glycogen-loading regimen prior to a major competition. In such a program, the carbohydrate intake is sharply limited during vigorous training, beginning about 1 week before the event. Then, 3 days before the event, the diet is supplemented with carbohydrate-rich food. Although evidence from laboratory tests has suggested that glycogen loading may increase muscle glycogen and endurance, endurance during competition was not improved significantly and aerobic performance decreased or was not improved. Endurance is affected by the minimum glycogen level and its rate of utilization rather than by initial glycogen level. Well-trained athletes, such as marathoners who finish in 2.5 to 3 hours, probably do not require a glycogen-loading regimen. While they are likely to deplete glycogen stores, they are also better able to utilize free fatty acids as their principal energy source. In such cases, a high carbohydrate diet without glycogen loading may be preferred. It should also be noted that the glycogen-loading regimen is potentially harmful for the runner undergoing cardiac rehabilitation.

Vitamin and Mineral Supplementation

There is no evidence that vitamin supplements improve the performance of healthy athletes with a history of continuing good dietary habits. Specifically, studies have found no improvement in performance following supplementation with vitamin B, C, or E. Many iron supplements also are of no value to athletes and may cause gastrointestinal complaints. Rather than being a manifestation of iron deficiency, borderline low hemoglobin levels in endurance athletes may be a physiologic adaptation to training to prevent sludging of red blood cells during exercise and hemoconcentration.

Concentrated Sugars

One popular but potentially harmful nutritional practice promoted for athletes seeking maximum performance is the use of concentrated sugars such as honey, candy, and soft drinks. Digestion and absorption of these foods competes with muscle metabolism for the blood supply, resulting in a diminished blood supply to the working muscles. These foods may also cause a surge in the release of insulin, leading to subsequent hypoglycemia.

Fluids

Fluid ingestion is effective in regulating body temperature and preventing dehydration during prolonged activity. Water is the essential ingredient; other fluids consumed during or just prior to exercise should be palatable and dilute, with a sugar content of less than 2.5 percent and electrolytes not in excess of 10 mEq sodium and 5 mEq potassium per liter. Frequent free access to fluids during exercise is preferable to the consumption of large amounts of fluid all at once.

The Pre-Event Meal

Timing. It is recommended that athletes in training consume at least three meals per day. The timing of the pre-event meal is important for participants in middle- and long-duration events, however. Consumption of the pre-event meal must be timed so as to allow it to be a source of energy, but not so as to cause the athlete to have a full stomach, which will impede performance in events of longer duration and which will endanger the participant in contact sports with a high potential for trauma. Therefore, to allow for gastric emptying, the athlete should eat at least 3 hours prior to the event.

Content. For short-duration events, the content of the pre-event meal is not significant, since the energy used comes from substances synthesized long before the meal. For longer-duration events, however, this meal should be low in protein and fat, which are less digestible and delay gastric emptying, and relatively high in carbohydrates for increased utilization. Generally, the pre-event meal should not include coffee or tea, flatulence-producing foods, or alcohol, in order to avoid diuretic effects, gastric discomfort, and impairment of fine coordination, respectively. The physician must not forget, however, that a particular food may have a psychologic benefit for an athlete even though it has no physiologic benefit.

CHAPTER 5

Food Additives, Toxins, and Hazards

Adverse effects of food may occur from certain kinds of processing or cooking, commercial additives, environmental contaminants, and natural toxins, in addition to risks encountered with eating. Environmental contaminants include infecting microorganisms, parasite infestations, and poisons, some of which are toxins produced by microorganisms. Certain plant and animal foods may generate natural toxins. Some individuals are intolerant of specific foods or additives. Finally, foreign bodies and formation of bezoars are some of the acute and chronic risks that may accompany eating. The toxic effects of alcohol are covered in Chapter 17, and the hazards of food faddism are discussed in Chapter 6.

FOOD PROCESSING AND COMMERCIAL ADDITIVES

Human beings have the capability to process food in addition to collecting, consuming, and storing it. Heating and adding salt are two common techniques for food processing that also enhance flavor. Food additives are

Table 5-1. TECHNICAL EFFECTS
OF FOOD ADDITIVES

Antioxidant
Coloring agent
Emulsifier
Flavoring agent
Moistening agent
Nutrient
Preservative

Table 5-2. MOST POPULAR FOOD ADDITIVES
IN THE U.S.

Type	Amount/Year (lb)
Sucrose	102
Sodium chloride	15
Corn syrup	8
Dextrose	4
Leavening, pH agents	
Yeast, bicarbonate, citric acid	9
Pepper, mustard, MSG	
Miscellaneous, ≈ 2000 agents	1

included in processing because of their presumed benefit. Almost 3000 different substances are classified as direct additives, purposely added to foods (Tables 5-1 and 5-2). The FDA defines food additives as "substances added directly to food, or which may reasonably be expected to become components of food through surface contact with equipment or packaging materials, or that may otherwise affect the food without becoming part of it."

Heating (Cooking)

The aim of cooking is to give foods appropriate texture, tenderness, taste, and flavor. Cooked meat is easier to chew than uncooked meat, and thus is more digestible. Although cooking coagulates muscle proteins, making them less readily digested, the meat becomes more tender as its collagen is converted into gelatin. While fruits and green vegetables may be eaten raw, cereals, roots, and legumes are not easily digested unless cooked. Heating causes the starch within plant cells to swell, bursting the insoluble and undigestible cell wall fiber. Trypsin inhibitors in soybeans and nuts are destroyed by cooking.

Some cooking methods themselves may produce hazards, however. For example, broiling and barbecuing have been linked by some investigators with an increased risk of cancer, while frying may generate toxic byproducts.

Preservatives

Fresh foods decompose by autolysis due to their lytic enzymes and also by the action of putrefactive bacteria and fungi in the environment. Foods may be preserved by heating, drying, salting, pickling, and fermenting, as well as the widespread refrigeration and preservation of foods in cans or plastic packages; however, none of these methods should be permitted to remove essential nutrients.

Sodium chloride, acetic acid, ethyl alcohol, and sucrose are among the most widely used chemical preservatives. The concentrations of preservatives allowed—usually less than 1 percent of toxic levels—are controlled by legislation. Sulfur dioxide and hydroxybenzoates are preservatives frequently added to fruits and vegetables, beer, meat, sauces, and spices. Propionic acid is used in bread and flour, and sodium nitrate and nitrite are used in curing meats. The adverse effects of nitrites and reactions to sulfites are discussed on pages 112–113. Radiation also can be used to preserve food, but its use is restricted in the United States.

Coloring and Flavoring Agents

Organic dyes are among the natural coloring agents; however, most agents are synthetic and are added to improve the appearance of food. Color additives such as tartrazine (yellow dye #5) are also added to drugs and may cause adverse symptoms in intolerant persons. Only five synthetic coloring agents are approved at present; the rest are natural pigments. Synthetic chemicals may mimic the flavors of fruits and vegetables. For example, benzaldehyde, N-propylacetate, and diethyl sulfite yield the flavors respectively of almond, pear, and peppermint. Monosodium glutamate (MSG) enhances the flavor of meat and is added to many sauces. Flavoring agents constitute the largest number of food additives permitted by regulation.

Sweeteners

Sweeteners include the nutritive sweeteners cane or beet sugar (sucrose) and corn syrup and the artificial (non-nutritive) sweeteners saccharin (has interim status as an additive), cyclamate (banned in the United States in 1969), and aspartame (N-L-α-aspartyl-L-phenylalanine methyl ester).

Antioxidants

The tocopherols, ascorbic acid, and artificial antioxidants such as butylated hydroxyanisole (BHA) or butylated hydroxytoluene (BHT) are among the antioxidants used to prevent rancidity of fat, especially in frying. Antioxidants also inhibit formation of free radicals in vivo and the carcinogenic action of polycyclic hydrocarbon carcinogens.

Other Additives

Other additives include emulsifiers (which modify surface tension to produce uniform dispersion within food components) and stabilizing agents such as glyceryl monostearate, flour improvers (bleaching agents), acids, humectants (chemicals that bind water), thickeners, polyphosphates, and micronutrients added as enrichments or fortification.

TOXICITY OF FOOD ADDITIVES

No additive may be used in food for human consumption unless its safety is ensured, no injury will result, and its use will be beneficial. No chemicals may be added before being thoroughly tested for toxicity in laboratory animals. Occasionally substances once approved are removed from use owing to newly demonstrated toxicity, as in the case of cyclamate, which was formerly used as an artificial sweetener in soft drinks. Later tests showed that rats given very high doses of cyclamate developed tumors of the urinary bladder.

The Food and Drug Administration

Legislation to protect consumers from toxic additives was first proposed in 1906, and in 1938 the Federal Food, Drug, and Cosmetic Act established the Food and Drug Administration (FDA). The FDA's areas of responsibility include

- food-borne infection
- nutrition
- environmental contaminants
- naturally occurring toxicants in food
- pesticide residue
- commercial food additives
- food labeling

GRAS Substances

Permissible additives are on a list of "generally recognized as safe" (GRAS) substances. About 700 of these additives, in use for years, never have been investigated intensively for toxic effects. The list includes such common items as sugar, pepper, mustard, cinnamon, MSG, BHA, and sulfur dioxide. If new evidence indicates that a listed compound is unsafe, it may be removed.

The Delaney Clause

A proviso of the 1958 Food Additive Amendment, the Delaney Clause, states: "No additive shall be deemed safe if it is found to induce cancer when ingested by man or animal." New additives must be tested for efficacy, quantitation, and safety (including teratology) in several species of animals—one nonrodent—over a lengthy period. Use of an approved new additive is periodically reviewed.

The Delaney Clause is controversial because methods to detect residues of additives have become much more sensitive since its passage. Interpretations of findings and the actual threat of carcinogenesis are thus unclear.

Monosodium Glutamate

Although MSG can generate symptoms in up to 25 percent of individuals, it has not been banned, because the symptoms are transient, lead to no permanent damage, and can be avoided. Reactions to MSG have been named the "Chinese restaurant syndrome"—numbness at the back of the neck radiating down the arms and back, palpitations, and general weakness occurring 10 to 20 minutes after eating and lasting from 1 to 3 hours. Other symptoms reported include flushing; facial pressure; a burning sensation over the upper trunk, neck, and shoulders; and chest pain felt as tightness, stiffness, tingling, warmth, or numbness, which may be severe. Headache, dizziness, and lightheadedness also are common; the headache resembles migraine and may not be part of the syndrome. Bronchospasm may occur up to 14 hours later. The threshold is 3 to 4 g (a portion of wonton soup contains 3 g of MSG). MSG has been withdrawn from infant foods, as those who ingest it may become irritable, cry, scream, shiver, or develop abdominal pain or delirium.

Nitrates

The addition of nitrates to meats prevents bacterial spoilage, especially by Clostridium botulinum. Although nitrates have been shown to cause cancer in rats, there has been no definite link to cancer in humans. For this reason, the use of nitrates has been restricted rather than banned. Levels of nitrates occurring naturally in some vegetable (beets, celery, lettuce, carrots, and spinach) are higher than those permitted to be added to bacon, other meats, and smoked fish. Nitrites formed from nitrates in cooked vegetables left to stand at room temperaturre can react with secondary amines to form carcinogenic nitrosamines as follows:

$$NO_2^- + H^+ \rightarrow HNO_2$$
nitrite

$$HNO_2 + H^+ \rightarrow H_2NO_2^+$$

in aqueous
acidic
solutions
pH 2.5–3.5

$$H_2NO_2^+ + NO_2^- \rightarrow N_2O_3 + H_2O$$
nitrous
anhydride

$$N_2O_3 + R_2NH \rightarrow R_2N - N = O + HNO_2$$
2° amines   nitrosamines

The reaction takes place in the digestive tract. It may also occur during frying, especially in bacon, when volatile nitrosamines escape into the air. Addition of ascorbate in foods tends to inhibit formation of nitrosamines in the digestive tract and also reduces the level of nitrites needed to inhibit growth of C. botulinum.

Sulfiting Agents

Various sulfiting agents (sodium or potassium metabisulfite, or bisulfite sulfur dioxide, or sodium sulfite) are used in wine making, in the milling of corn, and to prevent browning in the processing of fruits and vegetables. They also have a preservative effect, conserving carotene and vitamin C in foods, but they destroy thiamin. Foods with high sulfite levels (up to 3000 ppm) include dehydrated apples, apricots, bleached raisins, pears, peaches, and potatoes, as well as restaurant salads, shellfish, pickles, sausages, cheese mixtures, and fruit juices. Worldwide, the average sulfite level in wines ranges between 100 and 400 ppm; the maximum permitted by the FDA is 350 ppm. The acceptable daily intake of sulfites for a 70 kg adult is 50 mg, although most persons in the United States probably consume no more than 10 to 15 mg per day. Because the United States Department of Agriculture is the regulatory agency for fresh foods, it rather than the FDA is responsible for restricting the use of sulfites in fruits and vegetables.

Adverse effects of sulfites include the onset within minutes of flushing, bronchospasm, and hypotension. From 5 to 10 percent of asthmatic patients are at risk for this reaction. As of August 8, 1986, the FDA banned sulfiting agents for raw fruits and vegetables. Foods containing 10 ppm or more of sulfites must be so labeled.

ENVIRONMENTAL CONTAMINANTS

Food Poisoning

At least 30 species of worms, protozoa, bacteria, and viruses may cause illness when found in food, far exceeding the hazards of natural or manmade toxic agents. Meat, poultry, eggs, and milk from infected animals are the sources of these pathogens. Contamination may occur at the source of production, in storage and preparation, or when the food is served.

Bacterial food poisoning (Table 5–3) is usually a brief, self-limiting illness. However, in the aged, the very young, and those with debilitating diseases, severe dehydration and loss of electrolytes may cause death. Ninety-seven percent of all reported foodborne bacterial illness results from mishandled food in food service establishments or in the home. The diagnosis is established by examination and culture of the suspected food and stools of the patients and food handlers.

Salmonella

Salmonellae, most frequently Salmonella typhimurium, are the most common cause of bacterial food poisoning and are especially widespread in poultry and other animals. Salmonella enteritis remains the most frequent foodborne illness reported to the Centers for Disease Control (CDC), with most cases occurring in children under age 5. The illness is usually an acute gastroenteritis with diarrhea and vomiting, accompanied by fever and headache. The incubation period is 12 to 36 hours, with symptoms persisting for 1 to 7 days. Treatment is usually unnecessary, and antibiotic therapy may extend the period of fecal shedding of bacteria for up to 4 weeks.

Table 5–3. BACTERIAL FOOD POISONING:
PATHOGENICITY OF INFECTING MICROORGANISMS

Pathogen	Invasion	Toxin
Salmonella, E. coli sp.*	None	Some
Shigella, E. coli sp.	Local	None
Campylobacter jejuni	Local	Some
S. typhosa, Brucella	Generalized	None
C. perfringens, V. parahaemolyticus, B. cereus	None	Yes

*Some serotypes produce an enterotoxin.

Mice and rats infected with salmonellae excrete the organisms in their feces, and thus may contaminate food within their reach. Food handlers are more likely to become infected themselves than to contaminate food. However, to reduce risk of the disease, use of raw eggs should be discouraged, dried egg products pasteurized, meat products rinsed and thoroughly cooked, and food preparation areas kept clean and cleaned after exposure to poultry; scrupulous handwashing at all stages of food handling should be mandatory. These hygienic practices also should be encouraged at home.

Clostridium perfringens

This anaerobic organism (the "cafeteria germ") forms heat-resistant spores in soil and dust. Infection typically occurs following consumption of meat cooked the previous day that has cooled under conditions that permit surviving spores to generate vegetative forms. The individual ingests a virtual broth culture of the bacteria, which multiply in the gut, producing an enterotoxin. Incubation is 8 to 48 hours. Diarrhea may be accompanied by abdominal pain and vomiting, but fever is uncommon.

Shigella

Shigellosis is an acute bacterial disease of the lower colon, sigmoid, and rectum, with abrupt onset of diarrhea, abdominal cramps, and occasionally fever. Stools may contain blood, mucus, and pus. The incubation period ranges from 1 to 7 days, but is usually less than 3 days. The human gut is the only significant reservoir of this disease, and most cases are spread from person to person, especially in institutions. Susceptibility is higher in young children. The pathogenic effects are characterized by invasion of the epithelial cells of the intestinal tract, producing toxic products that diffuse into the circulation. Antibiotic therapy can shorten the course of the disorder.

Staphylococcus

In certain situations illness is caused by the presence of the bacterial toxin in the food. Staphylococcus aureus is the second most often reported cause of foodborne illness, and foods are readily contaminated by carriers. Some strains produce a powerful enterotoxin that is resistant to heat and is not inactivated by boiling for as long as 30 minutes. Ingestion of contaminated food (meats, desserts, salads) may be followed in 2 to 6 hours by vomiting and diarrhea.

Botulism

Botulism is a severe, often fatal form of food poisoning. Clostridium botulinum forms heat-resistant spores. If these spores are not destroyed by adequate heating, vegetative forms grow anaerobically to produce a potent toxin. The lethal dose for mammals is less than 1 μg per kg. Poisoning symptoms are eye muscle weakness, difficulty swallowing, and finally paralysis of the muscles of respiration and death in from 1 to 8 days. More than 90 percent of cases have involved home-canned vegetables, fruits, or pickles. Other sources of outbreaks have been restaurants (sautéed onions), fish and fish products, and commercial products such as vichyssoise, peppers, mushrooms, and smoked whitefish. Infant botulism has been attributed to consumption of honey by infants under 1 year old. The incubation period for botulism ranges from 6 hours to 8 days but is most commonly 12 to 24 hours. Nausea, vomiting, and constipation are early symptoms; fever is absent. The disorder is treated by lavage of the gastrointestinal tract or emetic, but if ingestion has occurred 12 hours or more before the start of therapy, this is ineffective. Respiratory support by mechanical ventilation with tracheotomy and antitoxin therapy are required. Mortality is 20 to 25 percent.

Unpasteurized Milk and Milk Products

Brucellosis, which is characterized by symptoms of undulant fever, lymphadenopathy, splenomegaly, and rash, is caused by consumption of cream or cheese made from unpasteurized cow's or goat's milk containing Brucella. Responsible organisms are B. melitensis and B. abortus. Ingestion of unpasteurized dairy products also is associated with illness due to group C streptococcal infections, staphylococcal enterotoxin, salmonella, Escherichia coli, Mycobacterium tuberculosis, Campylobacter fetus jejuni, and Listeria monocytogenes (meningitis and sepsis).

Campylobacter

Recently recognized as a cause of enteritis, Campylobacter infection is characterized by severe abdominal pain and profuse, watery diarrhea with blood. Diarrhea may develop in 3 to 5 days and may persist for 1 to 3 weeks. Reported outbreaks have been associated with consumption of raw milk or contaminated water. Campylobacter fetus jejuni may be a more common cause of infectious diarrhea than salmonella or shigella, especially in the 10- to 29-year-old age group. Erythromycin is the treatment of choice.

Cholera

Cholera, rare in the United States, is caused by Vibrio cholerae, present in contaminated water and food. V. cholerae produces a toxin that causes *severe* secretory diarrhea, developing in 24 to 72 hours. The main goal in patient management is compensation for massive fluid and electrolyte losses. Metabolic acidosis is directly related to loss of bicarbonate in the stool.

Other Pathogens

Most pathogenic bacteria and viruses are excreted in human feces, some in urine. Transfer of pathogens by flies and small rodents, or by human hands to foods or food utensils, spreads infection. Such infections include dysenteries and acute gastroenteritis often caused by viruses and E. coli. All such pathogens are destroyed by heat in food that has been properly cooked and handled. Hazards are undercooked food and food that may become contaminated after cooking, especially when improperly stored and then warmed. Pathogen carriers have been responsible for many disease outbreaks.

E. coli serotypes are associated with severe watery diarrhea, often in young children, and "traveler's diarrhea." Advice for avoiding "traveler's diarrhea" is "Boil it, cook it, peel it, or forget it!" Other pathogenic bacteria include V. parahemolyticus, which can cause profuse diarrhea 12 to 18 hours following consumption of raw or undercooked seafood; Enterobacteria yersinia enterocolitica, which causes gastroenteritis and mesenteric adenitis (yersiniosis); and Bacillus cereus, a spore-bearing saprophyte that produces an enterotoxin (especially in rice) that causes vomiting and diarrhea.

Viruses do not multiply in foods, but if contaminated food is consumed, a virus may multiply in the intestinal tract. This may be important in young children (see Chapter 8).

Sewage may contaminate drinking water. Amebic and bacillary dysentery, viral gastroenteritis, poliomyelitis, and infectious hepatitis are spread by the fecal route. Hepatitis A, found worldwide, is the virus most commonly associated with food infection, usually by fecal-oral transmission. Common source outbreaks in food or water often result from direct contamination by an infected food handler. Raw or incompletely cooked molluscs are a potential source of hepatitis. Norwalk virus is another common cause of outbreaks of gastroenteritis; myalgias are common.

In patients with an immune system compromised by disease or treatment or both, opportunistic organisms normally present in soil and water and found in raw salads may become invasive and cause infection. It may be advisable for such patients to exclude salads from their diets.

Parasites

Among the numerous parasites that may enter the body with food or as contaminants are Ascaris lumbricoides (roundworm); Trichuris trichiura (whipworm); cestodes, including Taenia sp. (tapeworm) and Echinococcus granulosis (tapeworm causing hydatid cyst); protozoa (Entamoeba histolytica and Giardia lamblia); and liver flukes. Raw salad is a potential source of infection from liver flukes, roundworms, whipworms, and Giardia lamblia. These may be more common contaminants of salad crops grown in areas using human night soil as fertilizer.

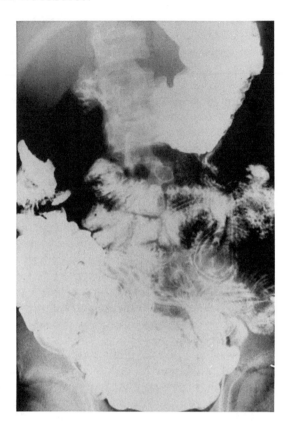

Figure 5–1. Radiograph with contrast of the gastrointestinal tract of a 17-year-old boy with growth retardation attributable to ascariasis (case 5a). The barium outlines the gut of the adult worms.

Roundworm

Roundworm infection is most common among children 1 to 5 years of age and is especially prevalent in subtropical and tropical regions. Infection occurs exclusively as a result of swallowing mature embryonated ova acquired from soil contaminated by human feces (as a result of consuming dirt, raw vegetables, or polluted water). A heavy worm burden may generate signs of protein-energy malnutrition or stunting (Case 5a; Fig. 5–1). Infestation is diagnosed by examination of the stool and is effectively treated with piperazine.

CASE 5a: ASCARIASIS

A 17-year-old boy was referred for evaluation of delayed puberty and failure to gain weight. He and his family were poor historians, and he was socially withdrawn. Despite apparently eating well, he failed to gain weight. His height (160 cm) and weight (31.4 kg) were below the 5th percentile. He was pale, appeared 5 or 6 years younger than his age, and lacked secondary sexual characteristics.

He underwent an extensive endocrine-metabolic workup, and was evaluated for a possible malabsorption syndrome. Radiographs with contrast media of the small intestine showed the presence of multiple worms (Fig. 5–1). The stool was positive for ascaris ova. A follow-up interview revealed that the patient was aware of having passed worms in his stool.

His bone age was 13 years, and laboratory values indicated mild hypochromic, microcytic anemia. Zinc levels were normal.

The patient was treated with Vermox, and within 2 months a high calorie, high protein diet with multivitamin supplements had increased his weight 5 kg.

LESSON:

This patient indicates the importance of careful history taking and shows that even in the United States parasitic infection may be a cause of retarded growth. Anorexia nervosa was negated by the absence of characteristic personality features, and his depression was assumed to be secondary to malnutrition and lack of growth.

Whipworm

Significant whipworm infection may cause blood-streaked diarrhea, abdominal pain, tenesmus, and weight loss. Anemia and failure to thrive may result.

Pig and Beef Tapeworms

Consumption of undercooked pork or beef and raw salads may cause infection with Taenia solium and T. saginata tapeworms. Adult worms develop in the gut following ingestion of cysts, and worm segments may be passed in the feces. Individuals infected with T. solium may further infect themselves with ova passed in the feces that can develop into larval forms that penetrate muscle and brain to form cysts, resulting in cysticercosis.

Fish Tapeworm

Fresh-water fish that are consumed raw may contain the tapeworm Diphyllobothrium latum. D. latum competes with the host for vitamin B_{12}, and infection with this tapeworm may lead to megaloblastic anemia.

Other Parasites

The larvae of Trichinella spiralis (ingested in undercooked pork or wild game meat) may penetrate the tissues and cause fever and muscle pain, the symptoms of trichinosis. The condition is prevented by proper cooking of meat.

Echinococcus is commonly derived from direct contact with dogs and sheep. The liver is most often affected by hydatid cyst, with the lungs the next common site.

Amebiasis may present as bloody diarrhea with varying degrees of fever, flatulence, and pain. Recommended treatment is metronidazole 20 to 40 mg daily for 5 to 7 days.

Giardia may cause failure to thrive in infants and malabsorption in adults. Giardia infection often develops from drinking contaminated water when hiking. Metronidazole is again the drug of choice.

Noninfective Environmental Contaminants

Food may also be contaminated by pesticides, radioactivity, trace minerals, antibiotics, and hormones. The bulk of chemical fertilizers consists of phosphorus, potassium, and nitrogen, with nitrate and phosphate major contributors of water pollution. Pesticide and herbicide residues in food are rarely responsible for acute poisoning. Chlorinated hydrocarbons accumulate in adipose tissue and are only slowly eliminated from the body.

Organic chemical contamination is found mostly in foods with a high fat content, such as meats, dairy products, and fish. Inorganic elements may be translocated into plants. The major environmental contaminants affecting the general population are industrial chemicals found in food and water. However, the long-term effects of continuous low-level exposure to toxic substances are difficult to ascertain. Possible carcinogenic or potential long-term health effects such as birth defects and reproductive disorders associated with chemical residues need to be evaluated to determine acceptable daily or weekly intake over a lifetime.

Polychlorinated biphenyls (PCBs) have been broadly dispersed in the environment over the past 50 years. These agents are almost ubiquitous in fish and to a lesser extent in other lipid-rich foods such as meat and poultry. Symptoms of PCB exposure—acne, eye irritation, diminished growth, and fatigue—have been observed in Japan.

Trace Minerals (See Also Chapter 2)

Mercury. The alkyl derivatives of mercury are highly toxic and produce an irreversible encephalopathy. Sources include carnivorous fish from polluted waters and seed grain that has been treated with mercurial fungicide. Fish from inland lakes in some parts of the United States, as well as canned tuna, swordfish, and pike may also have high levels of mercury. Concentrations of mercury in blood or hair can be measured, with amounts under

100 nM (20 μg per liter of whole blood) considered satisfactory. Symptoms of methyl mercury poisoning (Minamata disease in Japanese fishermen) include paresthesias; constriction of visual fields; impaired speech, hearing, and coordination; and mental retardation. Poisoning by inorganic mercury salts has been known for many years. For example, workers in the felt hat industry were sometimes intoxicated by mercuric nitrate used in treating the felt. Those unfortunates who developed "hatter shakes" were immortalized in *Alice in Wonderland* by the Mad Hatter.

Cadmium. Cadmium poisoning is a recognized industrial hazard. The substance accumulates in the body, with its highest concentration in the renal cortex. In Japan, Itai-itai disease, a severe and often fatal osteomalacia with aminoaciduria, has been associated with cadmium poisoning. The cadmium originated in rice grown on land irrigated with waste water from a mine. Thus, cereals, fruits, and vegetables grown in contaminated soil may have high cadmium levels. Levels greater than 1 mg per kg are not uncommon in shellfish and may be even higher in "brown" meat from crabs and lobsters. Individual weekly intake of cadmium should not exceed 400 to 500 μg, or about 1 μg per kg body weight per day. Cigarette smoking is a major source of cadmium.

Lead. Lead is present in trace amounts not only in food, but also in drinking water, especially water that is soft and slightly acidic. Where alcohol is made illegally (moonshine), lead contamination from automobile batteries used in the distilling process is common. The principal sources of lead contamination in food probably are lead from gasoline and solder. In children with pica, ingestion of flaking lead-based paint is also a source of contamination.

Owing to scant knowledge of the rates of accumulation of heavy metals in the body, provisional tolerable—rather than acceptable—weekly intakes have been determined for mercury, lead, and cadmium.

Antibiotics

Infectious diseases in farm animals are treated with antibiotics, which, when incorporated into animal feed, also promote growth. Penicillin and tetracycline are used in rearing livestock and poultry, as well as in food preservation. However, antibiotic residues may create the potential for harmful allergic reaction or the buildup of antibiotic-resistant bacteria. Antibiotic levels and the specific compounds permitted are therefore regulated by the FDA.

Steroids

Steroid sex hormones act as anabolic agents in beef cattle. In the United States, use of estrogens in beef production was banned in 1972, and many other countries today do not permit use of hormonal feed additives. The use of diethylstilbestrol (DES) is now restricted to earlier stages of cattle raising so that hormone residues are eliminated from tissues by the time the beef is marketed.

Radioactivity

Fallout from a nuclear explosion or an accident in a nuclear power plant can result in contamination of food supplies, affecting cereal crops, vegetables, and fruits eaten directly by humans, as well as grasses and shrubs eaten by cattle, consequently contaminating meat and milk. Potentially dangerous strontium-90 and cesium-137 are monitored in samples of milk from various countries. In such an emergency, canned foods are safe to consume.

TOXINS IN FOOD

Anyone can be affected by naturally occurring toxic substances in food. Most of these natural toxins are of vegetable origin. Such substances may

- reduce the nutritive value of other food constituents
- disturb normal physiologic function
- promote the development of cancer
- cause hallucinations, intoxication, and even death

Some persons are genetically predisposed to intoxication by certain substances or are intolerant to normal food constituents (inborn errors of metabolism).

Dietary Fats

Some unconventional sources of dietary fat may be toxic. Erucic acid (C22:1ω9) may constitute 50 percent of the fatty acid content of rapeseed and mustard oils, and may be harmful. Despite suspicions, there are no data to indicate that *trans* isomers of fatty acids in usual doses are toxic. Additional uncommon fatty acids include cyclopropene fatty acids in cottonseed oil and epoxy oils in soybean and sunflower oil.

Inborn Errors of Metabolism

Inborn errors of carbohydrate, fat, or protein metabolism predispose to toxicity. These disorders include galactosemia, fructose intolerance, and disturbed metabolism of branched chain fatty acids (Refsum's disease) with accumulation of phytanic acid (see Chapter 8). Amino acid toxicity is found in phenylketonuria. Amino acid imbalance and antagonism may lead to disorders such as leucine-induced hypoglycemia, cystinuria, and Hartnup's disease. Diseases involving the urea cycle lead to a marked reduction in protein tolerance, generating ammonia intoxication at higher protein intake.

Enzyme Inhibitors

Enzyme inhibitors are found in potato tubers, pineapple, and lima beans. Obesity has been treated with the α-amylase inhibitors in kidney beans (starch blockers) (see Chapters 6 and 16). The nutritive value of soybeans is improved by heat treatment owing to inactivation of the proteolytic enzyme inhibitor. Trypsin inhibitors are the most widely distributed inhibitors of proteolytic enzymes. Solanine, a nonprotein inhibitor of cholinesterase, may be found in abundance in potatoes, tomatoes, eggplants, sugar beets, and apples.

Goitrogens

Common toxicants in human food, the goitrogens are present in a variety of plants, such as cabbage, Brussels sprouts, cauliflower, grape seed, and mustard seed. Glucosinolates, the active agents, are split into isothiocyanates and oxazolidines, which competitively inhibit iodination of thyroxin.

Lectins

Lectins agglutinate red blood cells and may be responsible for the toxicity of raw legumes.

Effects on Vitamin Availability

Some substances may adversely affect the availability of vitamins. For example, thiaminase is found in the viscera of various fish. Thiamin inactivity effect has been attributed to some fruits and vegetables, such as blueberries, black currants, red beets, Brussels sprouts, and red cabbage. Niacin inhibitors are found in some cereals. A pyridoxine antagonist has been described in flax seed and a pantothenic acid inhibitor in pea seeds. Avidin, a biotin antagonist, occurs in raw egg white. However, adverse effects generally do not occur when these foods are consumed by healthy individuals in normal quantities in a mixed diet.

Toxins With Specific Biologic Action

Biogenic amines such as tyramine, phenylethylamine, histamine, and tryptamine are vasoactive and are found in some fruits (bananas, avocados, pineapple, plantains, and tomatoes), pickled fish, and chocolate. Fermented products such as aged foods or cheeses also may contain amines, produced by bacterial decarboxylases, that attack amino acids. Psychoactive substances include caffeine, other xanthines, and, of course, ethanol (see Chapter 17).

Alkaloids

Certain alkaloids in plants may induce acute or chronic poisoning. Cyanogenic glucosides give rise to hydrogen cyanide—cassava and almonds are classic examples.

Seafood Products

Various seafood products may be hazardous (Table 5–4). Microorganisms such as marine algae often produce intoxication. Three categories of toxins are found in fish: those in muscle, viscera, skin, or mucus, which are responsible for most cases of fish poisoning; those in gonads; and those in the blood. Most common worldwide are ciguatera, scrombroid, and puffer fish poisoning (tetrodotoxin).

Ciguatera Fish Poisoning. Ciguatera fish poisoning is caused by a microscopic plant, gambierdiscus toxicus, that lives on the surface of coral algae and passes its toxin up the food chain to larger fish such as red snapper and barracuda. The poison is stable against heat and cooking. Its symptoms include tingling of lips and tongue, abdominal and muscle pain, weakness, nausea, vomiting, and watery diarrhea. Death from ciguatera poisoning is rare.

The mechanism of action of ciguatoxin appears to be more complex than cholinesterase inhibition. The liver usually is the most toxic part of the fish, and large fish are most likely to be poisonous. More than half of all fish-related food poisoning in the United States is associated with ciguatoxin.

Scrombroid Poisoning. The symptoms of scrombroid fish poisoning (scrombroidosis) resemble a histamine reaction: flushing, headache, dizziness, burning mouth and throat, abdominal cramps, nausea, vomiting, and diarrhea. Urticaria and pruritis are common; treatment is symptomatic. Persons taking isoniazid are especially susceptible. This toxin may consist of histamine and other heat-stable substances thought to be formed by the decarboxylation of histidine by marine bacteria (Proteus, Klebsiella) acting on fish flesh. Bacterial growth is inhibited by chemicals or refrigeration.

Paralytic and Neurotoxic Shellfish Poisoning. Toxin derived from dinoflagellates ingested by molluscs is the cause of this type of poisoning. The

Table 5-4. FISH AND SHELLFISH POISONING

Type	Incubation	Duration	Source	Geographic Location
Ciguatera	1–6 hr	days–mo	Barracuda, red snapper, grouper	Hawaii, Florida
Scombroid	min–hr	few hr	Tuna, mackerel, bonito, mahi-mahi	Hawaii, California
Paralytic shellfish	<30 min	hr–days	Mussels, clams, oysters, scallops	New England West Coast, Alaska
Neurotoxic shellfish	min–hr	hr–days	Mussels, clams, oysters, scallops	Florida

dinoflagellates impart a red or reddish-brown discoloration to water—"red tide." Paralytic poisoning is characterized by paresthesias of the face and extremities, nausea, vomiting, and diarrhea. Unabsorbed toxins should be purged or lavaged. The neurotoxin—saxitoxin—is heat stable and acts to block sodium channels of the nerve membrane. One of the most potent low molecular weight poisons known, saxitoxin survives conventional cooking.

Mycotoxins

Compounds produced by molds and fungi may contaminate various foodstuffs and are widespread in the environment. For example, various strains of Penicillium produce mycotoxins, some of them neurotoxins.

Ergotism. Ergot alkaloids produced by a parasitic fungus that grows most often on rye are the cause of this disorder. The ergot alkaloids lead to vasoconstriction. This disease has been eliminated in the United States by the centralized milling of flour and strict quality control of cereals.

Aflatoxins. Derived from common molds of aspergillus strains, aflatoxins are the most potent naturally occurring carcinogens in foods. Peanuts and corn are among the many foods that may be contaminated with this toxin. Risk of intoxication is reduced by strict control of food storage.

Mushrooms. Several species of mushrooms produce mycotoxins. Some are polypeptides, others are alkaloids, with muscarine the best known. Hallucinations and gastrointestinal symptoms may follow ingestion. The most potent toxicants are found in Amanita phalloides, and may be fatal.

Other Toxins

Susceptible persons who consume broad beans are subject to favism, with symptoms of fever, jaundice, hemolysis, hepatomegaly, and splenomegaly. The disease is caused by deficiency of glucose-6-phosphate dehydrogenase. Fava beans contain substances that oxidize glutathione to its disulfide, which cannot be reduced, inducing hemolysis.

Lathyrism is characterized by paresthesias, spastic paralysis, and death. Outbreaks are associated with famine when large quantities of lathryus meal are consumed.

Jamaican vomiting sickness is caused by consumption of unripe ackee fruit, producing severe hypoglycemia in children. The fruit contains a water-soluble substance (α-,amino-β-,methylene cyclopropyl-propionic acid) that causes accumulation of branched short chain fatty acids.

Nutmeg, mace, and dill contain myristicene, which may have toxic effects on the central nervous system and which also cause vomiting and abdominal pain.

The Mexican plant peyote, containing mescaline, and the hemp plant cannabis indica (marijuana) are examples of plants purposely consumed for their psychic effects.

SENSITIVITY, INTOLERANCE, ALLERGY, AND ADVERSE REACTIONS

A wide range of symptoms affecting virtually any body organ or system may be associated with food "allergy," when a portion of ingested food is absorbed as large molecules and retains its antigenicity (see also Chapter 8). When the highly sensitized patient develops prompt and violent symptoms, allergy is obvious. Urticaria, wheezing, asthma, abdominal pain, vomiting, diarrhea, and coma may occur. Onset usually is within 2 hours of eating and often is provoked by relatively uncommon foods. The usual type of allergy, however, is manifested by mild, varied symptoms delayed hours or days after eating, and is induced by foods consumed practically every day. The obvious allergy is mediated by specific immune mechanisms involving IgE and specific IgG action against food allergens. Immunologic mechanisms responsible for the hidden allergy may include IgA, IgG, IgM, and IgD, and may involve lymphocytes, mast cells, basophils, eosinophils, and complement. High protein foods that have been ingested from infancy often cause allergy. Milk, eggs, nuts, and wheat frequently have been linked to food sensitivity.

Because no immunologic or antigenic effects can be demonstrated, food allergy may in many instances be more correctly termed "food intolerance."

Food Intolerance

Milk intolerance most often is due to lactose intolerance resulting from deficient lactase activity in the intestinal mucosa (see Chapters 1 and 21). Undigested lactose is hyperosmotic, a good substrate for intestinal flora enzymes that form lactic acid and gas, causing flatulence and diarrhea. Oligosaccharides in beans and legumes not split in the intestinal tract are digested by anaerobic microorganisms, producing gas, flatulence, dyspepsia, and diarrhea. Gluten enteropathy is discussed in Chapter 21.

Diagnosis of Food Allergy

Diagnosis depends on amelioration or disappearance of allergic manifestations when suspected foods are eliminated, and obvious aggravation or reappearance of manifestations on reintroduction of those foods. Elimination diets omit foods known to be frequent causes of allergy; then trial ingestion seeks to determine what food or foods may be responsible for the allergy.

Skin tests may be used to detect food allergens, but no test clearly and conclusively identifies such allergens.

Treatment of Food Allergy

Avoidance of allergenic food is the basis of treatment. The time required to develop tolerance to the food after the period of avoidance depends on the type of sensitization and the patient's age. As years of avoidance reduce sensitization, the food may be reintroduced in small amounts. While there is no drug that effectively and safely relieves food allergy symptoms, disodium cromoglycate serves as a preventive.

FOOD-DRUG INTERACTIONS

Certain drugs adversely influence nutritional status, while the effects of other drugs are markedly altered by the ingestion of specific foods and of alcohol, as well as by the timing of meals.

Drugs Influencing Nutritional Status

Many drugs cause nutritional depletion or have diet-related side effects; some examples are provided. Psychotropic drugs, such as phenothiazine and benzodiazepine tranquilizers, and antidepressant drugs, such as monoamine oxidase (MAO) inhibitors, tricyclics, and lithium carbonate increase the potential for obesity. Conversely, some of these tranquilizers may at times have sedative effects, and in underweight patients may undermine interest in food; patients may not be awake to eat at mealtimes.

Nausea, vomiting, and food aversions are common with cancer therapeutic drugs, especially in combination with radiation therapy (see also Chapter 24). Digoxin may provoke serious anorexia, at times with nausea and vomiting. In addition to methotrexate, the antibacterial trimethoprim and the diuretic triamterene are mild folate antagonists. Cholestyramine may bind fat-soluble vitamins, which therefore should be administered to resin users (especially vitamin K).

Adverse Effects of Food-Drug Combinations

Some foods and alcoholic beverages have harmful interactions with drugs; for example, oral hypoglycemic agents and ethanol. Another especially well-known example is the relationship between tyramine and monoamine oxidase inhibitors. Aged cheese, Chianti wine, and chicken livers contain high levels of tyramine, which stimulates the sympathetic nervous system and may increase blood pressure. Normally tyramine is destroyed quickly in tissues by monoamine oxidases. However, patients taking monoamine oxidase inhibitors (used for treating depression) who eat large portions of such foods may have alarming reactions, including headache, severe nausea and dizziness, severe hypertension, and occasionally cerebral hemorrhage or cardiac failure.

Foods Affecting Drug Absorption and Bioavailability

Drug absorption and bioavailability may be affected by food components or by the timing of food and drug intake. For example, some forms of dietary fiber adsorb drugs and reduce their absorption. Drug absorption can be delayed when drugs are taken with food or within 1 or 2 hours following a meal. For example, absorption of L-dopa is diminished when it is taken with a high protein meal. Milk and liquid formulas reduce absorption of penicillin and cephalexin; milk reduces absorption of tetracycline; and meals generally reduce absorption of erythromycin. Meals delay absorption of cephalexin, metronidazole, digoxin, and aspirin. By contrast, milk and meals promote absorption of some derivatives of erythromycin, as well as propranolol, coumadin, hydrochlorothiazide, and diazepam.

Patients therefore should be cautioned to

- read drug labels and package inserts
- follow physicians' orders concerning timing of drug intake and foods or beverages to be avoided
- inquire about drugs in relation to foods and beverages consumed in large amounts, or if particular foods cause unusual symptoms

FOOD ACCIDENTS

Formation of bezoars, ingestion of foreign bodies, aspiration of foreign matter into the respiratory tract, and choking are among the common food hazards reviewed here. Although the very young and the elderly are the most frequent victims of food accidents, all such accidental occurrences require swift intervention.

Bezoars

Bezoars are insoluble aggregates of ingested material that form in the gastrointestinal tract (see also discussion in Chapter 21). The lactobezoar, a protein coagulum found in the infant's stomach as a result of mixing powdered milk with insufficient water, is the most common food-related bezoar. Clinical symptoms include diarrhea, vomiting, dehydration, and fever, and there may be an abdominal mass and distention. A characteristic mass is apparent on radiographic examination. Rehydration by intravenous fluids brings spontaneous resolution in 60 percent of patients. Surgery may be indicated in those with severe obstruction or perforation.

Phytobezoars (of plant origin) are less common and may include fiber, skin, seeds, leaves, roots, and stems that form a compact, insoluble mass. The combination of gastrointestinal stasis and ingestion of nondigestible plant material—especially coconut, celery, pumpkin, grape skins and stems, prunes, or raisins—is the usual cause. Symptoms include pain, nausea, vomiting, and weight loss, with constipation or diarrhea. Diagnosis is usually by radiography. Intestinal obstruction, gastrointestinal ulceration, perforation, and peritonitis are potential complications. Bezoars may be removed endoscopically or surgically.

Ingestion of Foreign Bodies

Fish, chicken, and meat bones; poorly chewed food; and fruit pits are commonly ingested foreign bodies. The denture-wearing adult is a potential victim because dentures make it difficult to detect sharp or hard objects in food. Perception of the oral cavity may also be reduced by consumption of excessive alcohol—the "martini–olive pit" syndrome.

Eighty to 90 percent of swallowed bodies pass intact through the gastrointestinal tract without causing injury. Those that remain may result in obstruction, hemorrhage, abscess, or perforation. Bones are especially likely to cause perforation. Sphincters and areas of acute angulation are most susceptible to injury: the cricopharyngeus, pylorus, and ligament of Treitz; the ileocecal region (three fourths of perforations occur at this site); or areas of preceding lesions or disease, including strictures, rings, webs, pyloric stenosis, diverticulae, or tumors.

Foreign body ingestion is clinically manifested by abdominal pain, nausea, vomiting, abdominal distention, bleeding, and fever. There may be a leukocytosis with left shift or iron deficiency anemia. Initial diagnosis may be in error because of nonspecific symptoms, but radiography may prove useful. Removal is indicated if a foreign body has not been eliminated in 72 hours. Objects lodged in the intestinal tract should be removed endoscopically. Surgery is rarely indicated in the absence of perforation, obstruction, or bleeding within the gastrointestinal tract.

Aspiration of Foreign Bodies

Occurring most frequently in children between the ages of 1 and 3, aspiration is a leading cause of mortality in children under age 6. Almost 93 percent of aspirated bodies are organic, with nuts and seeds the most common. Aspiration into the main stem bronchus is the problem in most cases. While early diagnosis and removal are essential, symptoms that mimic infections or allergies may make diagnosis difficult. Although many respiratory tract disorders are associated with coughing, wheezing, and decreased air entry, foreign body aspiration should be suspected in the young child with these signs. A history of foreign body aspiration has been reported in up to 85 percent of lower airway aspirations, and prompt removal by bronchoscopy is the treatment of choice. Educating parents to supervise food preparation and meal times of children under age 6, and minimizing their exposure to foods such as nuts and seeds helps to prevent aspiration accidents.

Choking

With about 3000 deaths per year, food choking is the sixth leading cause of accidental death in the United States. The victim's inability to speak is the cardinal symptom of choking. As breath is cut off, the victim becomes pale, then blue or black, evidences great distress, and will die within minutes unless the airway is cleared.

The Heimlich maneuver is a simple, effective method for saving the life of a person choking on a bolus of food. The technique will expel even small objects causing partial obstruction, as evidenced by stridor. The Heimlich maneuver forces the food bolus out from below, rather than attempting to remove it through the mouth. This is accomplished by pressing quickly upward just below the rib cage and elevating the diaphragm, which compresses the lungs and utilizes the increased interpulmonary air pressure to dislodge the food from the airway.

When victim and rescuer are standing, the Heimlich maneuver is performed as follows:

- Stand behind the victim and wrap your arms around his or her waist.
- Place your fist thumbside against the victim's abdomen, slightly above the navel and below the xiphoid.
- Grasp your fist with your other hand and press into the victim's abdomen with a quick upward thrust.
- Repeat several times if necessary.

The maneuver is performed in the same fashion when the victim is sitting, with the rescuer standing behind the victim's chair.

When the victim is unconscious:

- Lie the victim on his or her back, while you kneel astride the victim's thighs.
- With one hand on top of the other, place the heel of the lower hand on the abdomen slightly above the navel and below the xiphoid.
- Press the victim's abdomen with a quick upward thrust.
- Repeat several times if necessary.

When the victim is an infant:

- Straddle the victim over your arm with his or her head down and the jaw supported.
- Deliver four back blows forcefully with the heel of your hand between the infant's shoulder blades.
- Sandwich the infant between the two hands and turn, placing on the thigh.
- Perform four chest thrusts.

Or—

- Place the infant on the rescuer's lap for the back blows and the chest thrusts.

The following measures will reduce the risk of choking:

- Cut food into small pieces and chew slowly and thoroughly.
- Avoid talking and laughing when chewing and swallowing.
- Avoid excessive intake of alcohol before and during meals.
- Restrict children from walking, running, or playing with food or foreign objects in their mouths.
- Keep foreign objects away from infants and small children.

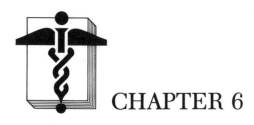

CHAPTER 6

Fads, Myths, and Quackery

Fads, myths, and quackery abound in the field of nutrition (Table 6–1). The most prevalent dietary fads relate to weight reduction, while myths, especially concerning vitamins, also are common. Publication of books about these dietary fads and myths, and subsequent promotion of them on TV talk shows, are time-tested ways to help quackery endure.

A fad is a temporary fashion that a group of people enthusiastically fol-

Table 6-1. AREAS OF FOOD FADS/MYTHS/QUACKERY

Vitamins/minerals
Weight reducing diets
Food combinations or eliminations
Special foods
Natural foods
Organic foods
Youthful foods
Pesticides
Food preservatives, additives, processing, and storage
Fertilizers, chemical vs. natural
Faulty diet
Subclinical nutritional deficiency
Super health
Stress needs
Popular magazines of the supermarket/beauty parlor distribution
Radio/TV, especially talk shows
Nutrition "counseling" services: biochemical, optimal, holistic
Nutritional assessment services: muscle, hair, saliva, body chemistry
Orthomolecular psychiatry
Enzymes
Spurious vitamins
Hypoglycemia, sugar
Caffeine
Fiber
Zen macrobiotic movement
Fruitarians
Supernutrition
Vegetarianism

low. While fad diets are not necessarily harmful, they usually promise quick results and make a number of non–fact-based claims. An important feature of some fad diets is a special product sold by the originators of the diet that must be purchased because of its unique weight loss properties.

A myth is an invented, imaginary story, a belief accepted uncritically, while a quack is a fraudulent pretender to medical skill and knowledge. Much too often, fad diets have elements of both myth and quackery.

FOOD FALLACIES

Folklore is a common source of "nutrition nonsense," as shown by the following false claims:

False	Facts
Starchy foods are fattening.	Starchy foods have no greater effect on body weight than any other source of similar calories (see Chapter 4).
Grapefruit and cottage cheese are slimming.	There are no special foods that lead to weight loss. Bulky foods with low caloric density may induce satiety so that less food actually is eaten.
Cheese is constipating.	Cheese is no more constipating than other low residue foods and is an excellent source of nutrients (see Chapter 4).
Hot food is better for you than cold food.	Temperature of food affects its sensory appeal, not its nutritional value.
Raw vegetables generate gas.	Beans are a vegetable that produces gas when eaten in large quantities. (See Chapters 2 and 4 for vegetables as sources of vitamins.)
Orange is too acid for infants and young children.	Orange juice is well tolerated by many infants over 3 months of age and is an excellent source of vitamin C, which may be deficient in milk formulas.
Adolescent acne results from eating too much chocolate, peanut butter, cheese, potato chips, nuts, and french-fried potatoes.	Foods do not cause acne; rather, acne depends on heredity and hormone balance.

FOODS AND THEIR INFLUENCES ON BEHAVIOR AND HEALTH

Among the food substances that are claimed to influence behavior positively or negatively are caffeine, sugar, lecithin, and certain amino acids.

Caffeine, a pharmacologic agent usually consumed as a beverage, influences sleep patterns.

Sugar has been implicated as a cause of aggression and hyperactivity, without convincing evidence. (Similar behavioral effects have been attributed to meat, also without confirming evidence.)

Lecithin has been claimed to improve memory, while some amino acids, such as tryptophan, have been suggested as treatment for insomnia, pain, depression, and hypertension. Some of these benefits have been demonstrated in laboratory animals, but the efficacy of these substances in humans remains under investigation. For this reason, any use in human subjects must be considered experimental.

Hypoglycemia

Hypoglycemia has been proposed as a cause of mood swings, nervousness, and irritability resulting from fluctuations in blood sugar, generally without substantiation relating symptoms to a measured low level of blood glucose. Control of reactive hypoglycemia, when demonstrated, is by frequent meals and avoidance of simple refined sugars. Other regimens have proved effective only anecdotally. Relief of hypoglycemia is not a panacea for increasing energy and improving sex life. Substitution of fructose for glucose or sucrose to prevent hypoglycemia is not scientifically sound.

VITAMINS

Among the many vitamin myths are claims that these substances are "insurance" against the effects of a poor diet, and that everyone should take some vitamins. (See Chapter 2 for more information about vitamins.)

Vitamin supplements are efficacious in individuals who have inadequate or restricted intake, malabsorption, increased requirements, or excessive loss. Supplements are *not* needed by healthy individuals with usual dietary intakes.

Among the more popular unsubstantiated claims for vitamins are the following:

- Riboflavin prevents or treats cataracts and glaucoma.
- Vitamin C prevents colds.
- Megadoses of niacin and other B vitamins prevent or cure schizophrenia and induce optimal health.

Megadoses

Although various individuals may recommend megadoses of vitamins to prevent or treat medical conditions, their use is generally not warranted.

Chapter 14 presents a complete discussion of vitamin deficiencies, some of which may require large doses of vitamins in their treatment, as well as vitamin toxicities and other side effects of excessive vitamin ingestion.

Vitamin E

Vitamin E heads the list of those touted to prevent or cure everything from acne to underarm odor, including

- prevention of senility and atherosclerosis
- promotion of fertility and sexual potency
- restoration of physical charm, especially to the skin

Vitamin E has also been proposed for the prevention or treatment of

- hypertension
- Buerger's disease
- diabetes mellitus
- varicose veins

and as an aid to promote wound and burn healing without scars. Proponents urge that to optimize its effects, vitamin E should be taken daily starting at an early age. (See Chapters 2 and 14 for discussions of the physiologic function of vitamin E and its value in treating hemolytic anemia of premature infants, preventing retrolental fibroplasia in premature infants, and treating intermittent claudication as well as abetalipoproteinemia, a rare etiology of malabsorption syndrome.)

Orthomolecular Psychiatry

Begun as a treatment for schizophrenia using massive doses of niacin, orthomolecular psychiatry gradually developed into treatment using additional B vitamins—B_6, B_{12}, and folic acid. The regimen is based on the theory that mental illness may be due to vitamin deficiencies resulting from some persons' exceptionally large vitamin needs. Linus Pauling has added ascorbic acid to the vitamins used. Up to 20 g of nicotinic acid has been used with a variety of adverse effects on skin, gastrointestinal tract, liver, blood sugar, and uric acid.

Spurious Vitamins

"Vitamins" B_{17} (laetrile) and B_{15} (pangamic acid) are nonvitamin quack remedies. (No new vitamins have been discovered since vitamin B_{12} in 1948.) "Laetrile" and "vitamin B_{17}" are trade names for the chemical amygdalin, which is abundant in kernels of peaches and apricots and contains 6 percent cyanide by weight. Laetrile is claimed to control cancer in combination with "metabolic therapy," a program that includes enzymes, enemas, megadoses of vitamins, pangamic acid, and a vegetarian diet. Metabolic balance is sought by means of the severely restricted diet, multiple high dosage nutritional supplements, live cell injections, animal gland extracts, enzymes, colonic irrigations, and coffee enemas. Chronic and fatal cyanide poisoning may result, especially from oral intake.

A compound marketed as a dietary supplement and drug for treatment of a variety of conditions, pangamic acid is a patented substance promoted as a "nondrug, nonfuel nutrient." It has been used in the Soviet Union to treat arteriosclerosis, pep up athletes, enliven the elderly, and prolong life. Additionally, it is supposed to reduce serum levels of lactic acid and cholesterol, normalize blood glucose, and improve oxygen utilization. However, there is no scientific evidence for any of these benefits, as they have never been tested in human subjects.

NONVITAMIN MYTHS AND QUACKERY

Some nonvitamin myths about food claim that

- specific combinations of foods cause or cure disease or cause obesity
- special foods increase vigor
- elimination of foods achieves health
- "natural" foods are better and prevent disease

Natural and Organic Foods

Natural foods are defined as those grown without pesticides or fertilizers, and with no preservatives, processing, or packaging. It is claimed that fertilizers cause malnutrition, that modern processing and storage remove all nutritive value from food, and that we are in danger of being poisoned by food additives. In fact, there is no evidence that chemical fertilizers differ in their inorganic salt content from the same elements found in manure, soil, and plants.

Retail sales in the health food industry have reached $3 billion per year. Items labeled "organic," or "natural," or "health food," are priced higher— often double the cost—of comparable ordinary food. It is unlikely that there is any difference in the nutritive value of foods grown organically or with fertilizer, except that the pesticide content of organic food apparently is higher! It may also be questioned whether labels are truthful, for the premium prices that can be charged increase the potential for fraud.

Among the natural foods that are claimed to restore youthfulness are

- blue-green manna (spirulina)—blue-green algae, a perfect protein, but intake is only 1.5 g daily
- ginseng—said to improve coordination and mental powers
- green magma—a powder from barley grass juice that, mixed with cold water, "brings the blossom of youth to your face"
- anazyme—a "cure" for arthritis that can be combined with green magma, selenium, and zinc to restore youthfulness to the skin
- linseed oil capsules—not only good for the skin, but may rid the body of adverse effects of processed foods
- water—100 percent electrically structured to "restore the life force electrical balance of our body"
- yogurt—claimed to increase longevity
- bee pollen—claimed to provide nature's as yet undiscovered nutrients in compact form
- superoxide dismutase (SOD)—promoted as "the fountain of youth in an easy-to-take pill form"

The enzyme SOD is derived from bovine erythrocytes, molds, and liver extract, and when ingested probably is totally inactive because it is digested by proteases. As is the case with many biologic products, the recommended dosage of SOD is too low to have any effect. However, breakdown products of ingested proteins may be allergenic. The major effect of many of these products is merely as a placebo.

SOURCES OF NUTRITION INFORMATION

Popular magazines, especially those written for women, are a major source of nutrition information. Unfortunately, much of what is published is unreliable. A 1982 review by the American Council on Science and Health of nutrition coverage in 19 major magazines indicated that *Parents Magazine*, *Redbook, Reader's Digest*, and *Good Housekeeping* presented accurate information, while *Vogue, Woman's Day, Family Circle*, and *Ladies Home Journal* were intermediate or inconsistent sources. *Cosmopolitan, Harper's Bazaar*, and *Prevention* were judged to be unreliable sources of nutrition information.

Because authors and editors are under no obligation to prove that what they publish about nutrition is true, the American consumer is advised to "shop" carefully for correct information. **It is legal to publish material that has been proved false, and a great deal of published nutrition information is simply wrong.**

Textbooks or other publications from scientifically reputable organizations prepared by nutrition professionals, or derived from governmental

Table 6-2. HINTS ON HOW TO RECOGNIZE (NO GUARANTEE)

Fads/Myths/Quacks	Facts/Truths/Science
Information cited as testimonials and anecdotes	Controlled, confirmed studies
Reported in popular magazines	Published in scientific journals
Unknown or made-up institutes	Bona fide academic institutions
Dramatic, emotional appeal	Factual, detailed, specific
Promissary	Cautious
Outlandish claims (hogwash)	Sensible
Advertised in all popular media	Modest advertising
Costly	Covered by health insurance
Mail order remedies	Usually requires referral, prescription
Catchy titles	Less flashy
No advanced degrees	M.D., Ph.D., D.D.S.—academic credentials (necessary but not sufficient)
Endorsed by celebrities	Rarely personalized
Door-to-door salesmen	Some respectable groups
Anti-establishment	Orthodox, establishment (academic, government, industry)

sources, are reliable guides to good nutrition. Although there may be disagreement on some issues, professionals' advice is at least safe. When in doubt, check with a knowledgeable physician or registered dietitian to help distinguish myth from reality (Table 6–2).

UNRELIABLE NUTRITION SERVICES AND PRACTICES

Because until 1982 no state laws or licensing standards regulated the practices of nutrition counseling services, anyone from a yoga teacher to a vitamin salesman could go into the business of nutrition counseling. As of early 1987, only 14 states had developed such regulations. Phrases such as "biochemical individuality," "optimal health," and "frank deficiencies" may be clues indicating promotion of the myth that everyone needs vitamin and mineral supplementation. Would-be nutritionists take advantage of the paucity of knowledge about long-range effects of subnormal body stores of vitamins or minerals that are not frankly deficient.

Inadequately trained practitioners lacking nutrition credentials may include diverse health professionals, naturopaths, and others such as those who staff "holistic" health centers. Many of these services conveniently sell their own brand of products, which they recommend for curing a disease or promoting health. Much of their misinformation is supported by strong conviction, rather than fact, but may seem convincing to the unsuspecting client. It should also be noted that orthodox nutrition services offered by medical centers and universities tend to be less costly than the balancing body chemistry and holistic clinics.

Food quacks assert that most disease stems from bad or faulty diets, and that most people are poorly nourished, suffering from subclinical and thereby unclassifiable nutritional deficiencies. While they offer no proof for their theories, scientific data to refute the claims unfortunately are scarce. In recent years, claims have been made that antioxidants (beta carotene, vitamin E, selenium, ascorbic acid, zinc) may prevent cancer and AIDS. An additional claim for which there is no evidence is that various types of "stress"—often meaning the strains of everyday life—increase the need for nutrients.

Nutritional Supplements

Nutritional supplements are available in door-to-door sales, in supermarkets, in drug and health food stores, and by direct mail. They are advertised and promoted in all popular media. With a market exceeding $1 billion per year, vitamin-mineral supplements outsell other supplements. The potential for harm from large doses of vitamins A and D is well established and the hazard from water-soluble vitamins is becoming increasingly visible as well. "Designer" products advocated by celebrities call for particular caution. In many instances of vitamin toxicity, however, the vitamin has been prescribed by a physician!

Unorthodox Nutritional Assessment

The unorthodox tools of nutritional assessment include

- muscle testing (applied kinesiology)
- hair analysis, which is useful for detecting excessive exposure to toxic heavy metals (lead, arsenic, mercury) rather than revealing nutritional deficiencies or metabolic disorders
- acupressure alarm points
- pulse diagnosis
- iridology (evaluation of the iris for healing strength)
- body chemistry balancing
- ionization
- saliva testing

Because the relationship between the hair concentration of a vitamin or trace element and the concentration in other body tissues is currently unknown, hair analysis is generally worthless for assessing vitamin status and of limited value for minerals. Also, there are problems with processing hair (it must be clean, not exposed to environmental contaminants, shampoo, and so on) and techniques for the trace mineral analysis have to be quality controlled and require facilities and skills found in only a few research laboratories.

DIETS

Weight Reduction

Weight loss diets are the most popular fad diets. They may work because they temporarily remove the dieter's choices and substitute what is generally fewer calories than the usual intake. Some of these diets are more nutritionally sound than others. (See Chapter 16 for recommended regimens for the management of obesity.) Popular weight loss diets are of five types:

- low carbohydrate
- high carbohydrate
- protein-sparing modified fast
- fruitarian (a type of monotonous diet, primarily of one component)
- additives to prevent growing fat

Low Carbohydrate Diets

A low carbohydrate diet typically restricts these compounds to less than 20 percent of calories ingested. Fat is similarly restricted in the low fat diet, and may in some instances be reduced to 10 percent of calories. Since salt and water are retained with ingestion of carbohydrate foods, there is fluid loss when such foods are restricted (see Chapter 1). Some types of low carbohydrate diets are

- the Stillman diet—high in protein and low in carbohydrate
- the Atkins diet—high in fat and with no carbohydrate
- the Scarsdale diet—high in protein, low in carbohydrate and fat

The Scarsdale diet requires daily consumption of 1000 calories for 2 weeks and then increases the calorie level. There is also a "drinking man's diet," which permits no carbohydrate but allows unlimited alcohol!

These diets all produce diuresis and may cause fatigue and lassitude. They are clearly unphysiologic and may be hazardous. For example, the high protein diet is bad for patients with renal disease and may raise cholesterol levels and induce vitamin deficiencies. The high fat diet induces ketosis and also promotes hyperlipidemia. Because of the increased renal solute load, the ketogenic diet results in fluid loss and may cause dehydration.

The High Carbohydrate Diet

Often recommended by physicians for the management of cardiovascular disease, obesity, and diabetes mellitus (see Chapters 16 and 18), the high carbohydrate diet is typified by the Pritikin regimen and other high fiber regimens. The regimen permits 3.5 oz of lean meat three times per week, emphasizes whole grain foods, and is low in fat (less than 10 percent of calories) and cholesterol (less than 100 mg per day). The Pritikin regimen also includes abstinence from tobacco, does not permit sugars or processed foods, and is accompanied by an exercise program. It contains some foods that are relatively unpalatable and that cause excessive flatulence and gas. While some aspects of the Pritikin program may be nutritionally sound, some essential nutrients—especially minerals—are made relatively unavailable because of binding to fiber. The regimen is not recommended for sick persons, children, or women of childbearing potential, and it may be contraindicated in the elderly.

The Protein-Sparing Modified Fast

The protein-sparing modified fast is a modification of a starvation regimen. This type of relatively more hazardous diet should be used only under strict medical supervision and when significant weight loss (more than 20 lb) is required. Starvation purportedly cleanses the bowel and "rests" gastrointestinal enzymes—neither of which, even if true, contributes to the management or prevention of obesity (nor to health promotion or disease prevention). Starvation regimens actually use up the lean body mass and are poorly tolerated in the elderly, the young, and the sick.

The liquid protein diet and the Cambridge diet are examples of the protein-starving modified fast. While these diets may result in weight loss, their risk unsupervised outweighs possible benefits. It has been found that the liquid protein diet contained low quality protein, was deficient in trace minerals, and led to sudden arrhythmias and cardiomyopathy in some dieters. The Cambridge diet provides only 330 calories and 33 g of quality protein per day along with the RDA of vitamins and minerals.

The Beverly Hills Diet

The Beverly Hills diet is a low protein/high fiber diet in which for 10 days one eats nothing but generous quantities (0.5 lb or more) of specified fruits, on certain days, in rigid order. This diet is nutritionally unsound, and serious nutritional deficits may occur. The regimen is followed by a high fat, high cholesterol maintenance diet. There is no scientific basis for the Beverly Hills diet, which invents a new human physiology. Its side effects may include severe diarrhea, muscle weakness, dizziness, and the risk of severe hypotension. A diet so low in protein may result in rapid loss of scalp hair after 5 to 10 weeks.

Starch Blockers

Starch blockers are ineffective, unsafe (potentially poisonous or allergenic), and expensive. They contain an α-amylase inhibitor derived from raw kidney beans.

Other Diet Fads

The Zen macrobiotic dietary regimen combines elements of Oriental philosophies with varying diet levels and other health recommendations. It consists of 10 different dietary prescriptions coupled with restricted fluid intake designed to achieve a balance of yin-yang, or positive-negative, polarity within the body. The diet varies from -3, approximating the Western diet (the most harmful), to $+7$, consisting only of brown rice. Numerous deaths have been reported in individuals who adhered to diet 7, with nutritional deficiencies especially noted in children. Serious deficiencies of iron, calcium, protein, vitamin C, riboflavin, and vitamin B_{12} result from prolonged adherence to this diet. Pregnant women who follow this regimen are also at increased risk. A recent variant requires consumption only of raw foods, seriously limiting nutrient intake.

The fruitarian is another outlandish diet, resting on the belief that consumption of meat produces mucus, the breeding ground for disease. Fasting and consumption of natural laxative products, such as some fruits, are claimed to clear the intestine of mucus. Such diets are protein deficient and inadequate in many vitamins.

Supernutrition has been advocated by popular authors and talk-show nutritionists such as Adele Davis and Carlton Fredericks. Their books suggest special food regimens, are anecdotal, refer liberally to medical literature and "scientific" credentials, but do not necessarily reflect the truth. Among their more hazardous recommendations are toxic doses of fat-soluble vitamins and excessive potassium intake for renal disease patients.

Vegetarian and High Fiber Diets

There is no definitive proof that for the healthy population it is better to be a vegetarian or to adhere to a high fiber diet, or both, than to consume a more balanced diet (see Chapter 4). There is likewise no evidence that such diets cure ailments ranging "from arthritis to depression to vaginal infections," or that vegetarians are passive or nonaggressive. Possible health benefits of vegetarianism include low blood lipids, less heart disease and hypertension, reduced cancer rates, and lower body weight. However, these diets present varying problems when there is inadequate intake of protein, iron, and vitamin B_{12}. High fiber diets similarly are not panaceas correcting everything from appendicitis, cancer, and constipation to heart disease, hiatus hernia, and varicose veins. Although some individuals may indulge in vegetarian and high fiber diets as fads, for others they are sound diets that are based on religious or ethnic preferences, or that represent effective treatment for obesity or diabetes mellitus (see Chapters 16 and 18).

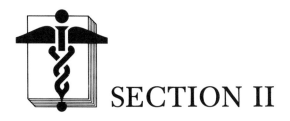

SECTION II

Nutrition Throughout
the Life Cycle

There is no finer investment for any community than putting
milk into babies.

Sir Winston Churchill, 1874–1965, radio broadcast, March 21,
1943.

While Section I concentrated on nutrients as molecules, as meals, and as potential hazards, Section II focuses on the provision of nutrients throughout life. This discussion includes the nutritional requirements of individuals at different ages and in both healthy and diseased states.

Chapter 7—**Pregnancy and Lactation**—deals with the nutritional requirements of pregnancy, how the prenatal diet influences fetal development, nutrition in specific problems of pregnancy, and various aspects of diet for the lactating woman.

Chapter 8—**Pediatric Nutrition**—focuses on the nutritional requirements of infants and children both in health and in disease states. The first part discusses breast feeding versus bottle feeding, vitamins, solid foods, adolescents, and the special needs of premature infants. The second half delineates parenteral and enteral nutrition, the provision of nutrition in specific disease states, and chronic pediatric nutrition problems.

Chapter 9—**Geriatric Nutrition**—discusses specific nutritional problems confronting older persons, including the psychosocial factors influencing nutrition, deficiencies, common illnesses, and those individuals at particular nutritional risk.

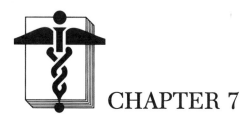

CHAPTER 7

Pregnancy and Lactation

147

Nutritional status before and during pregnancy contributes significantly to the well-being of the mother and her infant. Adult women who have had adequate childhood nutrition and were well nourished prior to conception are more likely to have uncomplicated pregnancies and deliver healthy babies. A healthy diet is likewise important for the lactating mother, as breast feeding provides advantages to both infant and mother. For these reasons nutritional assessment and advice are essential components of good antenatal care.

Because of the potential for delivering premature or growth-retarded infants, it is essential to recognize pregnant women who are at high risk for poor nutrition. Physiologic changes associated with pregnancy require that maternal diets provide increases in energy substrates, protein, vitamins, and minerals. In addition, the mother's nutrient intake during pregnancy may have specific influences on fetal development.

Specific health problems of pregnant women such as diabetes mellitus, anemia, hypertension, or hyperemesis need careful attention. Ideally, appropriate nutritional counseling should be provided before conception, but in any case at the first antenatal visit, throughout the pregnancy, and thereafter. Because of her concern for the health of the infant-to-be, the pregnant woman generally is quite compliant with dietary recommendations; however, this is often untrue for adolescents and among women of some socioeconomically deprived groups. It is important for the health professional to be able to assess which pregnant women may be at risk for not complying with dietary recommendations.

Because oral contraceptives are related to family planning, their effects on nutritional status are included in this chapter.

NUTRITIONAL REQUIREMENTS IN PREGNANCY

This section explains why pregnancy increases the body's requirements for specific nutrients, while Table 7-1 and the section further on entitled "Prenatal Diet" present the actual recommended increases in maternal intake.

Energy

Energy requirements of the pregnant woman increase minimally during the first trimester, but rise rapidly at the end of this period and continue to be increased throughout the rest of pregnancy. This demand is independent of that needed for activity levels, which may diminish. Assuming an unchanged

Table 7-1. ESTIMATED DIETARY NEEDS OF PREGNANT AND NONPREGNANT WOMEN

	Teenage 11–14 yr	Teenage 15–18 yr	Adult	Pregnant	Lactating
Calories	2200	2100	2000	+300	+500
Protein, g	46	46	44	+30	+20
Vitamin A, μg RE*	800	800	800	+200	+400
Vitamin D, μg	10	10	5	+5	+5
Vitamin E, mg αTE†	8	8	8	+2	+3
Vitamin C, mg	50	60	60	+20	+40
Vitamin B_1, mg	1.1	1.1	1.0	+0.4	+0.5
Vitamin B_2, mg	1.3	1.3	1.2	+0.3	+0.5
Vitamin B_3, mg NE‡	15	14	13	+2	+5
Vitamin B_6, mg	1.8	2	2	+0.6	+0.5
Folate, μg	400	400	400	+400	+100
Vitamin B_{12}, μg	3	3	3	+1	+1
Calcium, mg	1200	1200	800	+400	+400
Phosphate, mg	1200	1200	800	+400	+400
Magnesium, mg	300	300	300	+150	+150
Iron, mg	18	18	18	**	**
Zinc, mg	15	15	15	+5	+10
Iodine, μg	150	150	150	+25	+50

* Retinol equivalent: 1 μg RE = 1 μg retinol or 6 μg β-carotene
† α-tocopherol equivalent: 1 mg TE = 1 mg d-α-tocopherol
‡ Niacin equivalent: 1 NE = 1 mg niacin or 60 mg dietary tryptophan
**A supplement of 30–60 mg iron is recommended in pregnancy to be continued for 2–3 months after parturition during lactation.
(Adapted from the Recommended Dietary Allowances, Washington, DC, 1980.)

level of activity, calorie requirements usually increase about 15 percent, or 300 kcal, for the second and third trimesters. Provision of adequate calories is essential for placental development.

Protein

From the second month of pregnancy on, there is an increase in protein requirement of about 0.5 g per kg body weight per day. Protein content of the fetal, placental, and amniotic fluid compartments increases, and there are also similar increments in the uterus, blood protein, and breasts (Table 7–2). The total amount of protein added during pregnancy amounts to slightly less than 1 kg. Most measurements of nitrogen in maternal blood are reduced as a result of dilutional processes and losses owing to increased tissue anabolism and renal clearance (excretion of creatinine, urea nitrogen, uric acid, and amino nitrogen). There is a small increase in circulating α_1, α_2, and β globulins. If maternal protein intake is inadequate, the fetus will parasitize protein from the mother.

Carbohydrates and Lipid Metabolism

While fasting plasma glucose is reduced in pregnancy, glucose tolerance deteriorates as gestation progresses, and in late gestation a clear elevation in plasma glucose occurs in response to oral glucose challenge. Plasma triglycer-

Table 7–2. CUMULATIVE PROTEIN INCREMENT
IN FETAL AND MATERNAL COMPARTMENTS

	Cumulative Incremental Protein Contents (g)		
	End of 1st Trimester	End of 2nd Trimester	End of 3rd Trimester
Maternal	52	255	382
Blood proteins	10	100	135
Uterus	30	90	166
Breast	12	65	81
Fetal	4	207	543
Fetus	1	150	440
Placenta	3	55	100
Amniotic fluid	0	2	3

(Adapted from Pitkin, R.M.: Obstetrics and gynecology. In Schneider, H.A., Anderson, C.E., and Coursin, D.B. (eds): Nutritional Support of Medical Practice, ed 2. Harper and Row, Philadelphia, 1983, p. 494.)

ides increase by multiples of 2.5 to 4, and cholesterol and phospholipids rise about 25 percent, with lipid values tending to level off in the last trimester.

Iron

Iron requirements in pregnancy are substantial, with the term infant containing on the average 200 to 250 mg of iron and the placenta and cord about 50 mg. Maternal red cell volume increases 500 ml—representing 500 mg of iron—and thus total maternal iron requirements in pregnancy may range from 750 to 900 mg. Iron is transported from mother to fetus regardless of maternal status.

Serum iron values decrease with advancing gestation in unsupplemented women, a change that is associated with an increase in total iron-binding capacity and transferrin and a decrease in percent saturation of transferrin. Iron supplementation ameliorates or prevents these effects. Bone marrow iron stores also decrease in pregnancy.

Iron absorption increases from an average of 6.5 percent at the start of pregnancy to 14.3 percent near term in the absence of iron supplements. Such absorption has averaged only 8.6 percent with supplementation. In addition, iron supplementation reduces the usual decline in mean hemoglobin and hematocrit levels.

Calcium

More calcium than any other mineral is accumulated during gestation, mostly during the last trimester. The total accumulation of about 30 g is distributed as 27 g in the fetus and about 1 g each in the placenta and the maternal tissues. Almost all the fetal calcium is added during the last trimester. Intestinal absorption of calcium doubles early in gestation and remains high throughout pregnancy. This is accompanied by increased levels of dihydroxy vitamin D—the placenta, in addition to the kidney, can hydroxylate vitamin D.

Trace Minerals

There is a decline of approximately 25 percent in levels of plasma or serum zinc by the third trimester. This decrease reflects an increase in blood volume and a decline in serum albumin levels rather than an actual zinc deficiency. In association with an increase in ceruloplasmin, serum copper levels increase.

Vitamins

Especially during the third trimester, pregnancy demands sharp increases in folate intake as serum levels of this vitamin commonly fall at that time. The decrease may be due in part to increased urinary excretion of folic acid, but the principal reason for the rise in folate need is increased maternal erythropoiesis, resulting in the increase in red cell volume.

PRENATAL DIET

The pregnant woman's intake of calories, protein, calcium, iron, and folic acid should substantially exceed normal requirements (see Table 7–1). Most of this increase can be met by increasing food consumption to achieve a weight gain of 11 to 12.5 kg. However, iron supplementation is recommended to meet requirements for this mineral during pregnancy. There is some question whether folate, calcium, and pyridoxine need to be supplemented, but one or more of these nutrients may be included in commercial prenatal vitamin-mineral supplements often prescribed.

Calories

The increase in total caloric requirements in the sedentary American pregnant woman is about 56,000 kcal (and may range as high as 75,000 kcal), for an average of 200 kcal per day throughout pregnancy. However, weight gain in the first trimester is negligible, increasing and becoming constant in the second and third trimesters. Therefore, caloric intake usually remains level for the first trimester, with an increase of about 300 kcal per day in the later trimesters. An increase in carbohydrate intake usually satisfies the need for additional calories.

Protein

To meet increased protein requirements, the diet should include increased servings of the milk and meat groups. Excess intake should be approximately 30 g per day to meet the total protein accumulation during pregnancy of about 900 g. Most of this protein is deposited in the second half of pregnancy when approximately 5 g per day is added to fetal tissues.

Calcium

Calcium requirements exceed the prepregnancy intake by about 50 percent, an increase normally met by a higher intake of the milk foods group. Other foods rich in calcium include sardines, mackerel, and some vegetables (see Chapter 2).

Iron and Folate

Iron requirements rise sharply at the end of the first trimester because of the marked increase in maternal erythropoiesis. This increase, along with the greater growth rate of the fetus, accounts for the prevalence of anemia at this time in pregnancy. Meeting these needs requires absorption of about 6 mg of iron daily during the last half of pregnancy. A supplement of 30 to 60 mg per day of a ferrous sulfate is recommended to meet this absorption requirement plus account for an iron loss of 1 mg per day. There is some controversy over whether similarly increased needs for folate can be adequately supplied by the diet or whether folate supplement should be prescribed. (See Chapter 2 for dietary sources of folate.)

Food Cravings

There may be altered taste and smell sensations in pregnancy with accompanying cravings for substances that are sweet, sour, or sharp tasting.

Pica

Pica is a craving for unnatural foods, the persistent compulsion to ingest unsuitable substances with little or no nutritional value. In pregnancy it usually involves consumption of dirt, clay, laundry starch, or ice. It is not clear whether this practice causes iron deficiency by binding iron and preventing absorption or whether iron deficiency is a cause of pica. Other nonfood substances ingested have included burnt matches, hair, stone or gravel, charcoal, soot, toilet bowl air fresheners, cigarette ashes, mothballs, antacid tablets, milk of magnesia, baking soda, coffee grounds, and even tire innertubes. Pica is an ancient practice, especially notable in pregnant women, particularly among Southern black women. In a recent study at the Medical College of Georgia, 16 percent of the pregnant women interviewed admitted practicing pica.

WEIGHT GAIN IN PREGNANCY

The average woman's weight gain in pregnancy ranges between 10 and 12.5 kg. The fetus is the major single contributor to the weight gain, with increases also added by the amniotic fluid and placenta and increases in maternal blood volume, interstitial fluid, and uterine and breast size (Table 7–3). Approximately 3 kg may be added to maternal adipose tissue.

The usual pattern of weight gain begins with approximately 0.65 kg at 10 weeks' gestation; 4 kg at 20 weeks; 8.5 at 30 weeks; and 12.5 kg at 40 weeks (Fig. 7–1). Since half of this total is in the products of conception, and most of this weight is added in the second half of pregnancy, many women feel they are becoming fat before midpregnancy is reached. Fat stores may be noticeable on the hips, upper arms, thighs, abdomen, and back. The maximum rate of fat storage occurs in midpregnancy, providing a store of calories for the third trimester and lactation.

Weight gain in the second trimester results largely from increased maternal blood volume, size of breasts and uterus, and adipose tissue. The third trimester brings growth of the fetus, placenta, amniotic fluid volume, and fluid retention in the legs and pelvis. Moderate fluid retention and some edema are considered normal physiologic changes of pregnancy. However, excessive, especially sudden weight gain and fluid retention, particularly in late pregnancy, may be an ominous sign of toxemia of pregnancy.

Weight gain in pregnancy is variable and is dependent on factors such as age, parity, and body habitus. The pattern of weight gain can be plotted on a grid, where any deviation from normal may be a sign of fluid retention or excessive food intake. Failure to gain weight indicates inadequate nutritional intake. If the woman does not gain a normal amount in the first trimester

Table 7–3. COMPONENTS OF WEIGHT GAIN
IN FETAL AND MATERNAL COMPARTMENTS

Component	kg	lb
Fetal	5	11
Fetus	3.3–3.5	
Placenta	0.6–0.65	
Amniotic fluid	0.8	
Maternal	6–8	13–17
Extracellular fluid	1.2–1.8	
Other tissue (fat)	2–3	
Uterus	0.9	
Breast	0.4	
Blood	1.25–1.8	
Total	11–13	24–28

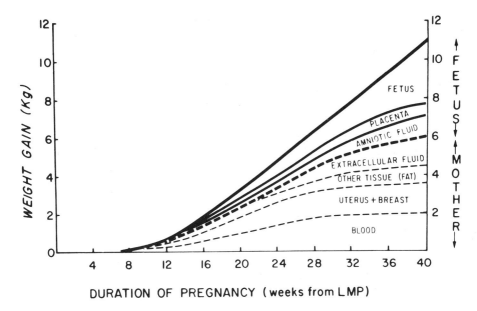

Figure 7–1. Pattern and components of cumulative weight gain during pregnancy. Total weight gain is assumed at 11 kg. (From Pitkin, R.M.: Nutritional support in obstetrics and gynecology. Clin Obstet Gynecol 19:49, 1976, with permission.)

(less than 1.35 kg or 3 lb), the chances of fetal prematurity increase from 3.9 percent to an average of 7.5 percent. The incidence of premature labor rises to between 10.4 and 11.8 percent in women with 81 to 95 percent of ideal body weight (IBW), and reaches 22.2 percent in those with 80 percent or less of IBW. If weight gain in the first trimester is normal, failure to gain appropriate weight in the second trimester raises the potential for premature labor from 3.9 to 7.3 percent.

ASSESSMENT OF NUTRITIONAL STATUS

The first step in the nutritional assessment of the pregnant woman is the evaluation, as early as possible, of her prepregnancy nutritional status. The elements of this evaluation are similar to those of the usual nutritional assessment: history, including diet history; physical examination; and appropriate laboratory values (see Chapter 3).

Of special interest in the history:

- Has the woman had a previous pregnancy?
- If so, were there complications (hypertension, hyperemesis, anemia, and so on)?

- What were the durations of previous pregnancies?
- What were infants' birth weights and heights? Any low birth weights?
- Any abortions?
- Any developmental abnormalities?

Particular attention in the diet history should be given to alcohol consumption, prior use of oral contraceptives, vitamin intake, and use of hormones or anticonvulsants. A 24- or 48-hour diet history should be obtained and analyzed. A complete blood count and urinalysis are essential components of the assessment for all pregnant women; however, if the history and physical examination indicate possible nutritional deficiencies, appropriate additional laboratory tests should be ordered.

Nutritional Risk Factors

Nutritional risk factors that might adversely influence the outcome of pregnancy should be identified. Women at risk of nutritional deficiency in pregnancy include

1. adolescents (within 3 years of menarche, and especially within 1 year)
2. women significantly above or below IBW (see Chapter 3)
   a. low prepregnant weight (less than 85 percent of IBW)
   b. obese (exceeding 120 percent of IBW)
3. women with low income or food purchase problems
4. women with histories of frequent conception (three or more pregnancies within 2 years)
5. women with histories of low birth weight infants
6. women with histories of inadequate weight gain in pregnancy, possibly with poor calorie and protein intake
7. women with such diseases as diabetes mellitus, tuberculosis, anemia, malabsorption syndromes (Crohn's disease, pancreatitis), or other metabolic disorders
8. women who smoke, have depression, or are addicted to drugs or alcohol
9. food faddists, vegetarians, or women exhibiting pica or excessive vitamin intake

The pregnant adolescent has increased needs for calcium, protein, and calories to provide for her normal growth as well as her requirements for pregnancy and the requirements of the fetus. Women whose weight is significantly lower than ideal, as well as those whose weight gain is inadequate, are at risk of having low birth weight infants. (Adverse effects of some specific nutritional practices on fetal development are covered on pages 162–166.) The underweight mother-to-be may be at increased risk for toxemia. She should be counseled to gain weight prior to pregnancy, but if this is not possible, she should be encouraged to gain somewhat more weight during pregnancy than may be recommended for one whose prepregnant weight was normal. Such weight gain may be achieved only with use of enteral supplements in addition to the usual meals (see Chapter 11). Obese women face increased risk of developing diabetes mellitus, hypertension, and thromboembolism during pregnancy. Rather than limiting weight gain in pregnancy, obese women should gain the usual 24 pounds and defer attempts to lose weight until the postpartum period.

THE PREGNANT ADOLESCENT

Because girls continue to grow even after the age of 17, pregnancy before this age competes with nutrients required for growth. Common problems of the pregnant adolescent include

- hypertension
- premature labor
- low birth weight infants
- high neonatal mortality
- iron deficiency anemia
- fetopelvic disproportion
- prolonged labor

Premature infants are most common among the youngest girls. Fetopelvic disproportion accompanied by increased rates of dystocia and cesarean section is very common before the age of 15.

The pregnant teenager's needs for added calories, protein, calcium, and iron exceed the requirements in adult pregnancies. Thus, pregnant girls between the ages of 11 and 14 need 2700 kcal per day, while those between 15 and 18 need 2400 kcal per day. Since the pregnant adolescent is vulnerable to the same fads as her nonpregnant peers (see Chapter 6), she should be counseled to maintain a nutritious diet and to avoid high calorie snack foods, bizarre diets for slimness, and similar risks. Iron and folate supplements should be prescribed, and consumption of 6 cups of milk—preferably skim milk—per day encouraged.

DEVELOPMENTAL NUTRITION

Explanations for abnormal births have been sought in all ages. Ancient beliefs associated such occurrences with punishment for past sins, copulation with animals or devils, or prophecies of the future. One hundred years ago, maternal environmental impression was considered an important factor in teratogenesis. After the turn of the century, genetic factors were found to be more important than environmental influences, and it was determined that the fetus was a parasite capable of drawing all needed nutrients from maternal tissues. The first nutritional manipulation to produce a congenital malformation was carried out in vitamin A–deficient sows in 1933. Sixty-five to 70 percent of today's developmental defects are unexplained. Nutritional factors may contribute to the pathogenesis of these defects, perhaps interacting with genetic factors.

Fetal Body Composition Versus Fetal Age

With the increasing survival rate of premature infants, knowledge of the body composition of the fetus at various gestational ages becomes more important in the feeding of such babies. As the fetus matures, the amount of water decreases and the amount of tissue increases. The percentage of fat increases about 10-fold from 24 weeks' gestation to term (Fig. 7–2). Both fetal skeleton and lean body mass increase markedly in late gestation. Copper retained also increases, growing sixfold from 24 weeks to term, or approximately 0.05 mg per kg per day.

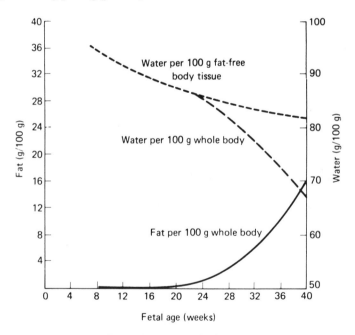

Figure 7–2. Percentages of fat and water in the human fetus in relation to fetal age. (From Hurley, L.S.: Developmental Nutrition. Prentice-Hall, Englewood Cliffs, NJ, 1980, p. 28, with permission.)

Placental Transport of Nutrients

Glucose is the major fuel of the fetus, derived mainly by facilitated diffusion from the maternal circulation at a rate of 6 mg per min per kg, or about 18 mg per min at term. The placenta metabolizes glucose by the processes of glycogenesis and glycogenolysis and the production of pyruvate, lactate, and CO_2. Placental lactate can diffuse back to the maternal circulation or into the fetus.

By a process of active transport from maternal to fetal circulation, amino acids are transferred to the fetus, which synthesizes protein from them. In addition, the amino acids are concentrated by the placenta, which synthesizes and transfers protein to the fetus. The placenta also transaminates amino acids and can carry out gluconeogenesis.

Fatty acids are also transferred from the maternal to the fetal circulation. The placenta concentrates fatty acids and has a high concentration of arachidonic acid. Transfer of cholesterol is slow, and thus cholesterol levels are lower in the fetus than in the mother. The placenta synthesizes triglycerides, phospholipids, cholesteryl esters, and produces CO_2. The fetus synthesizes fat. Produced by the placenta, transferred and oxidized, ketones may protect the newborn against hypoglycemia. Ketone bodies also are transferred from maternal to fetal circulation.

Nutritional Practices Inducing Abnormal Fetal Development

Nutritional practices can induce a variety of abnormalities, including

- death with stillbirth or abortion
- birth defects
- low birth weight and length
- premature birth
- complications of pregnancy

Famine reduces fertility, a phenomenon observed in World War II, when birth rates in famine-affected areas fell by two thirds. Abortion and miscarriage rates rose fivefold, and neonatal deaths were more than three and a half times the normal rate. With frank starvation, infant birth weight declined by about 350 g (0.75 lb). Closely related to protein intake, birth weight increased with higher levels of protein consumption (Table 7–4).

When the maternal nutritional state was good or excellent, the physical condition of 94 percent of the infants was classified as superior or good; only 50 percent were so classified if the mother's nutritional status was fair; and only 8 percent attained that highest physical condition if the mother's nutritional state was poor (Fig. 7–3).

Table 7-4. PROTEIN INTAKE
AND BIRTH WEIGHT

Protein (g/day)	Birth Weight (lb)
<45	5.8
65–74	8.0
85+	9.2

Starvation has been associated with increased morbidity, mortality, prematurity, and abnormalities particularly of the central nervous system, including spina bifida, hydrocephalus, and cerebral palsy.

Malnutrition and the Brain

Brain growth and learning are affected by malnutrition. Brain size decreases, but the permanence and functional significance of this alteration, in terms of human ability, are unknown. The normal human brain has a growth

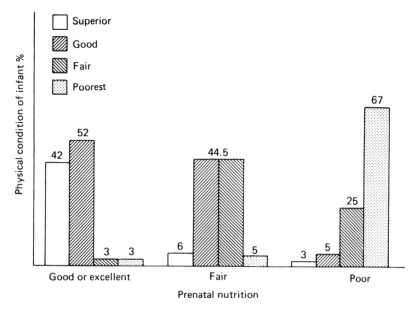

Figure 7–3. Correlation of prenatal nutrition of mother with condition of the infant at birth. Numbers over bars indicate percent of newborns in that category. (From Hurley, L.S.: Developmental Nutrition. Prentice-Hall, Englewood Cliffs, NJ, 1980, p. 84, with permission.)

spurt at birth; its final growth occurs up to 2 years of age. Weight of the brain at birth is 25 percent of its weight 2 years later (1200 g). Neonatal malnutrition has a more marked effect on body weight than on brain weight, with the former declining by 50 percent and the latter by 30 percent.

Approximately 75 percent of the brain DNA is present at birth, with 100 percent at 1 year (Fig. 7-4). Myelination takes place following birth; cholesterol content of the brain increases and water content decreases.

The brain is vulnerable to malnutrition during its growth spurt, with permanent effect on the number of cells appearing early, and similar effect on the size of cells noted later. Refeeding will bring permanent recovery unless the damage occurs during replication. The effects of malnutrition differ with respect to the various cell types, structures, and parts of the brain. Malnutrition reduces the rate of myelination by 25 percent in cholesterol content and concentration, 36 percent in cerebrosides and gangliosides, 26 percent in phosphatidylethanolamine and sphingomyelin, and 3 to 21 percent in RNA, protein, and DNA.

It is difficult to assess whether behavior reflects the specific effects of malnutrition, or whether apathy, for example, might be caused by sensory deprivation and lack of stimulation. Because learning is affected by factors other than nutrition, such as income and socioeconomic level, home environment, intellectual incentive, care and education, sanitation, infection, and family size, it is not known whether the effects of early nutritional deprivation are long lasting or bring irreversible decreases in intellectual capacity.

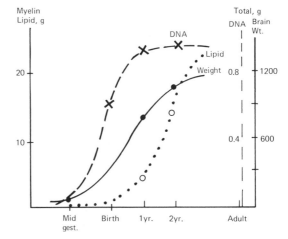

Figure 7-4. Relative increase in total brain weight, cellularity (DNA) and myelin lipid (cerebroside and sulfatide) of the human brain. (Adapted from Hurley, L.S.: Developmental Nutrition. Prentice-Hall, Englewood Cliffs, NJ 1980, pp. 96, 97, 98.)

ENZYME DEFICIENCY DISEASES

Phenylketonuria

Excessive levels of amino acids in the maternal circulation may have deleterious effects on the fetus. Infants born with phenylketonuria (PKU), with deficient phenylalanine hydroxylase, are usually treated with a low phenylalanine diet until they reach 6 years of age. These children develop normally but retain high levels of phenylalanine, and their future offspring may suffer from intrauterine growth retardation and microcephaly, with skeletal, cardiac, esophageal, spleen, and lung abnormalities. Mothers of infants with PKU frequently have abortions. The intelligence of offspring appears to be inversely related to mothers' phenylalanine levels. These outcomes suggest that women with PKU should follow a lifelong diet restricted in phenylalanine.

Galactosemia

Infants of mothers heterozygous for galactosemia, with deficient galactose-1-phosphate uridyl transferase, are subject to mental retardation and cataracts after birth that can be prevented by limiting exposure to galactose in utero via a low lactose maternal diet in pregnancy; the children must be maintained on a low lactose diet thereafter.

NUTRIENT EXCESSES

Ascorbic Acid

Excessive maternal intake of ascorbic acid may result in early abortion. Alternatively, it may result in so-called conditioned scurvy in the offspring. When placed after birth on diets of lower ascorbic acid content, the infants' excess catabolism of vitamin C may induce symptoms of scurvy.

Iodine

Maternal iodine excess may result in congenital goiter and hyperthyroidism, increased neonatal mortality, and mental retardation.

Vitamins

Some nutrient excesses (as well as deficiencies) have been shown to be teratogenic in animals, but their effects in humans are uncertain. Excessive maternal intake of vitamin A has been linked with anomalies of the urinary tract or central nervous system in some case reports. The defects were observed in the offspring of women who took 25,000 to 150,000 IU of vitamin A daily during the first trimester. Retinoids used to treat acne are teratogenic and their use is contraindicated in pregnancy.

While excessive maternal intake of vitamin D may be related to infantile hypercalcemia, severe cases probably are associated with excessive fetal sensitivity rather than with increased maternal intake. Offspring may develop a vitamin B_{12} dependency syndrome when the mother has taken an increased amount of this vitamin. Because of the potential harm that may result from vitamin megadoses, pregnant women should be strongly advised to use caution when taking vitamin supplements (see Chapter 6).

NUTRIENT DEFICIENCIES

- Essential fatty acid deficiency in the mother results in reduced infant survival, lower birth weight, and a decrease in cerebroside levels in the brain.
- Maternal vitamin D deficiency results in rickets and enamel hypoplasia in the infant, with increased susceptibility to dental caries.
- In the coumadin syndrome, prenatal vitamin K deficiency is produced when the mother is given anticoagulants. This results in a syndrome of malformations, including a hypoplastic nasal structure, mental retardation, and bone abnormalities. Such abnormalities are dose dependent and were observed when mothers at risk for thrombophlebitis were given oral anticoagulants.
- Inadequate maternal intake of ascorbic acid may lead to increased risk of premature birth.
- Vitamin B deficiency leads to increases in vomiting, prematurity, and stillbirth.
- Offspring of women with thiamin deficiency may have congenital beriberi.
- Folic acid deficiency may result in fetal death, abortion, brain abnormalities (neural tube defects), and small-for-date infants. Effects may persist through the first year of life.

MINERAL DEFICIENCIES

- Maternal iron deficiency may result in low hemoglobin in offspring.
- Maternal iodine deficiency results in endemic goiter or cretinism in offspring, defects that are prevented by sufficient iodine intake prior to conception.
- Zinc deficiency may be responsible for malformed or post-term infants, premature deliveries, and inefficient labor. Because zinc, unlike calcium, is not mobilized from maternal tissues (bone store), adequate provision to the fetus requires a constant maternal intake.

FETAL ALCOHOL SYNDROME

Recognized since 1973, this syndrome, which occurs as often as Down's syndrome, consists of small-for-gestational-age infants, dysmorphism (especially of the face and eyes, heart, joints, and internal genitalia), and mental deficiency. Facial features include a low nasal bridge, short palpebral fissures, indistinct philtrum, thin and reddish upper lip, short nose, small mid-

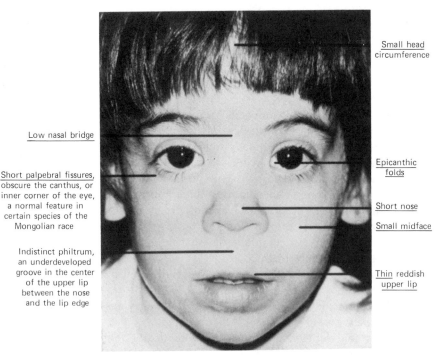

Figure 7-5. Facial features of a child with the fetal alcohol syndrome. (From Iber, F.L.: Fetal alcohol syndrome. Nutr Today 15:5, 1980, with permission.)

face, epicanthic folds, and small head circumference (Fig. 7–5). Infants show disproportionate growth retardation, with greater decrease in weight than in length, no catch-up growth, and increased perinatal mortality. They tend to be tremulous, irritable, and hyperactive, with impaired brain development and function. Incidence of the syndrome has been estimated at 30 to 50 percent of the offspring of alcoholic mothers, defined as those who ingest more than 3 ounces of alcohol per day during pregnancy. Since no safe level of alcohol intake during pregnancy has been established, it is recommended that women avoid alcohol during pregnancy.

CAFFEINE

It is uncertain whether caffeine has detrimental effects in pregnancy. When variables such as alcohol intake, smoking, age at pregnancy, and previous pregnancy history are controlled, heavy coffee consumption has minimal if any apparent adverse effect on late pregnancy outcome. However, it is recommended that coffee consumption during pregnancy be limited.

SPECIFIC PROBLEMS OF PREGNANCY

Anemia

Iron deficiency anemia and megaloblastic anemia caused by folate deficiency are the most common gestational anemias (see also Chapter 15). Other types, such as sickle cell or other hemolytic anemias, may overlap the pregnancy period. Clinicians should suspect anemia in patients with a history of the condition, complaints of fatigue and weakness, menorrhagia, history of pica, previous multiple births, or poor intake of iron, folate, protein, or vitamin C. Anemia can be prevented in the normal woman who is seen early in pregnancy by

- monitoring hemoglobin and hematocrit every 2 months, but not less often than every 3 months
- repeating tests at biweekly intervals when laboratory values are borderline
- recommending a diet high in protein and iron, containing adequate vitamin C
- supplementing with folate and iron
- evaluating the patient for the practice of pica

The anemic patient (hemoglobin less than 10 g per dl, hematocrit less than 30 percent) should have the peripheral smear evaluated and serum iron and total iron-binding capacity measured and their ratio calculated. Treatment with appropriate iron supplementation and re-evaluation in 1 month should follow, the iron given as ferrous iron in divided doses with meals. Iron therapy should be continued when the desired hemoglobin level has been reached. The patient who fails to respond to oral iron may require increased folic acid supplementation, and at times parenteral iron may be needed.

A diagnosis of folate deficiency may be suggested by

- a precipitous drop in hemoglobin
- macrocytosis and poikilocytosis
- hyperlobulated neutrophils
- low white cell and platelet counts
- circulating megaloblasts
- high serum iron levels

A bone marrow biopsy will confirm the diagnosis.

When folate deficiency is found, it is important to rule out other micronutrient deficiencies, especially of vitamins C and B_{12}. Patients with folate deficiency anemia should take 10 to 15 mg of folic acid daily along with supplemental iron.

Diabetes Mellitus

Obstetric complications that threaten the pregnant diabetic patient include an increased incidence of polyhydramnios, abortion, and premature or postmature delivery. Additional risks are toxemia and increased incidence of congenital abnormalities and neonatal mortality. A diabetic expectant mother in poor insulin control often delivers a large infant; therefore, obstetric difficulties such as dystocia are common. Presence of diabetes mellitus is suggested by

- persistent glycosuria
- family history of diabetes mellitus
- history of large babies (>4000 g)
- history of stillbirth
- history of repeated abortions
- recurrent candidiasis

Depending on the severity of her disease, a pregnant diabetic patient normally is seen every week or two, with measurements of blood glucose, urine glucose and acetone, and microscopic examination of the urine performed at each visit. The standard prenatal diet generally remains unchanged, with the usual iron and folate supplement given, body weight followed, and sodium intake restricted if hypertension develops. Referral to a dietitian for counseling and use of the usual diabetic exchange list are routine (see Chapter 18). The patient should be encouraged to eat her meals at the same time every day.

The size of the fetus is monitored by ultrasound because of the potential for macrosomia. Prior to delivery, amniocentesis with fluid analysis for fetal lung maturity should be performed, and placental function may also be evaluated.

Hypertension

When any of the following signs appear—usually after the 24th week of pregnancy—hypertension is diagnosed:

- systolic blood pressure >140 mm Hg
- a rise in systolic blood pressure of 30 mm Hg
- diastolic pressure of >90 mm Hg
- a rise of 15 mm Hg in diastolic pressure

(These findings should be verified by repeated measurement.)

- significant proteinuria
- significant edema of face and hands
- sudden, excessive weight gain

Severe hypertension is marked by systolic blood pressure of 160 mm Hg or diastolic of 110 mm Hg, proteinuria exceeding 5 g per 24 hours, oliguria, cerebral or visual disturbances, pulmonary edema, or cyanosis. The pregnant patient with antecedent hypertensive vascular disease may manifest a systolic blood pressure exceeding 200 mm Hg, with retinal exudates and hemorrhages, and cardiomegaly.

Sudden excessive weight gain suggests abnormal fluid retention. Headache and blurred vision are ominous signs. The sodium content of the diet should be decreased and the patient advised to rest. Hospitalization usually is recommended. While the degree of sodium restriction is controversial, the following guidelines may be helpful:

mild—2 g sodium diet

more severe symptoms or lack of improvement—1.5 g sodium diet

These amounts are reached by combining the daily guide for pregnancy (Table 7-5) with a low salt diet for pregnancy (Table 7-6).

Gastrointestinal Symptoms

Nausea and vomiting are common in early pregnancy. Measures to combat this condition include taking vitamin B_6 (100 mg tid), Coca-Cola syrup, and small meals primarily composed of carbohydrate. Constipation, heartburn, or hyperacidity may also occur, symptoms that result from atony of the gastrointestinal tract with smooth muscle relaxation. Increased fluids, moderate exercise (walking), and a high fiber diet may help to overcome constipation. Small, frequent meals, often omitting fluids, and milk between meals may also be helpful.

Table 7-5. DAILY GUIDE

Milk 3–4 glasses	Vegetables and Fruits 4–5 servings
Low fat	Dark green leafy or dark yellow
Skim	Turnip greens
Canned	Collard greens
Buttermilk	Mustard greens
Chocolate	Carrots
Powdered	Squash
Lean Meat 2–3 servings	Pumpkin
Any fresh *lean* meat:	Sweet potatoes
Beef	1–2 fruits (or juice) or other
Fish	vitamin C foods
Chicken	Orange
Pork	Grapefruit
Game	Cantaloupe
Liver (try to have at least once a	Tomato, tomato juice
week)	Cabbage, raw
or substitutes for meat:	Watermelon
Eggs (2)	1–2 other fruits or vegetables
Cheese	Such as potatoes, okra, green
Peas	beans, corn, butter beans,
Beans	peas, peaches, apples, grapes
Bread and Cereal 3–4 servings	Fat—no more than 1 tsp at each meal
Lightbread	Use only *one* at each meal:
Cornbread	Margarine
Biscuits	Butter
or	Vegetable oil
Cereals: Grits, oatmeal, rice, dry	Shortening
cereal, cream of wheat	Fatty meat
(A serving of cereal is ¹⁄₂ cup)	Mayonnaise (salad dressing)

Hyperemesis Gravidarum

Pernicious vomiting in early pregnancy may indicate hyperemesis gravidarum. Such patients should be hospitalized and fed intravenously to maintain nutritional status (see Chapter 12).

THE LACTATING WOMAN

Modest deficiencies in maternal nutrition are more likely to affect the mother's own nutrient stores rather than the nutritional quality of her milk, which tends to sustain adequate levels of calories, proteins, vitamins, and minerals. Malnourished mothers, however, may have a diminished volume of milk. In addition, when the maternal diet is deficient in water-soluble vitamins, the milk may be vitamin-deficient as well.

Table 7-6. LOW SALT DIET FOR PREGNANCY

Do not use these foods:

A. Salt in cooking

B. Salt at the table

C. Meats high in salt:

Bacon	Hog dogs
Fat back	Head cheese
Sausage	Souse meat
Ham	Canned meat
Ham hock	Canned fish: tuna, salmon, sardines
	Luncheon (sandwich) meats—bologna

D. Fat drippings from any of the high salt meats listed above

E. Canned soups and packaged soup mixes

F. Snack foods:

Potato chips	Peanut butter
Pig skins	Popcorn
Crackers	Pickles
Salted peanuts	Catsup, mustard, meat sauces
Pretzels	

Do *not* use any home remedies or medicines not prescribed by your doctor.

To make your foods taste better you can use:

Pepper	Stew beef
Lemon juice	Cinnamon
Vinegar	Garlic
Onion	*Dry* mustard
Neck bones	Vanilla extract
Orange juice	

(Adapted from the Maternity and Infant Care Project #506, April, 1972.)

Requirements

Compared with nonlactating women, the RDA for many nutrients is increased for lactating women, and in some cases exceeds that recommended for pregnancy (see Table 7–1). Major increases are in calories (+500 kcal per day), proteins (+20 g per day), and calcium (+400 mg per day). The caloric increment is even greater when the period of lactation exceeds 3 months. By this time, fat stores accumulated during pregnancy are depleted, while the requirements of the growing infant increase. Consumption of slightly less than 1 quart of whole milk per day is sufficient to meet increased needs for calories, protein, and calcium. Calcium needs are probably best met with calcium supplements for women who do not drink milk. The lactating woman's iron requirements are only slightly above normal; however, the iron supplement given during pregnancy should be continued several months postpartum to assist in restoring depleted iron stores.

Oral Contraceptives and Lactation

The usual estrogen/progesterone oral contraceptive diminishes milk supply, while progesterone alone reduces milk protein content. The lactating woman normally is advised to choose an alternate form of contraception.

Metabolism and Lactation

Lactation increases the basal metabolic rate about 60 percent, while the energy content of human milk itself ranges from 67 to 77 kcal per 100 ml. About 90 kcal are required for the production of 100 ml of milk. Milk output commonly ranges from 850 to 1200 ml per day, with a protein content of 1.2 g per dl. The 2 to 4 kg of body fat stored during pregnancy provides 200 to 300 kcal per day during a lactation period of 100 days, or about one third the cost of an average milk production of 850 ml per day. Women with high milk production may lose as much as 1 g of calcium per day.

Advantages of Breast Feeding

In the absence of contraindications, the physician or prenatal counselor should explain the advantages of breast feeding to the pregnant woman, and recommend this method of infant feeding (see Chapter 8).

Gastrointestinal Symptoms in the Infant

Certain foods consumed by the mother may tend to cause flatulence or diarrhea, or both, in the breast-feeding infant. However, each woman is different and should determine from experience which foods may upset her infant.

ORAL CONTRACEPTIVES

The use of oral contraceptives is accompanied by changes in some nutrients. Adverse effects may include
- impaired glucose tolerance
- increases in plasma lipids (total cholesterol, triglycerides)
- HDL cholesterol decrease
- decline in postheparin lipolytic activity
- changes in coagulation factors, renin activity, and blood pressure

Many of these effects are associated with excessive quantities or particular types of estrogen or progestogen; metabolic effects of the various components tend to be dissimilar in healthy young women.

Users of oral contraceptives generally have systolic blood pressure 2 to 3 mm Hg higher than nonusers, with no apparent difference in diastolic pressure. The degree of pressure elevation may in some measure be related to the amount of progestogen in the pill.

Oral contraceptive use has also been associated with myocardial infarction, thromboembolism, stroke, and hyperlipidemia. Triglyceride concentrations appear to increase with increasing estrogen potency. Thus, the net effect of an oral contraceptive depends on its formulation. Oral contraceptive use should be monitored in women who present with cardiovascular risk factors (see Chapter 19). The effects of these agents may also vary with age and basic metabolic and nutritional status.

Additional changes observed in women who use oral contraceptives may be summarized as follows (control values versus mean treatment values):

- increase in circulating vitamin A (43, 63 μg per dl)
- decrease in vitamin B_{12} (37, 22 ng per dl)
- decrease in leukocyte ascorbic acid (26, 19 mg per dl)
- increase in iron (94, 116 μg per dl)
- increase in copper (118, 300 μg per dl)
- decrease in calcium (9.9, 9.4 mg per dl)
- decrease in phosphorus (4.4, 3.9 mg per dl)
- decrease in zinc (96, 69 μg per dl)

Estrogen effects include increases in levels of thyroid hormone, plasma cortisol, aldosterone, renin, angiotensin, insulin, and growth hormone.

Folic acid is the only vitamin deficiency noted, reflected in slight but statistically significant decreases in hemoglobin, hematocrit, and RBC count with elevated RBC indices. Overt megaloblastic anemia is rare in oral contraceptive users and may represent a defect in absorption of folate or sequestration of folate with a binder protein.

No unusual incidence of fetal abnormalities has been observed in children born to mothers who had been oral contraceptive users. However, there may be an increased risk for such abnormalities if the mother continues to take the pill after becoming pregnant.

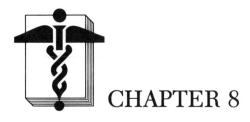

CHAPTER 8

Pediatric Nutrition
DRUCY BOROWITZ, M.D.

Nutrition has a central role in pediatrics, both in well child care and in the management of sick children. Growth and feeding are vital concerns in infancy and childhood. A term infant should double its weight in 4 to 6 months, triple it by the end of the first year, and double it again by age 6 years. A second growth spurt occurs in adolescence. Thus, the nutritional requirements of this rapidly growing child clearly differ from those of the adult.

Feeding is a main sphere of parent-child interaction—a source of both joy and frustration. Infancy is the only time in the human life cycle when a single food comprises the entire diet. Furthermore, infants and young children are completely dependent on others to feed them. There are thus specialized needs in the pediatric population, and parental interest is high, as is reflected in the many questions asked concerning feeding. This area presents physicians with an opportunity to educate themselves and their patients about nutritional needs and goals.

Since illness increases metabolic requirements, nutrition is especially important in the sick child. Nutritional inadequacies are inevitable when illness is superimposed on a person whose needs already are maximal. The malnourished child is more susceptible to illness, and the ill child is at high risk for becoming malnourished. The physician can break this cycle by applying nutritional knowledge to patient management.

INFANT REQUIREMENTS

Water

The body composition of the infant is 70 to 75 percent water, compared with that of an adult, which is 60 to 65 percent water (see Fig. 1–2). Infants therefore need to drink 10 to 15 percent of their body weight as water, versus only 2 to 4 percent for adults. Fortunately, infant foods tend to have a high water content.

Calories

Infants' caloric requirements also are high, with newborns needing approximately 100 to 120 kcal per kg per day. This need decreases to about 80 to 100 kcal per kg per day by the end of the first year. For the average newborn, 55 kcal per kg per day fills basal metabolic needs, 35 kcal per kg per day are for growth, and 10 to 25 kcal per kg per day are for activity. The very active baby may require even more calories.

Caloric intake depends on both parental and infant factors. Infants tend to regulate their intake to meet caloric needs. If fed dilute formula they will increase the volume consumed at each feeding; however, when fed a calorie-dense formula they may increase the volume to satisfy thirst, thereby taking in more calories than necessary. Thus parents play a major role in controlling caloric intake by regulating frequency and amount of feedings until the infant is sufficiently mature to feed himself or herself.

In practice, the best indicator of adequate calorie intake is normal growth rate as shown by a standard growth curve (Fig. 8–1). Such curves should be a part of every child's medical record and updated at each routine visit. Height, weight, and head circumference should follow similar percentiles. Weight may shift from one percentile channel to another at some point in the first year, and this is not a matter for concern. However, lack of growth, crossing several percentile lines, or "falling off the growth curve" are worrisome signs that should be investigated. (See "Failure to Thrive," p. 228.)

Parents should be shown the growth charts, as anxious or uncertain parents may be reassured when shown a normal growth curve. It is important to stress that the 95th percentile is not equivalent to 95 on a test. Growth charts record the normal distribution of sizes in the population; thus growth **rate** is more significant than absolute values for growth parameters.

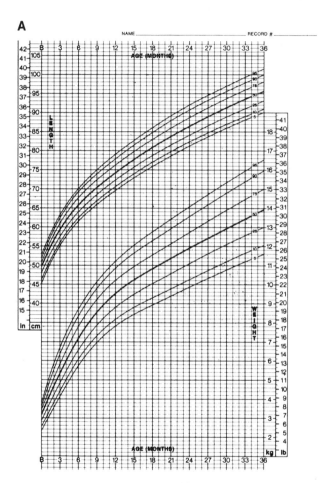

Figure 8-1. Standard growth curves for children. Curves are NCHS percentiles. *A*, Girls, birth to 36 months, length and weight for age. (*Figure continues on next page.*) (Figure 8-1*A–H* from Ross Laboratories, Columbus, Ohio, 1982, with permission.)

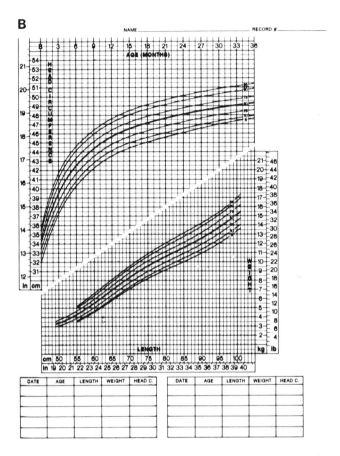

Figure 8-1B. Girls, birth to 36 months, head circumference for age and weight for length. (*Figure continues on next page.*)

Protein

Most of the healthy adult's protein intake is used to maintain lean body mass, while the infant uses a large proportion for growth. For this reason, protein requirements are expressed per unit of caloric intake during the first year of life. The requirement is approximately 1.6 g protein per 100 kcal for the first 6 weeks, decreasing to 1.4 g protein per 100 kcal thereafter. Since both human milk and commercial formulas meet these needs, protein intake will be adequate in a healthy infant who is taking the breast or the bottle well. Solid foods supply additional protein as milk intake decreases.

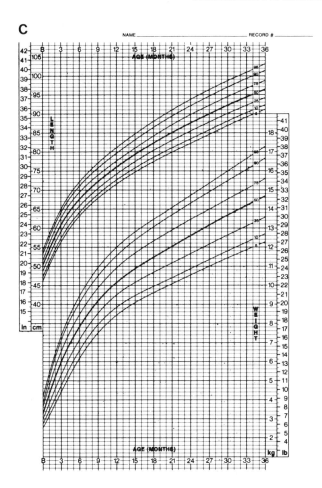

Figure 8-1C. Boys, same as *A.* (*Figure continues on next page.*)

BREAST FEEDING

Because of its biochemical, immunologic, psychologic, and socioeconomic advantages over commercial formulas, breast feeding is the best way to nourish a healthy term infant (Table 8–1).

Biochemical Advantages

We will present an overview of human milk content, since many factors affect the concentrations of its constituents. The content varies not only with

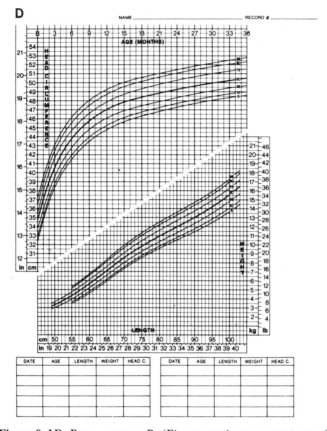

Figure 8-1D. Boys, same as *B*. (*Figure continues on next page.*)

the duration of lactation but also during a feeding, with more fat present at the end of the feeding. Different mothers have different proportions of breast milk nutrients, and even the milk of an individual mother changes in content during the course of a day.

Colostrum, Transitional Milk, and Mature Milk

Colostrum is secreted in the early postpartum period. It is high in protein (especially immunoglobulins), fat-soluble vitamins, and minerals, and relatively low in fat. In the second postpartum week, a transitional milk is produced in which concentrations of lactose, fat, and water-soluble vitamins increase to the levels seen in mature milk. In addition, a greater volume of milk is produced at each feeding. Even the components of mature milk change over time. For example, after 3 months of lactation, immunoglobulins account for only a small portion of breast milk proteins.

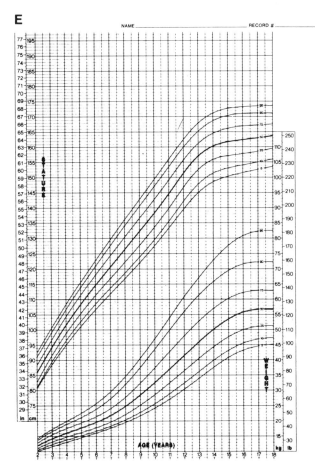

Figure 8–1E. Girls, 2 through 18 years, stature and weight for age. (*Figure continues on next page.*)

Water

Water is the major component of human milk. Even infants in a hot, humid climate or in the desert can be adequately hydrated with human milk alone. In practice in developed countries, water may be offered to babies during hot weather.

Fat

Fat is the major nonwater nutrient of human milk and accounts for 30 to 55 percent of its calories. It is present in small globules which are emulsified by phospholipid complexes and are partially digested by breast milk lipase. Infants have less pancreatic lipase and bile salts compared with adults. These

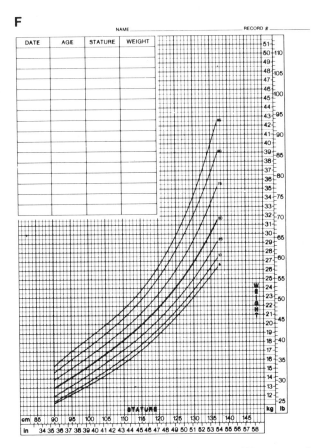

Figure 8–1F. Girls, prepubescent, weight for stature. (*Figure continues on next page.*)

factors in human milk therefore aid in the digestion and absorption of fat, the major source of calories for growing infants. In addition, human milk has a high concentration of beta-monopalmitin. This monoglyceride aids in micelle formation, is rapidly absorbed, and does not interfere with calcium absorption as does the free palmitate of cow's milk.

The amount of fat (and therefore calories) in human milk cannot be increased significantly by adding fat to the mother's diet. However, changes in the mother's diet can alter the breast milk fat profile. When a mother is calorie deficient, the lipids in her milk will reflect those in her depot fat, which is mobilized along with other compounds stored in fat, such as pesticides and environmental contaminants. A mother who has had a major exposure to toxins should take care not to become catabolic during lactation, since this may release large amounts of these toxins into her milk.

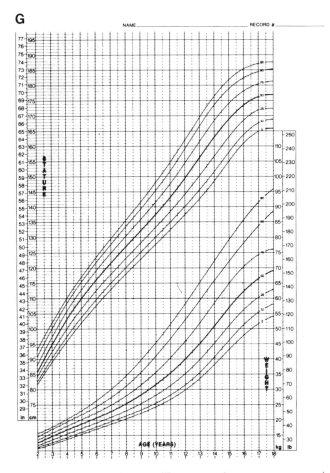

Figure 8–1G. Boys, same as *E.* (*Figure continues on next page.*)

Cholesterol. Human milk has more cholesterol than formula has, and breast-fed babies have higher serum cholesterol values than do formula-fed babies, although both groups are equivalent at the end of the first year of life. The serum cholesterol level for optimal growth and physiologic function during the first year of life is unknown. Some have speculated that the cholesterol in breast milk is necessary for formation of cell membranes. The function of the cholesterol is not clear, nor is there a rationale for the lower cholesterol content in commercial formulas.

Autopsy Studies. Some autopsy studies of patients who died during the first two decades of life showed a reduced frequency of fatty streaks and atherosclerotic plaques in the arteries of those who were breast fed. No studies have demonstrated an alteration in the incidence of atherosclerotic cardio-

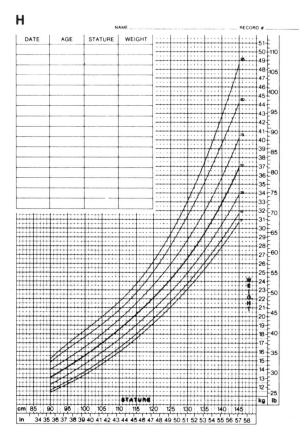

Figure 8-1H. Boys, same as *F*.

vascular disease later in life in those who were breast fed. However, it is difficult in a study to control for all the factors that contribute to atherosclerosis over an entire human lifetime.

Protein, Amino Acids, and Carnitine

The proteins in human milk are of two categories: casein and whey proteins. By definition, caseins (curds) are insoluble in an acid environment such as the stomach. The clear fluid left after the milk clots is whey. The ratio of whey to casein in human milk is 60:40, compared with a 20:80 ratio in cow's milk.

The whey-to-casein ratio is important because of the difference in digestibility of these proteins and in their amino acid composition. Cow's milk has higher concentrations of phenylalanine and tyrosine than does human milk. Human infants have a relative inability to metabolize these aromatic

Table 8-1. CHARACTERISTICS OF HUMAN MILK
AND BREAST FEEDING

A. Biochemical
 1. Water: content high
 2. Fat: easily absorbed
  a. emulsified by phospholipids
  b. partly digested by breast milk lipase
  c. high concentration of beta-monopalmitate
 3. Protein: casein-to-whey ratio = 60:40
  a. easily digestible
  b. appropriate amino acid profile
 4. Carbohydrate: primarily lactose
 5. Minerals: low renal solute load
B. Immunologic
 1. Cellular components
  a. macrophages
  b. lymphocytes (T, B, and null)
 2. Humoral components
  a. secretory IgA
  b. complement
  c. lysozyme
  d. lactoferrin
  e. promotes colonization with Lactobacillus bifidus
  f. others
C. Psychologic
 1. Promotes mother-child bonding (effect on father-child bonding?)
 2. Lactation versus sexual role
D. Socioeconomic
 1. Inexpensive
 2. Decreased maternal fertility during lactation

amino acids early in life. The cysteine content of human milk is higher than that of cow's milk, whereas cow's milk has large amounts of methionine. The methionine-to-cysteine ratio of human milk is almost 1:1, more akin to plant proteins than to other mammalian milks. Human babies are deficient in certain enzymes needed to metabolize these sulfur-containing amino acids. It is important to note that the distribution of amino acids in human whey proteins is not the same as that found in bovine whey proteins. The same is true for human versus bovine casein proteins.

In the newborn period many enzyme systems must become established. This usually occurs without incident, except for those babies with inborn errors of metabolism such as tyrosinemia or phenylketonuria (PKU). The most common example of this enzyme immaturity is the physiologic jaundice of the newborn, which is attributable to a decreased capacity to conjugate bilirubin. Although the amino acid profile of cow's milk apparently is harmless, human milk seems more optimal for the metabolic development of the infant.

Taurine, another sulfur-containing amino acid, is present in large amounts in human milk, but is not found in cow's milk nor, until recently, in most formulas. Taurine is not incorporated into proteins, but is conjugated to bile acids. Infants have a higher percentage of taurocholic acid than do adults, who have primarily glycholic acid. Taurine also has a role in neural tissue. Taurine-deficient kittens develop retinal degeneration and blindness, akin to retinitis pigmentosa. Neonates, especially those born prematurely, cannot synthesize taurine, and thus, for them, it is an essential nutrient.

Carnitine transports free fatty acids into mitochondria, where they are oxidized to release energy. The biosynthesis and storage of carnitine is limited in infants. Carnitine is present in human and cow's milk, but not in soy milks unless it is added during processing.

Carbohydrate and Minerals

The predominant carbohydrate of breast milk is lactose. To balance its high lactose concentration, the mineral content of human milk is low to maintain isotonicity and lessen the osmotic load to the neonatal gut. Cow's milk contains three times the sodium, chloride, calcium, and magnesium of human milk, and eight times the phosphorus. Large amounts of phosphorus may cause hypocalcemia. The low levels of minerals in human milk present a solute load that the neonatal kidney is able to handle. Thus, the content of human milk seems designed to provide adequate nutrients without placing undue stress on the immature organism.

Immunologic Advantages

One of the most significant advantages of breast feeding is the protection it affords against infection; this cannot be duplicated by infant formula, for fresh human milk contains both cellular and humoral factors.

There are approximately 4000 white blood cells per mm^3 of human milk. Most of these are macrophages that phagocytose and kill microorganisms. The remainder of the cells are lymphocytes (T, B, and null cells) with some polymorphonuclear leukocytes and epithelial cells. Milk cells do not survive freezing to $-23°C$ or heating to $63°C$.

These cells produce humoral factors such as complement, lysozyme, lactoferrin, and an interferon-like substance. The most important of these factors is secretory IgA, an antibody active against bacteria and viruses that is resistant to proteolytic enzymes and low pH, and therefore remains intact in the gastrointestinal tract, where it acts at the mucosal surface. (In some animals it is absorbed by the intestinal mucosa, but this is not the case in full-term human infants.) IgA production in milk is greatest during the first 3 months of lactation, when the infant's immune system is least effective. Antibody activity is increased by lysozyme, which increases during lactation.

Lactoferrin inhibits bacterial growth by depriving fastidious microorganisms, such as Escherichia coli and Candida, of iron. Giving supplemental iron to a breast-fed baby may interfere with this mechanism.

Breast feeding promotes gut colonization with Lactobacillus bifidus. When this gram-positive anaerobe, rather than E. coli and bacteroides, predominates in the gut flora, the growth of staphylococci, shigella, and protozoa is suppressed. In addition, E. coli enteric infections are less likely.

These and other anti-infective properties of human milk are most important in children in less developed countries. Enteric infections are the leading cause of infant mortality worldwide. In countries where the water supply is poorly regulated and where infant diarrhea is common, breast feeding should be strongly encouraged. It has been argued that breast-fed babies have fewer hospitalizations for infections in the United States, but the data are not clear cut.

Psychologic Advantages

Breast feeding can be a wonderfully intimate experience for the mother and baby, which contributes to mother-child bonding. Along with this comes a disadvantage—the father may feel excluded. In addition, because in our society breasts have a greater role as sexual objects than as functioning organs, lactation may cause conflicts for some parents. Awareness of these problems and counseling if necessary can be helpful.

Socioeconomic Advantages

Human milk is less expensive than infant formula; its cost is only the extra nutrients the lactating mother needs. Breast feeding decreases fertility and is probably the most widely used form of birth spacing worldwide. This protection is not absolute, however. Couples should use more reliable methods of contraception during lactation if they wish to avoid pregnancy.

Disadvantages

Are there reasons to discourage breast feeding?

- Galactosemia is an absolute contraindication. Infants with this disease cannot metabolize galactose: lactose, a glucose-galactose dimer, is present in high concentrations in human milk.
- The use of human milk for very low birth weight infants is discussed in the section on "Nutrition and Premature Infants," p. 203.
- When either a mother or child is seriously ill, the initiation or continuation of breast feeding is a matter of judgment.
- The role of breast milk in transmission of viruses such as herpes, cytomegalovirus (CMV), AIDS, and hepatitis B is currently being defined. Each case must be reviewed before a mother is discouraged or encouraged to breast feed.
- In the case of maternal metabolic diseases, such as poorly controlled diabetes mellitus, breast feeding may be contraindicated.

Drugs

Any drug the mother takes may pass into her milk. The degree of ionization of the drug as well as its concentration in maternal serum affects its secretion. Mothers with impaired renal or hepatic function may have higher concentrations of drugs in their milk. In general, nursing mothers should avoid taking drugs, since controlled studies of secretion and effects on infants are not available. Most information about specific drugs is anecdotal. Mothers who must take antithyroid drugs (especially radioactive iodine), lithium, cimetidine, and most anticancer drugs should not nurse. One good source of information on drugs and breast milk is the statement of the Committee on Drugs of the AAP, published in *Pediatrics*, volume 72, pages 375 to 383, September, 1983.

Practical Aspects

Preparation

Like "natural" childbirth, breast feeding is neither automatically successful nor painless. Not all mothers see a pediatrician before their child is born, and instruction in preparation for breast feeding may not be sought from the obstetrician. When the opportunity arises, the mother should be instructed to prepare her nipples by rubbing them with a rough terry cloth towel after showering. She should also roll her nipples between her thumb and forefinger daily. Even with such preparation, the strong suck of the newborn may be painful.

The First Few Days

During the first 3 to 4 days of life, the baby should be allowed to suck frequently, but for no longer than approximately 5 to 10 minutes per breast at each feeding to prevent nipple soreness. The baby will receive colostrum until the **transitional milk** begins to flow. At this stage the mother's breasts may become engorged and be warm, tight, and painful. Now it is important to continue to put the baby to each breast. It may be necessary for the mother to express some milk first if her breasts are very engorged, so that the baby may latch on more easily. Applying warm compresses, wearing a tight-fitting nursing brassiere 24 hours a day, and, in selected cases, using aspirin and codeine will relieve this short-lived problem.

Many breast-feeding mothers ask how they can tell if the baby is receiving any milk. In a world where each ounce of formula consumed by a baby can be measured, it is easy to understand why this question troubles parents and professionals. The mother will begin to see milk in the corners of the baby's mouth, or milk leaking around the nipple, as the baby sucks. Milk may also drip from the other breast. The baby may spit up milk. Once milk production has been established, the baby may suck for approximately 10 to 15 minutes per breast at each feeding. Uterine contractions may be noticeable at feeding times in the first few weeks.

Cracked or Sore Nipples and Plugged Ducts

Cracked or sore nipples are common during the establishment of nursing. Nipples should be dried in the air before the brassiere is refastened. Nipple creams may be used but are not necessary. The clinician should check the position of the nursing couple. If the baby is poorly positioned, or if he or she sucks only the nipple and not the entire areola, this problem will be exacerbated. Poor position may also lead to plugged ducts, which may result from insufficient rest or poor maternal fluid intake. Warm showers, breast massage, and continued breast feeding will alleviate this problem and prevent the development of full-blown mastitis.

Environment and the "Let Down" Reflex

Breast feeding should be done in a comfortable position with few distractions. Drinking just prior to a feeding reminds the mother to keep herself well hydrated and will also aid the "let down" (milk ejection) reflex. In this hypothalamic–pituitary–end organ reflex, oxytocin causes the mammary myoepithelium to contract. This is sensed as a tingling in the breasts, but the sensation may not be apparent until many weeks postpartum. This reflex can be inhibited centrally by cold, pain, or emotional stress. Let down may be elicited in a lactating woman merely by hearing her baby cry.

Assessment

Most infants lose weight immediately after birth, and breast-fed babies may not regain their birth weight until 2 weeks postpartum. If an infant has lost a significant amount of weight, the clinician should observe the nursing couple. If this observation and the physical examination are unremarkable, reassurance and close, frequent follow-up are called for. The mother should be encouraged to rest and her diet and fluid intake evaluated. It is important to assess the mother's motivations to breast feed, as this will influence patient management. Infant formula supplements may be necessary at times.

Successful Establishment of Breast Feeding

As in any relationship, it takes time for each partner to get used to the other. It usually takes at least 2 to 3 weeks before all runs smoothly for the breast-feeding couple. This should be emphasized to mothers, and they should be encouraged to call with any problems or questions. Patience and persistence in the first few weeks are the keys to successful establishment of breast feeding. Ineffective suckling or an inadequate frequency of nursing results in incomplete emptying of the breast. Each breast-feeding session should last long enough for the baby to empty the breast. Once lactation is established, the breast can adapt to a wide range in nursing frequency.

Relief Bottles

After the first few weeks, when the milk supply is well established, the baby may be offered a bottle of expressed breast milk or formula if the mother desires. Use of a "relief bottle" has several purposes. It enables the mother to rest for a longer period of time, since someone else can feed the baby, and it gives the father an opportunity to share in one of the most joyful interactions a parent can have with a newborn. It may also relieve any feelings of exclusion the father may have. In addition, if the mother plans to return to work, the baby will become accustomed to taking both bottle and breast, thus facilitating the continuance of breast feeding at that time.

Weaning

Human milk is a complete diet for a child, at least through the first 6 months of life. After this period, babies should not be denied the experience of eating solids. Weaning may be done at any time, although logical times are when the child begins to bite or to drink from a cup. Some mothers may go on to breast feed their toddlers. Whether the mother chooses to breast feed her infant for a brief or an extended period, this form of feeding should be encouraged.

INFANT FORMULAS

Infant formulas have evolved dramatically since their introduction in the first half of this century. Specialized formulas are available for babies with specific requirements, but those commonly used fall into two groups: cow's milk based and soy protein based. Both provide 20 calories per ounce (0.67 kcal per cc).

Cow's Milk Based

Three major cow's milk–based formulas are currently available (Table 8–2). These products use heat-treated, dialyzed bovine milk as a base, with added vegetable oils and vitamins. Cow's milk protein is altered in an attempt to decrease its potential antigenicity, since the infant's intestinal mucosa is permeable to intact protein.

Approximately 1 percent of infants develop cow's milk protein–induced intestinal injury. This syndrome may include fever, vomiting, failure to thrive, anemia, and diarrhea, which may be heme positive. The intestinal mucosa will heal and all symptoms will resolve when cow's milk proteins are removed from the diet. Beta-lactoglobulin is thought to be responsible, although other cow's milk proteins may play a role. Allergic symptoms such as

Table 8-2. COW'S MILK–BASED STANDARD INFANT FORMULAS

Brand Name	Protein	Carbohydrate (mg/100 ml)	Lipid	kcal/oz kcal/cc
Enfamil	Whey:casein = 60:40	Lactose	Soy oil, coconut oils	20/0.67[†]
Similac	Whey:casein = 20:80[*]	Lactose	Soy oil, coconut oils	20/0.67[†]
SMA	Whey:casein = 60:40	Lactose	Oleo, oleic, coconut oil, soy oils	20/0.67[†]

Brand Name	Na	K	Ca	P	Fe
Enfamil	19	73	46	32	0.11[‡]
Similac	22	81	51	39	0.15[‡]
SMA	15	56	44	33	1.2[§]

[*] Also available in a whey-predominant formulation.
[†] Also available with 24 kcal/oz (0.80 kcal/cc).
[‡] Similac with Iron and Enfamil with Iron have 1.2 mg Fe/100 ml.
[§] Lo-iron SMA has 0.15 mg Fe/100 ml.

rhinitis, wheezing, and skin rashes also may be linked to the ingestion of cow's milk protein. However, the vast majority of infants tolerate cow's milk proteins without any ill effects.

Of the three formulas, SMA and new formulation Enfamil have a 60:40 whey-to-casein ratio, similar to the ratio in human milk. Similac has introduced a whey-predominant formula, but standard Similac is still casein predominant. As noted earlier, cow's milk whey is not identical to human whey. Recently, all infant formulas have been supplemented with taurine and carnitine.

All three formulas have lactose as their carbohydrate, and since vegetable oil is their lipid source, they lack the cholesterol content of human milk. Although cow's milk is dialyzed to lower its mineral content, these products still contain more sodium than does human milk. SMA has the lowest sodium content. In one study, infants fed low sodium milk for 6 months had lower blood pressure at the end of the study than those fed standard formulas. However, it is not known whether this difference will persist over time.

Soy Based

The major soy-based formulas are listed in Table 8–3. The protein in soy, similar to other plant proteins, is incomplete (see Chapter 1). These formulas are supplemented with methionine, and taurine and carnitine have been

Table 8–3. SOY-BASED STANDARD INFANT FORMULAS

Brand Name	Protein	Carbohydrate	Lipid	kcal/oz kcal/cc
Isomil*	Soy	Corn syrup solids, sucrose	Soy and coconut oils	20/0.67
Nursoy	Soy	Sucrose	Oleo, oleic, coconut, and soy oils	20/0.67
Prosobee	Soy	Corn syrup solids	Soy and coconut oils	20/0.67
Soyalac†	Soy	Corn syrup sucrose	Soy oil	20/0.67

Brand Name	Na	K	Ca (mg/100 ml)	P	Fe
Isomil	32	95	71	51	1.2
Nursoy	20	74	63	44	1.2
Prosobee	24	82	63	50	1.2
Soyalac	28	78	69	48	1.2

* Also available without sucrose as Isomil SF.
† Also available with tapioca dextrins and sucrose instead of corn syrup as i-Soyalac.

added to some. Some practitioners believe that all infants with a strong family history of allergies should be fed soy formula prophylactically if they are not breast fed. Unfortunately, not all long-term studies show a reduction in allergic symptoms in patients fed the soy formulas. Soy has been given to children with cow's milk–induced intestinal injury; however, a similar syndrome may be induced by soy protein. Some children are sensitive to both proteins. Soy formulas are not appropriate for low birth weight infants or as a treatment for infant colic.

The four major soy formulas also have vegetable oil as their lipid. None use lactose as a carbohydrate. Isomil, Nursoy, and Soyalac contain sucrose and glucose polymers; Prosobee and Isomil SF are sucrose-free. Nursoy and I-Soyalac do not use corn syrup solids as a carbohydrate source and may be used for patients with a known history of corn allergy. Since soy-based formulas are lactose-free, they are often used temporarily after a bout of diarrhea, which may induce a transient lactase deficiency.

Soy formulas have an even higher mineral content than cow's milk–based formulas.

Practical Aspects

Formulas come in three forms: ready-to-feed, powder, and liquid concentrate. Ready-to-feed formula is the most expensive, but is also the most convenient. Powdered formula is usually reconstituted with one unpacked, level measuring tablespoon of powder per 2 ounces of water. Concentrated liquid is usually mixed in a 50:50 ratio of concentrate to water. Except in special circumstances, formula should always be prepared according to directions. Either dilute or concentrated formula may cause severe metabolic abnormalities. Any infant with abnormal serum electrolytes of unknown origin should have a diet history taken emphasizing the method of formula preparation.

Many pediatricians continue to recommend sterilization of bottles and all equipment used for formula preparation. In our society, with its reliable water supply, clean technique may be used instead. Bottles may be made individually, or a 24-hour supply can be prepared. Good handwashing prior to preparation is mandatory, and equipment such as a can opener or measuring spoons and cups should be thoroughly cleaned and used exclusively for formula preparation. Opened cans of concentrated formula or prepared bottles must be covered and refrigerated, and should be discarded after 48 hours. A bottle taken from the refrigerator should be discarded if not used within 1 hour. Bottles need not be warmed, but some infants dislike refrigerator-cold formula.

Formula may be replaced with fresh cow's milk during the second half of the first year of life. Some authorities recommend waiting until after the first birthday. Unmodified cow's milk is not fed to infants because of its high renal solute load owing to its protein and mineral content and its potentially harmful protein. In addition, cow's milk has negligible iron. The child should be consuming iron-rich foods, such as fortified infant cereals or meats, before cow's milk becomes a major part of the diet. Infant formula is much more expensive than cow's milk. Milk intake should be limited to no more than 1 quart per day.

VITAMINS

Opinions concerning vitamin use in infants range from full multivitamin supplementation for all infants, to no use at all. The recommendations of the American Academy of Pediatrics are summarized in Table 8–4.

All infants, regardless of gestational age or planned mode of feeding, should receive vitamin K shortly after birth to prevent hemorrhagic disease of the newborn.

Breast-Fed Infants

Breast-fed infants receive adequate amounts of all water-soluble vitamins, provided that the mother's nutritional status is good. Vitamin A deficiency is extremely rare in breast-fed infants, and these babies do not require additional vitamins E or K. The need for vitamin D supplementation is controversial. Because of the low content of vitamin D in human milk, it would seem that a breast-fed baby would receive much less than the 400 IU per day RDA of vitamin D; however, rickets is uncommon in breast-fed infants. Of course, infants who receive adequate sunshine do not need vitamin D supplements. Dark-skinned babies, or those born in the winter in northern latitudes, may benefit from a supplement during breast feeding.

Increased bioavailability of vitamin D may explain the antirachitic properties of breast milk. This is certainly the case with iron, which is present in breast milk only in small amounts. The iron is avidly absorbed, perhaps aided by lactoferrin. Although infants exclusively fed human milk until the age of 1 year may not show evidence of iron deficiency, it is advisable to begin other sources of iron by age 6 months. Since one mechanism of milk's anti-infective properties is to deprive fastidious organisms of iron, it has been argued that giving iron supplements to breast-fed infants may do more harm than good. Since fluoride does not cross into breast milk, some infer that young infants do not require it. However, unerupted teeth are mineralizing during the first 6 months of life. The AAP therefore recommends that breast-fed infants begin fluoride supplements shortly after birth, but recognizes that this supplementation could begin at age 6 months.

Table 8-4. GUIDELINES FOR USE OF SUPPLEMENTS
IN HEALTHY INFANTS

Child	A-D-C Drops	Fluoride*	Iron	Multivitamin-Multimineral
Term Infant				
Breast-fed	+[†]	+	0	0
Formula-fed[‡]	0	+[§]	0	0
Older Infant (> 6 mo)				
Normal	0	+[‖]	0	0
High risk	0	+[‖]	+	+

* See Fluoride Schedule.

[†] Most practical form of vitamin D for breast-fed babies requiring supplements.

[‡] Babies fed homemade formulas based on evaporated cow's milk will need supplements of vitamin C and iron; those fed homemade formulas based on goat's milk will need supplements of folate and iron.

[§] Fluoride should be given to babies solely fed ready-to-feed formula or those fed any formula prepared with nonfluoridated water.

[‖] Unless they consume enough fluoridated water to provide 0.25 mg fluoride/day (see Fluoride Schedule).

Fluoride Schedule

A. Dosage of Fluoride, mg/day

Age	Concentration of Fluoride in Water (ppm)		
	> 0.7	0.3-0.7	< 0.3
2 wk-2 yr	0	0	0.25
2-3 yr	0	0.25	0.50

B. Dosage Equivalence of Fluoride to Fluoridated Water

Fluoride	Volume of Water (ml)		
	1 ppm	0.7 ppm	0.3 ppm
0.25 mg	250	357	750
0.50 mg	500	714	1500

(Adapted from *Pediatric Nutrition Handbook*, AAP, Evanston, IL.)

Formula-Fed Infants

Proprietary formulas have adequate amounts of all vitamins but do not contain fluoride. If concentrated or powdered formula is prepared with fluoridated water, no supplements are needed. If the water supply contains less than 0.3 ppm of fluoride, or if the infant receives ready-to-feed formula, 0.25

mg per day of fluoride should be given; this may be started shortly after birth or at age 6 months.

Term infants are born with iron stores adequate to sustain them for 3 to 4 months, and during this time no exogenous iron is necessary. After this time infants require additional iron. All of the cow's milk–based formulas come in two varieties: one with less than 1 mg iron per quart and one with approximately 12 mg iron per quart.

Home-prepared formulas are used infrequently. Evaporated cow's milk, diluted with water and augmented with sugar, should be supplemented by vitamin C and iron. Goat's milk has been used as a formula base for infants with food sensitivity, but it is deficient in folate, which must be provided as a supplement.

Practical Aspects

Liquid vitamin drops are available in limited formulations. Vitamins A, D, and C are present in fixed formulations for historic reasons and can be dispensed with or without fluoride. Multiple vitamin preparations are available with or without fluoride and with or without iron. Folate is not present in the liquid multivitamins and must be provided as a crushed tablet if needed. Fluoride and vitamin C are available as single supplements in liquid form.

Although the therapeutic index for vitamins is high, acute poisonings have been reported, especially with iron. Vitamins should not be prescribed unless they are needed (see Chapters 6 and 14).

ADDITION OF SOLIDS

Solid foods are usually added to a baby's diet during the first half of the first year. The exact timing varies among infants, as does the achievement of other developmental milestones (Table 8–5).

Infant Readiness

In the past, infants only several weeks old were fed solids; this amounts to nothing more than force-feeding. Newborns have a tongue-thrusting reflex. They suck fluids by compressing the nipple between their tongue and palate and "stripping" the nipple by thrusting their tongue forward. Until this reflex wanes and the infant is able to manipulate his tongue consciously (usually between the ages of 3 and 6 months), solids will be spit out unless they are placed far enough back on the tongue to slide easily into the esopha-

Table 8-5. FEEDING SKILLS AT DEVELOPMENTAL AGES
UP TO 2 YEARS*

Age	Skills
Newborn	Rooting reflex
	Suck and swallow pattern (uses tongue thrust for suck)
	Palmomental reflex
2-3 mo	May have established a feeding pattern
	Parents better able to distinguish hunger cry from other cries
	Holds up head
	Begins to recognize hands
4-5 mo	Sits with support
	Brings hand to mouth
	Able to manipulate tongue; tongue thrust disappearing
	Becomes excited with feeding preparations
6-7 mo	Sits unsupported
	Up and down chewing
	Can hold a bottle
	Can drink from a cup if it is held at his lips
	Feeds self biscuit
8 mo-1 yr	Good eye-hand coordination makes self-feeding easier
	Use of cup and spoon more accurate
	Rotary chewing beginning
about 15 mo	Continued maturation of biting, chewing, and swallowing
	Uses spoon without help
	May have words for water or bottle
	Indicates desires by pointing
	Food preferences begin
about 18 mo	Easily feeds self
	Uses cup skillfully
about 2 yr	Uses spoon skillfully
	Good rotary chewing
	Speech improving

*Pediatrics is a developmental specialty. Not only do nutrient requirements change at different times of life, but feeding skills also follow a developmental sequence.

gus. Furthermore, an infant should be able to control his head and trunk before feedings of solids are instituted. The infant will then be able to turn the head away when sated. If the introduction of solids is delayed past the time of developmental readiness, feeding problems may ensue.

Added Calories and Nutrients

The added calories of solids are not needed until the second half of the first year of life. Solid foods constitute a minor portion of the baby's total caloric intake until the end of the first year. They represent a new, exciting experience for an infant and add nutrients to the diet.

Iron

The most important nutrient is iron, and iron deficiency is the most prevalent deficiency state among children in the United States. As noted earlier, fetal iron stores are depleted by age 3 to 4 months in term infants. Human milk and iron-fortified formula will provide some iron, and since infant cereals are a good source, they are usually the first solids to be introduced. Infant cereals contain approximately 1 mg iron per tablespoon dry cereal.

Iron Deficiency. The incidence of iron deficiency anemia in the United States in children aged 6 to 24 months (defined as hemoglobin less than 11 g%) has been estimated to range between 3 and 24 percent. The clinical signs of iron deficiency include irritability, lack of interest in surroundings, anorexia, and poor weight gain (see Chapter 15). Prolonged, severe iron deficiency may result in koilonychia, atrophy of the tongue papillae, gastric achlorhydria, and altered small bowel structure and function. Some studies have demonstrated marked improvement in cognition and behavior in previously iron-deficient children whose iron stores have been repleted. Because of the prevalence of iron deficiency and its potential effects on development, the importance of maintaining adequate iron must be emphasized. Monitoring of hemoglobin or hematocrit several months after formula or human milk has been discontinued and during the second year of life should be routine.

Introduction of Foods

Foods should be introduced one at a time, and each tried for 3 to 5 days before a new food is begun. This enables parents to identify more easily those foods that cause constipation, diarrhea, or a rash. Single-grain cereals such as rice (least allergenic), barley, and oatmeal are typically introduced first. Strained fruits and yellow vegetables such as squash and carrots are then added. These foods are rich in vitamins A and C and have a flavor and texture that most babies will accept easily.

Green vegetables, meats, and egg yolk are added next. To reduce the possibility of food intolerance and allergy, citrus, seafood, nut butters, chocolate, nitrate-containing vegetables, and egg whites are not introduced until the end of the first year.

Combination foods may be introduced after tolerance to single-ingredient foods is established. Use of desserts providing "empty" calories should be discouraged. High protein baby foods should be encouraged if formula or milk intake is low. Babies do have taste preferences, and if one refuses a food, it should be set aside and offered again later.

Food Preparation and Storage

Infant foods may be prepared commercially or at home. Commercial products do not contain added salt, and neither salt nor sugar should be added to home-prepared foods. Milk will meet the infant's sodium requirements. Uneaten foods may be covered and stored in the refrigerator for 2 to 3 days. Before serving, baby food should be spooned from the original container into a dish to prevent the remainder from being contaminated with the enzymes and bacteria of the baby's saliva. Average serving size is only a few tablespoons to start with.

Transition to Table Foods and Self-Feeding

As the baby gets older, foods with coarser textures are added (mashed as opposed to pureed). When the child is able to manipulate objects and wants to feed himself or herself, finger foods are added: crackers, hard cheese sticks, bananas, and partially cooked strips of vegetables. Foods that may cause choking should be avoided. These include nuts, corn, popcorn, raw vegetables, stringy foods, and foods with seeds. Children can eat spicy foods, although very "hot" foods may cause discomfort. Use of a cup should be encouraged.

Self-feeding is a messy but important developmental step for infants, who slowly make the transition from infant foods to the wide variety of table foods that other family members eat toward the end of the first year.

TODDLERS AND PRESCHOOL-AGE CHILDREN

Toddlers and preschool-age children are notorious for having strong food preferences. It is not uncommon for children in this age group to pick a few foods and eat these exclusively, day in and day out, for long periods of time. They may then switch their preferences, refusing to eat foods that were formerly favorites. In addition, many parents complain that their children "hardly eat enough to survive."

These two common problems are in line with normal development. Toddlers are experiencing autonomy for the first time, and it is natural that they should exercise their newfound powers at meals. Parents should be counseled to expect a narrowing of the child's diet. It is futile to try to alter food preferences at this growth stage, and attempts to do so only result in tension and conflict. Parents should continue to offer the child a variety of foods and should be neither miffed if he or she refuses a food nor surprised if a formerly rejected food is accepted.

The amount of food that children eat is small. Thus, parents need to be reminded that a child's portion may be only one fourth to one fifth of an adult's portion. "A few bites of sandwich" may be an adequate serving for a toddler. Parents can be shown the leveling off of the rate of weight gain on standard growth charts. The average child will gain only 5 to 6 pounds in the second year and will lose much of the baby fat. Weight gain in the third to sixth years is only 4 to 5 pounds per year. It is difficult for parents to adjust to this decreased caloric need after the emphasis on first-year feeding with its attendant rapid increases in weight.

The health care professional should continue to monitor the child's diet to see if it is distributed reasonably well among the four food groups (see Chapter 4). If the diet has severe imbalances, iron, calcium, or multiple vitamin supplements may be prescribed (Table 8–6). Caloric adequacy can be assessed by continuing to measure height and weight and plotting these on growth charts.

ADOLESCENT NUTRITION

Marking the second and final exponential growth spurt, adolescence is also a time of increased nutritional needs. Caloric intake is 60 to 80 kcal per kg per day, depending on the relative size, growth velocity, and activity of the teenager. Prepubertal boys and girls have similar body composition. At the end of this growth spurt, girls have proportionately more fat than boys, while boys may gain twice as much lean body mass as girls. Calcium and iron requirements increase greatly. Calcium intake should be approximately 1200 mg per day, almost equal to that of a lactating woman. Iron intake should be 18 mg per day. The vitamin requirements of a 13-year-old are equal to those of an adult. Unfortunately, many adolescents eat nutrient-sparse junk foods, and although their caloric intake may meet their needs, vitamins and minerals may be insufficient (see Table 8–6).

Nutritional Counseling

As with other age groups, nutritional counseling of adolescents must be keyed to developmental issues. Adolescents are body conscious and want to fit into the group. They have emerging sexual drives. Areas of concern may be acne, weight reduction diets, sports participation, and birth control. Physicians can initiate discussions by noting patients' height and weight and asking if they are satisfied with these measurements. A brief diet history may be obtained by recall.

Dr. Judith Wurtman, of the Department of Nutrition and Food Science at Massachusetts Institute of Technology, notes that although no experimental study has convincingly shown that diet influences the state of one's complexion, there is certainly no evidence that a poor diet helps it. Therefore one can state without bending scientific proof that a diet of soft drinks, french fries, candy and potato chips is not going to improve the condition of the skin, and some alternative foods with nutritional value can be suggested.

This statement is taken from Dr. Wurtman's chapter in *Textbook of Pediatric Nutrition* (R.M. Suskind, ed., Raven Press, New York, 1981).

Weight Reduction Diets

Adolescents on weight reduction diets are especially prone to fad diets (see Chapter 6). In its most extreme form, this may be manifested as anorexia nervosa or bulimia (see Chapter 16). Many teenagers have a distorted body image and will perceive themselves as obese despite evidence to the contrary. Use of extreme hypocaloric diets should be discouraged. Teens with a significant amount of weight to lose must be on realistic, balanced diets over a long period of time and must increase their energy expenditure. Young teenagers probably do not have the cognitive maturity or independence concerning food intake at home to be very successful with weight reduction diets. Increased activity should be their goal. There is some evidence that weight loss should not be attempted prior to the completion of puberty. Older teens may be more successful with weight loss. At any age, adolescents do best in a group setting. Parents should also receive dietary guidance. Weight loss, difficult to achieve for adults (see Chapter 16), is even more so for body-conscious obese teenagers who are prone to erratic, impulsive eating.

Sports Participation

Many teenagers present to a pediatrician for medical assessment prior to sports participation. This is the time to dispel myths concerning the need to take massive amounts of vitamins and protein to achieve peak athletic performance (see Chapter 4). Active adolescents who weigh significantly less than expected for height may need to greatly increase their caloric intake in a balanced way. They may be counseled to eat four or five meals a day, rather than constantly snacking. They should also be counseled against use of protein-predominant diets, or drugs such as anabolic steroids, growth hormone, or cyproheptadine. Teenagers involved in weight-class sports such as wrestling or junior football should be made aware of the fact that attempts to reduce weight by short-term dehydration will affect their performance adversely.

Table 8-6a. RECOMMENDED DIETARY ALLOWANCES, REVISED 1980

Age (yr) and Sex Group	Infants		Children			Males			Females		
	0.0–0.5	0.5–1.0	1–3	4–6	7–10	11–14	15–18	19–22	11–14	15–18	19–22
Weight, kg	6	9	13	20	28	45	66	70	46	55	55
lb	13	20	29	44	62	99	145	154	101	120	120
Height, cm	60	71	90	112	132	157	176	177	157	163	163
in	24	28	35	44	52	62	69	70	62	64	64
Protein, g	kg × 2.2	kg × 2.0	23	30	34	45	56	56	46	46	44
Fat-soluble vitamins											
Vitamin A, μg RE[a]	420	400	400	500	700	1000	1000	1000	800	800	800
Vitamin D, μg[b]	10	10	10	10	10	10	10	7.5	10	10	7.5
Vitamin E, mg αTE[c]	3	4	5	6	7	8	10	10	8	8	8
Water-soluble vitamins											
Vitamin C, mg	35	35	45	45	45	50	60	60	50	60	60
Thiamin, mg	0.3	0.5	0.7	0.9	1.2	1.4	1.4	1.5	1.1	1.1	1.1
Riboflavin, mg	0.4	0.6	0.8	1.0	1.4	1.6	1.7	1.7	1.3	1.3	1.3
Niacin, mg NE[d]	6	8	9	11	16	18	18	19	15	14	14
Vitamin B$_6$, mg	0.3	0.6	0.9	1.3	1.6	1.8	2.0	2.2	1.8	2.0	2.0
Folacin,[e] μg	30	45	100	200	300	400	400	400	400	400	400
Vitamin B$_{12}$, μg	0.5[f]	1.5	2.0	2.5	3.0	3.0	3.0	3.0	3.0	3.0	3.0

Table 8-6a. RECOMMENDED DIETARY ALLOWANCES, REVISED 1980 — Continued

Age (yr) and Sex Group	Infants		Children			Males			Females		
	0.0-0.5	0.5-1.0	1-3	4-6	7-10	11-14	15-18	19-22	11-14	15-18	19-22
Minerals											
Calcium, mg	360	540	800	800	800	1200	1200	800	1200	1200	800
Phosphorus, mg	240	360	800	800	800	1200	1200	800	1200	1200	800
Magnesium, mg	50	70	150	200	250	350	400	350	300	300	300
Iron, mg	10	15	15	10	10	18	18	10	18	18	18
Zinc, mg	3	5	10	10	10	15	15	15	15	15	15
Iodine, µg	40	50	70	90	120	150	150	150	150	150	150

* Retinol equivalents: 1 retinol equivalent = 1 µg retinol or 6 µg β-carotene.
† As cholecalciferol: 10 µg cholecalciferol = 400 IU vitamin D.
‡ α-tocopherol equivalents: 1 mg d-α-tocopherol = 1 αTE.
§ 1 NE (niacin equivalent) = 1 mg niacin or 60 mg dietary tryptophan.
‖ Folacin allowances refer to dietary sources as determined by Lactobacillus casei assay after treatment with enzymes ("conjugases") to make polygluta-myl forms of the vitamin available to the test organism.
** The RDA for vitamin B_{12} in infants is based on average concentration of the vitamin in human milk. The allowances after weaning are based on energy intake and consideration of other factors, such as intestinal absorption.

Table 8-6b. ESTIMATED SAFE AND ADEQUATE DAILY DIETARY INTAKE

Age, yr	Infants		Children			
	0.0–0.5	0.5–1.0	1–3	4–6	7–10	11+
Vitamin K, µg	12	10–20	15–30	20–40	30–60	50–100
Biotin, µg	35	50	65	85	120	100–200
Pantothenic acid, mg	2	3	3	3–4	4–5	4–7
Copper, mg	0.5–0.7	0.7–1	1–1.5	1.5–2	2–2.5	2–3
Manganese, mg	0.5–0.7	0.7–1	1–1.5	1.5–2	2–3	2.5–5
Fluoride, mg	0.1–0.5	0.2–1	0.5–1.5	1–2.5	1.5–2.5	1.5–2.5
Chromium, mg	0.01–0.04	0.02–0.06	0.02–0.08	0.03–0.12	0.05–0.2	0.05–0.2
Selenium, mg	0.01–0.04	0.02–0.06	0.02–0.08	0.03–0.12	0.05–0.2	0.05–0.2
Molybdenum, mg	0.03–0.06	0.04–0.08	0.05–0.1	0.06–0.15	0.1–0.3	0.15–0.5
Sodium, mg	115–350	250–750	325–975	450–1350	600–1800	900–2700
Potassium, mg	350–925	425–1275	550–1650	775–2325	1000–3000	1525–4575
Chloride, mg	275–700	400–1200	500–1500	700–2100	925–2775	1400–4200

Adapted from Recommended Dietary Allowances, 9th Rev. Ed., 1980. National Academy of Sciences, Washington, DC, p. 178.

PEDIATRIC NUTRITION   203

Contraception and Pregnancy

The most frequently used form of birth control among teenagers is oral contraceptive pills. These pills may increase the need for some B vitamins and vitamin C (see Chapter 7). Furthermore, many teenage girls who begin taking oral contraceptive pills will gain weight. A full diet history should be taken when the pill is prescribed; if the diet contains few vitamin-rich foods, a multiple vitamin supplement may be ordered. Anticipatory guidance concerning caloric intake and potential weight gain may prevent noncompliance with birth control.

Teenage pregnancy has become more prevalent in recent years. The pregnant or lactating teenager has the highest overall nutritional requirements of any healthy human being, and for this reason should be followed closely in a high-risk obstetric setting to monitor the health of both mother and fetus (see Chapter 7). A complete, detailed diet history should be taken, and a vitamin supplement containing both folate and iron prescribed. Frequent, personal nutritional counseling is essential.

NUTRITION AND PREMATURE INFANTS

Since the early 1960s, when neonatal intensive care became a reality, pediatricians have been able to care for younger, smaller, and sicker infants. Babies acquire stores of fat and other nutrients during the third trimester of pregnancy (see Chapter 7). When premature infants are born before amassing adequate stores, the physician must supply them. This can be achieved by the intravenous or enteral route, depending on the baby's gestational age and clinical status.

Parenteral Nutrition

Parenteral feeding, an important breakthrough in the case of premature infants, requires constant monitoring, attention to detail, and adjustment (Table 8–7).

Central Venous Access

Because of the low fluid volumes tolerated by the premature infant, especially with pulmonary or cardiac disease, central venous access is usually necessary to provide concentrated calories. Jugular or subclavian lines or an umbilical venous catheter with its tip distal to the liver may be used. These lines should not be used for medications, blood products, or blood drawing.

Table 8-7. TOTAL PARENTERAL NUTRITION FOR
PREMATURE INFANTS

A. Mechanical factors
  1. Central line placement at or near right atrium
  2. Use good dressing technique
  3. Use for TPN alone
B. Major nutrients
  1. Calories: aim for at least 90 kcal/kg/day
     Increase for:
     a. sepsis
     b. cardiopulmonary distress
     c. cold stress
     d. other metabolic stress
  2. Carbohydrate: gradually increase while monitoring:
     a. dextrostix
     b. urine glucose
  3. Lipid: 10% or 20% preparations
     a. begin at 0.5 g/kg/day
     b. maximum is 4 g/kg/day (3 g/kg/day if < 1500 g infant) or 50% of total
        calories
     c. check serum for lipemia
     d. use with caution, if at all, in the presence of pulmonary hypertension or
        jaundice
  4. Protein: aim for 2-3 g/kg/day

Good dressing technique will prolong the life of the line and reduce infectious complications.

Caloric Requirements

Since caloric requirements of a premature infant are high and lipid stores are low, provision of adequate calories is most critical. A premature infant will require at least 50 to 75 kcal per kg per day to meet the resting energy expenditure. Nonstressed premature infants fed intravenously will grow if given in excess of 90 kcal per kg per day. A baby with increased needs, as for sepsis or cardiopulmonary distress, will require added calories. Because the stress of a cold environment will increase caloric needs, infant temperature should be servocontrolled in an isolette or warmer. Fat, at 9 kcal per g, is a more concentrated source of calories than carbohydrate (4 kcal per g). A combination of these energy sources is used, with fat accounting for no more than 50 percent of total calories.

Carbohydrate. Larger premature infants will tolerate 10 percent dextrose solutions, and the carbohydrate concentration can be increased daily by 2.5 percent. Serum and urine glucose should be monitored, and sudden glucose intolerance should prompt an investigation for sepsis. This is especially critical in patients with central lines. Very low birth weight babies often demonstrate hyperglycemia and glycosuria at average doses of glucose (5 to 6 mg per kg per minute). Because these infants are extremely sensitive to very small doses of insulin, use of insulin is not recommended.

Fat. Intravenous (IV) fat is available as a 10 percent or 20 percent emulsion. The latter is especially useful in small premature infants with fluid restriction. The manufacturers suggest a test dose of 0.1 ml per kg given over 10 to 15 minutes to watch for signs of acute intolerance. The emulsions may then be started at 0.5 g per kg per day and increased by 0.5 g per kg per day to a maximum of 4 g per kg per day (3 g per kg per day for babies less than 1500 g) not to exceed 50 percent of total calories. The infusion should be run as slowly as may be feasible, but no longer than 20 hours in order to give the serum a chance to clear. If spun serum is lipemic 4 hours after the infusion is discontinued, the dose is too high. Although this is a very insensitive screen, it requires only a small blood sample.

Problems. Numerous problems have been attributed to the use of fat emulsions. At autopsy some low birth weight babies were found to have fat globules in alveolar macrophages and capillaries and pigment deposition throughout the reticuloendothelial (RE) system. It is unknown whether the function of the RE system is affected. Infants with pulmonary hypertension may show changes in transcutaneous oxygen levels while intravenous fat is being infused; thus, IV fat should be used with extreme care, if at all, in these patients. The free fatty acids (FFA) released by the metabolism of IV fat will compete with bilirubin for binding sites on albumin. This occurs in vivo when the FFA-to-albumin ratio exceeds 6. Guidelines developed at Stanford University show that a slow infusion of intravenous fat begun in the second week of life when the bilirubin level is less than one half of the exchange level will not place premature infants at risk for kernicterus.

Protein

The optimal parenteral protein formulation for premature infants has yet to be defined. It will certainly differ from formulations currently available for adults, which do not contain cysteine or taurine. Premature infants have a diminished capacity to convert methionine to cysteine. Taurine also may be essential for premature infants. Tyrosine is present in the usual formulations in concentrations much lower than that required by the premature infant. Products formulated for adults also contain greater amounts of nonessential amino acids than are required, thus presenting an added, unnecessary metabolic load to these patients. Some amino acid mixtures formulated for infants are now available (see Table 8–11). Two to 3 g per day of protein provide adequate protein for growth without causing complications such as hyperammonemia and metabolic acidosis seen with higher intakes.

Table 8-8. INTRAVENOUS VITAMIN RECOMMENDATIONS FOR INFANTS AND CHILDREN

For infants <3 kg and children up to 11 yr:

| Infants | 1 kg | 30% of vial |
| Infants | 1-3 kg | 65% of vial |

MVI–Pediatric, 5 ml vial
Contains:

A (retinol), μg	700.0
D (ergocalciferol), μg	10.0
E (D-1-α tocopheryl acetate), μg	10.0
C (ascorbic acid), mg	80.0
B_1 (thiamin, HCl), mg	1.2
B_2 (riboflavin-5-phosphate Na), mg	1.4
Niacinamide, mg	17.0
B_6 (pyridoxine HCl), mg	1.0
B_{12} (cyanocobalamin), μg	1.0
Folic acid, μg	140.0
Dexpanthenol, mg	5.0
Biotin, μg	20.0
K (phytonadione), μg	200.0

INTRAVENOUS TRACE MINERAL RECOMMENDATIONS

Body Weight	<20 kg	>20 kg
Zinc	0.1 mg/kg	4 mg
Copper	0.02 mg/kg	1 mg
Manganese	0.002 mg/kg	0.8 mg
Chromium	0.14–0.2 μg/kg	10 μg

Intravenous vitamin and mineral requirements adapted from Kerner, J.A. (ed.): Manual of Pediatric Parenteral Nutrition. John Wiley and Sons, New York, 1983, pp. 148, 169.

Other Nutrients

The precise amounts of other parenterally delivered nutrients required by premature infants for optimal growth are unknown. General guidelines appear in Table 8–8. Some specifics of mineral requirements are discussed subsequently.

Enteral Feeding

The major challenge in the enteral feeding of premature infants is to provide nutrients needed for growth despite immaturities of digestion and absorption (Table 8–9). Premature infants have decreased gastrointestinal motility and their intestinal mucosa is very sensitive to injury, as with necro-

**Table 8-9. DEVELOPMENTAL FEEDING PROBLEMS
IN PREMATURE INFANTS**

A. Uncoordinated suck and swallow if < 32–34 wk gestation
B. Decreased gastrointestinal motility
C. Intestinal mucosa sensitive to injury (e.g., necrotizing enterocolitis)
D. Protein digestion and absorption relatively intact
E. Lipid
   1. Digestion limited by decreased pancreatic lipase
   2. Absorption limited by contracted bile salt pool
F. Carbohydrate
   1. Digestion limited by:
      a. Decreased pancreatic and salivary lipase activity
      b. Late acquisition of brush border lactase
   2. Digestion aided by brush border glucoamylase activity (greater than that of adults)
   3. Absorption is intact

tizing enterocolitis (NEC). Protein digestion and absorption are relatively intact, but fat and carbohydrate digestion and absorption are diminished compared with those of the term infant. Fat digestion is limited by the decreased activity of pancreatic lipase, and fat absorption is hindered due to the lower concentration of bile salts. Medium chain triglyceride (MCT) oil may be used as a fat source to circumvent these deficiencies. Carbohydrate absorption is intact, but its digestion is limited by decreased pancreatic and salivary amylase activity and the late acquisition of lactase activity. Brush border glucoamylase activity may be present at greater than adult levels. For these reasons, lactose is supplemented with glucose or glucose polymers for premature infants.

Gavage Feedings

Prior to 32 to 34 weeks' gestation, sucking and swallowing reflexes are not coordinated; therefore, young premature infants will require gavage feedings (that is, passive delivery of food to the gastrointestinal tract, usually by an orogastric tube). These are usually started in small amounts at less than full strength. Volume and concentration are slowly increased while monitoring for increased gastric residuals and blood and/or reducing substances in the stool. These tests are used as a screen for the development of NEC. Among the many factors contributing to the occurrence of NEC is hyperosmolarity; therefore, premature infants should never be fed a formula that is hyperosmolar to serum.

Table 8-10. FORMULAS FOR PREMATURE INFANTS

Brand Name	Protein	Carbohydrate (mg/100 ml)	Lipid	kcal/oz kcal/cc
Enfamil Premature	Whey:casein = 60:40	Lactose:glucose polymers = 40:40	MCT = 40% Soy = 40% Coconut = 20%	24/0.80
Similac Special Care	Whey:casein = 60:40	Lactose:glucose polymers = 50:50	MCT = 50% Soy = 30% Coconut = 20%	24/0.80
"Preemie" SMA	Whey:casein = 60:40	Lactose:glucose polymers = 50:50	MCT = 13% Coconut, oleic, oleo, and soy oils = 87%	24/0.80

Brand Name	Na	K	Ca	PO₄	Fe
Enfamil Premature	32	90	95	48	0.2
Similac Special Care	41	113	146	73	0.3
"Preemie" SMA	32	75	75	40	0.3

Composition of Available Formulas

Premature infants require at least 100 to 120 kcal per kg per day enterally for growth. There are three major premature infant formulas available. These have 24 kcal per ounce at full strength, a 60:40 whey-to-casein ratio, a mixture of long chain and medium chain triglycerides, and both lactose and glucose polymers as a carbohydrate source (Table 8-10).

Mineral and Vitamin Requirements

Premature infants have a greater mineral requirement than term infants since most of the minerals are incorporated into the fetus during the third trimester of pregnancy. Rickets of prematurity, seen during the second postnatal month, seems to be due to inadequate intake of calcium and phosphorus rather than to inadequate vitamin D. Premature infants also are deficient in iron. It is more difficult to measure zinc and copper status, but it is likely that relatively high amounts of these trace elements also are needed. The content of premature formulas reflects these needs to varying degrees.

The issue of iron supplementation is linked to that of vitamin E supplementation. Some infants are found to be vitamin E deficient, a condition manifested clinically as hemolytic anemia, thrombocytosis, and edema. Vitamin E is an antioxidant and stabilizes red blood cell (RBC) membranes (see Chapter 2). Iron is an oxidizing agent and will therefore aggravate the hemolysis seen in vitamin E–deficient babies. These babies should receive vitamin E first, then iron (for example, vitamin E 25 IU during hospitalization, and $FeSO_4$ 2 mg per kg per day at discharge). Vitamin E deficiency may contribute to pulmonary oxygen toxicity. Studies have not demonstrated that vitamin E prevents bronchopulmonary dysplasia. There may be some benefit of vitamin E prophylaxis in the prevention of retrolental fibroplasia. Recent reports, however, have linked pharmacologic levels of vitamin E to NEC and sepsis in premature infants. The use of an intravenous preparation of vitamin E (E-ferol) was linked to neonatal deaths, and this preparation has been withdrawn from the market.

Preterm and Term Human Milk

It is clear that pooled, term human milk is insufficient to support normal growth in very low birth weight infants. However, milk from mothers who have delivered prematurely differs from term milk in the initial few weeks after delivery. Preterm milk contains more sodium and protein and seems adequate to support weight gain and to maintain micronutrient status according to balance studies; however, it does not contain enough calcium, phosphorus, or magnesium to achieve intrauterine accretion rates or to prevent radiologic or biochemical evidence of rickets. Certainly the immunologic benefits of human milk cannot be duplicated by formula. Mineral supplements are now available commercially to be added to the breast milk of mothers of premature infants when the choice is made to pump the milk.

NUTRITION IN DISEASE STATES

Use of Parenteral Nutrition

Parenteral nutrition (see Chapter 12) can be instituted when the gastrointestinal tract cannot be used due to inflammation, surgical disorders, dysmotility, or major organ failure. The use of parenteral nutrition in premature infants is discussed earlier.

Fluid Volume

Fluid volume must be assessed on an individual basis since some factors will increase fluid needs (for example, fever, vomiting, diarrhea) and some will decrease them (for example, cardiac and renal failure). A rule of thumb in calculating average maintenance requirements follows:

Body Weight	Fluid Volume
0–10 kg	100 cc/kg/day
10–20 kg	50 cc/kg/day
> 20 kg	20 cc/kg/day

Formulations

Infants at least age 1 year and older children can begin parenteral nutrition with a solution of 5 percent dextrose and have this increased by 2.5 percent per day to a maximum of 35 percent dextrose, similar to the percentage used for adults (see Chapter 12). During this time serum and urine glucose should be measured, and sudden glucose intolerance should prompt a workup for sepsis. If a central venous catheter malfunctions, a peripheral infusion of 10 percent dextrose should be instituted to prevent rebound hypoglycemia. Protein can be initiated as a 1 percent solution of amino acids and increased by 0.5 percent per day to a maximum of 5 percent (final concentration). Recently an amino acid formulation specific for infants and young children has become available (Table 8–11; compare with Table 12–4). The nitrogen-to-calorie ratio should be 1:150 to 1:200 to ensure optimal utilization of protein. Intravenous fat can be used to supply added calories but should not contribute greater than 60 percent of the total calories. Term infants and children can receive 1 g per kg per day of IV fat initially, and the amount may be increased by 0.5 g per kg per day. Infants may receive up to 4 g per kg per day, but other patients should not receive more than 2 g per kg per day. Essential fatty acid deficiency can be prevented with 0.5 to 1.0 g per kg per day of the usual IV fat. Electrolytes, minerals, and vitamins are added according to individual needs. Guidelines appear in Tables 8–8 and 8–12, and Figure 8–2 provides a sample order sheet.

Table 8–11. COMPOSITION OF TrophAmine (McGaw)

Amino Acids, % of Total			
Essentials		*Nonessentials*	
Isoleucine	8.2	Alanine	5.3
Leucine	14.0	Arginine	12.2
Valine	7.8	Histidine*	4.8
Lysine	8.2	Proline	6.8
Methionine	3.3	Serine	3.8
Phenylalanine	4.8	Tyrosine*	2.3
Threonine	4.2	Taurine[†]	0.25
Tryptophan	2.0	Cysteine	<0.3
		Aspartic acid	3.2
		Glutamic acid	5.0
Available concentration, %	6		
Aliquot size, ml	500, 250		

*Considered essential for infants and young children.
[†]Possibly essential for the neonate.

Table 8-12. INTRAVENOUS ELECTROLYTE
RECOMMENDATIONS FOR INFANTS AND CHILDREN

Mineral	Daily Amount
Sodium	2–4 mEq/kg
Potassium	2–3 mEq/kg
Chloride	2–3 mEq/kg
Magnesium	0.25–0.5 mEq/kg
Calcium gluconate	100–500 mg/kg
Phosphorus	1–2 mmol/kg

Adapted from Kerner, J.A., Jr. (ed.): Manual of Pediatric Parenteral Nutrition. John Wiley and Sons, New York, 1983, p. 130.

Complications

The technical aspects and complications of parenteral nutrition are well described (see Chapter 12). The most serious chronic metabolic complication of parenteral nutrition is liver disease. Adults may develop a reversible steatosis; however, infants develop cholestasis, which may go on to chronic fibrosis. The features on liver biopsy are (1) bile stasis in canaliculi, hepatocytes, and Kupffer cells; (2) portal inflammation; (3) portal fibrosis; and (4) bile duct proliferation. Histopathologic abnormalities persist longer than serum transaminase, ammonia, and coagulation abnormalities after parenteral nutrition is discontinued. The hepatic disease can resolve but will persist and become severe if parenteral nutrition is continued.

The etiology of the hepatic disease is unclear, although every component of parenteral nutrition has been implicated. The patients at highest risk are premature infants. In some studies a higher incidence was found in patients who had gastrointestinal surgery. The longer the duration of total parenteral nutrition, the more likely the patient is to have hepatic complications.

Other chronic metabolic complications of long-term parenteral nutrition have included cholelithiasis, bone pain, and eosinophilia. Serum transaminases, alkaline phosphatase, ammonia, and bilirubin should be monitored on a regular basis along with complete blood count, serum electrolytes, total protein, albumin, triglycerides, cholesterol, and vitamin and trace mineral status as needed.

Hospital and Home Use

Parenteral nutrition may be used in the hospital or may be managed by the family at home with frequent outpatient monitoring. Parents or older children can be taught line care and simple monitoring.

PEDIATRIC PARENTERAL NUTRITION ORDER SHEET

BIRTH WT _____ KG   FLUID ROUTE:
AGE _____ CURRENT WT _____ KG PN FLUID # _____ CENTRAL ☐ PERIPHERAL ☐   START DATE _____   START TIME _____

DAILY FLUID REQUIREMENTS: _____ ml/kg/day or a total of _____ ml/day.   Supplied as: _____ ml of PN FLUIDS
                                                                                              _____ ml of LIPIDS
                                                                                              _____ ml of OTHER

PROTEIN REQUIREMENT:☆ (Check One)   FINAL DEXTROSE CONCENTRATION: (Check One)

☐ 0.5Gm/kg/day   ☐ 5%   Note: Dextrose supplies 3.4KCal
☐ 1.0Gm/kg/day   ☐ 10%   per Gram.
☐ 1.5Gm/kg/day   ☐ 12.5%
☐ 2.0Gm/kg/day   ☐ 15%
☐ 2.5Gm/kg/day   ☐ 17.5%
☐ 3.0Gm/kg/day   ☐ 20%

_____
Pharmacy Use Only
PROTEIN PERCENT CALCULATION:

$$\frac{Gms \times 100}{Total\ Grams/Day} \div \frac{ml}{Total\ PN\ Volume/Day} = \frac{\%}{Final\ Protein\ \%}$$

☐ 25%
☐ 30%

LABEL AS FOLLOWS/24 HOURS OF FLUID | CALCULATIONS/PREP/48HRS OF FLUID

(Protein) _____ %   _____ ml of _____

ADDITIVES: (Order as additive dose per kg per day ONLY.)   Dextrose _____ % _____ ml   _____ ml of D- -W

	STANDARD EXCEPT		
☐ STANDARD ADDITIVES ONLY	☐ ADDITIVES INDICATED BELOW	with these additives:	_____ ml of Sterile Water
Sodium Chloride 3mEq	_____ mEq NaCl	Sodium Chloride _____ mEq	_____ ml of _____ NaCl
Potassium Chloride 1mEq	_____ mEq KCl	Potassium Chloride _____ mEq	_____ ml of _____ KCl
Potassium (as Phosphate)☆ 1mEq	_____ mEq K Phos	Potassium (as Phosphate) _____ mEq	_____ ml of _____ K Phos
Heparin Sodium 1U/1ml	_____ U Heparin	Heparin Sodium _____ Units	_____ ml of _____ Heparin
Magnesium Sulfate 0.25mEq	_____ mEq Mag	Magnesium Sulfate _____ mEq	_____ ml of _____ Mag
Calcium Gluconate☆ 100mg-200mg	_____ mg Ca Glu	Calcium Gluconate _____ mg	_____ ml of _____ CaG
Pediatric Trace Element Package-A☆ 0.47ml (or)	_____ ml Ped TEP-A	Pediatric Trace Element Package-A _____ ml	_____ ml of Ped TEP-A
Pediatric Trace Element Package-B☆ 0.2ml	_____ ml Ped TEP-B	Pediatric Trace Element Package-B _____ ml	_____ ml of Ped TEP-B
H.V.I. Pediatric 1ml	_____ ml MVI Ped	M.V.I. Pediatric _____ ml	_____ ml of MVI Ped
	Other: _____	_____	_____ of _____
☆See reverse side for contents and additional information.	Other: _____	_____	_____ of _____
	Other: _____	_____	_____ of _____

TOTAL VOLUME: _____ ml ÷ 48 hrs =

FLOW RATE: _____ ml/hr

IV FAT EMULSION: ☐ 10% (1.1KCal/ml) ☐ 20% (2KCal/ml)   Desired Dose: _____ Gm/Kg/Day.

_____ ml, over _____ hours, at _____ ml/hour. Start (Date/Time): _____
(Dispensed in 60ml syringes as Intralipid or Liposyn.)

_____ Physician's Signature   _____ Date/Time   _____ Nurse's Signature   _____ Time Needed

_____
For Pharmacy Use Only

Calculations By: _____   Date & Time Prepared: _____   Prepared By: _____
Base Solution: _____ R.Ph.   Additives: _____ R.Ph.   Label: _____ R.Ph.   Lipids: _____ R.Ph.

PS 1632 8/84

Figure 8–2. Example of pediatric parenteral nutrition order sheet.

Use of Enteral Nutrition

The enteral route should be used for feeding whenever possible (see Chapter 11). Although parenteral nutrition can deliver the energy and nutrients needed for growth and metabolism, recent studies have shown that the structure and function of the gastrointestinal tract can be improved by intraluminal nutrition. Because parenteral nutrition bypasses digestion and absorption, these factors must be evaluated before choosing a defined diet.

Formulations

In some disease states protein hydrolysates may be used rather than intact proteins (for example, protracted diarrhea with mucosal injury, cystic fibrosis). If steatorrhea is a prominent symptom, MCT may be used (for example, liver disease, inflammatory bowel disease with terminal ileal dysfunction). Carbohydrates should be chosen based on the patient's needs (for example, lactose-free in children with mucosal injury, lactose- and sucrose-free if the injury is severe). If modular components are added, the nitrogen-to-calorie ratio should be assessed. A 1:150 nitrogen-to-calorie ratio has been reported to be more than adequate for recovery and growth of malnourished infants. Modular elements may cause hyperosmolarity.

A variety of products are available to fit each patient's needs. Infant formulas and modular components are listed in Table 8–13. Formulas for older children are similar to those used in adults (see Chapter 11).

Nasoenteral Tubes

Defined feedings can be delivered via nasogastric or nasojejunal tubes. Number 5 or 7 French silastic feeding tubes can be left in place for several weeks without problems. Nasoenteral tubes have caused airway obstruction in very small infants. Babies have had necrosis of the nasal alae from tubes that were taped in such a way as to exert pressure on the nose. If an infant inadvertently pulls out a tube, it can be replaced. The stylet should never be inserted into a tube in situ. Parents can learn to place nasogastric tubes in infants requiring home feedings; older children can learn self-intubation.

Gastrostomy and Jujunostomy Tubes

Gastrostomy or jejunostomy tubes may be inserted if prolonged feedings are necessary, as in patients with severe neurologic damage, or if the upper alimentary tract must be bypassed, as in patients with esophageal burns or severe gastroesophageal reflux.

Table 8–13. SPECIALIZED INFANT FORMULAS
AND MODULAR COMPONENTS*

Brand Name	Protein†	Carbohydrate	Lipid	kcal/oz kcal/cc
Pregestimil	Casein hydrolysate	Corn syrup solids, modified tapioca	LCT:MCT = 60:40	20/0.67
Nutramigen	Casein hydrolysate	Sucrose modified tapioca	Corn oil	20/0.67
Portagen	Sodium caseinate	Corn syrup solids, sucrose, lactose	LCT:MCT = 14:86	20/0.67
RCF	Soy	(Must be added)	Coconut, soy oil	(Varies with added CHO)
Polycose liquid	—	Glucose polymers	—	60/2.0
MCT oil	—	—	MCT from coconut	228/7.6

Brand Name	Na	K	Ca	PO₄	Fe
	(mg/100 ml)				
Pregestimil	31	73	63	42	1.3
Nutramigen	31	68	63	49	1.3
Portagen	31	83	63	47	1.3
RCF	30	71	70	50	0.15
Polycose liquid	2.5 mEq/100 ml	0.5 mEq/100 ml	30	6	—
MCT oil	—	—	—	—	—

*Specialized formulas for metabolic errors are not listed.
†All protein-containing products have added taurine.

Complications of Tubes

Gastric tubes of any type may obstruct the pylorus. Jejunal tubes can cause bacterial overgrowth of the small intestine or gastrointestinal perforation.

Increasing Volume and Strength

In general, continuous feedings are better tolerated than bolus feedings. The smaller and younger the patient, the more caution must be employed in advancing feedings. A ballpark figure for initiating feedings is 1 to 2 cc per kg per hour. Volume can be increased every 12 to 24 hours as tolerated. The initial formula is usually dilute. When the patient is tolerating approximately one third to one half of the desired total volume, the strength can be increased gradually. Hypertonic feedings should not be used for neonates and must be used with caution in older children. Never increase the volume and strength simultaneously.

Monitoring

Abdominal girth, gastric residuals, frequency of emesis and stool, stool consistency, blood, reducing substances, and pH are monitored for signs of intolerance; urine specific gravity values also are followed. The position of the tube tip and entry site should be checked frequently.

Oral Stimulation

Infants who are tube fed should be allowed to suck on pacifiers. Nonnutritive sucking has been shown to increase the tolerance of feedings, shorten the course of tube feedings, and improve the transition to nipple feedings. Older infants should be given oral stimulation to prevent later refusal of solids.

DISEASE STATES

Gastrointestinal Disease

Gastrointestinal disorders (see Chapter 21) may cause malnutrition in children not only because of the anorexia they produce but also because of malabsorption of nutrients. Five disease states are discussed here.

Infant Diarrhea

Acute. Acute diarrhea may be caused by certain strains of E. coli, rotavirus, or other viruses, as well as shigella, salmonella, Campylobacter, Yersinia, or Giardia. Usual outpatient management of acute uncomplicated diarrhea includes clear liquids for 12 to 24 hours followed by reintroduction of dilute formula, progressing to full-strength formula. Fruit juices are hyperosmolar and therefore may prolong diarrhea if they are not diluted (Table 8–14). Commercial products are available that are isosmolar and contain appropriate amounts of electrolytes (Pedialyte, Infalyte, Resol, Lytren). Prolonged hypocaloric intake should be discouraged. Some authors have argued that there is no need to change a child's usual diet in the face of uncomplicated acute diarrhea.

Table 8-14. OSMOLALITY OF FRUIT JUICES AND
FRUIT-FLAVORED DRINK

Product	Oxmolality (mOsm/kg H$_2$O)
Apple juice	654–734
Apple drink	699–816
Cranapple drink	1106–1212
Cranberry juice	888
Fruit punch	647–727
Grape drink	266–794
Grape juice	1167–1190
Orange drink	343–515
Orange juice	553–710

From Wendland, B.E., et al.: Oral fluid therapy: sodium and potassium content and osmolality of some commercial "clear" soups, juices and beverages. Can Med Assoc J 121:564, 1979.

Diarrhea may cause transient lactase deficiency. Many practitioners will use soy-based formulas (because they are lactose free) for a period of time following a diarrheal disease, although some studies have challenged the efficacy of this dietary manipulation. Breast-fed babies may be maintained on breast milk unless the diarrhea is severe or prolonged. Older children may be put on a BRAT diet (bananas, rice, apples, toast). These foods tend to be binding. In general, a high starch, low fat diet may be used. There are few controlled clinical trials to support the standard dietary management of acute diarrhea; however, empirical experience supports use of this therapy for *brief* periods of time in uncomplicated cases. The BRAT diet will not supply the child with the RDA of many nutrients and is not adequate for normal growth.

Chronic. Chronic infant diarrhea is a major public health problem worldwide. Severe diarrhea causes malnutrition, and malnutrition in turn prolongs diarrhea. Protracted diarrhea of infancy, which results in intestinal mucosal injury, is the most severe form of chronic diarrhea. It may result from cow's or soy milk protein–induced enteropathy, necrotizing enterocolitis, or other mucosal insults. At one time, most children with this disorder died of malnutrition. Currently, severe diarrhea is treated with bowel rest and total parenteral nutrition. Continuous elemental enteral feedings are then added slowly. An infant formula containing hydrolyzed casein as its protein, glucose and glucose polymers as carbohydrate, and primarily MCT oil as fat serves this purpose (see Table 8–13). Slow elemental feedings may stimulate mucosal renewal. Feedings should not be hyperosmolar, since this may aggravate or induce intestinal injury. Most children will require excess calories to recover, and intakes greater than 140 kcal per kg per day may be necessary in some cases.

Inflammatory Bowel Disease

Noninfectious inflammatory bowel disease can be divided into two categories: ulcerative colitis (UC) and Crohn's disease. In UC, inflammation is usually limited to the mucosa of the large intestine and terminal ileum. In Crohn's disease, the inflammation is transmural, and granulomas may be seen. Any part of the gastrointestinal tract may be affected (see Chapter 21).

Poor nutrition in patients with inflammatory bowel disease (IBD) may express itself in several ways. Children may have anemia due to (1) chronic gastrointestinal blood loss, (2) sulfasalazine-induced folate malabsorption, or (3) terminal ileal disease interfering with vitamin B_{12} absorption. These children may be underweight with poor energy intake due to disease-induced anorexia or to self-imposed dietary restrictions aimed to decrease diarrhea. Patients with IBD are no more likely to be lactase deficient than the general population. Many of these patients are Jewish, and lactase deficiency is common in that ethnic group; therefore, formal breath hydrogen testing may be indicated in these patients (see Chapter 20). Lactose-intolerant patients with IBD may improve when milk is removed from their diets. Mucosal injury, bacterial overgrowth in patients without an ileocecal valve, or a decreased bile salt pool in patients whose bile salt reabsorption is diminished due to terminal ileal dysfunction or absence may lead to steatorrhea and consequent loss of calories.

Up to 30 percent of patients with Crohn's disease and 10 percent of patients with ulcerative colitis may have short stature that is unrelated to steroid use or endocrine abnormalities. Growth failure in prepubertal patients is responsive to increased calories. Calories can be provided to outpatients via continuous nocturnal enteral feedings by nasogastric infusion. Although this technique is relatively new, it has been used successfully. In addition to experiencing improvement in their growth, some patients gain a sense of well-being and require fewer medications while receiving enteral feedings.

Total parenteral nutrition has been used to treat acute exacerbations of IBD. Bowel rest and provision of adequate calories may help control acute flares of disease activity and have resulted in improved surgical outcome.

Celiac Disease

Celiac disease is a lifelong intolerance to the gliadin fraction of gluten. Gluten is found in wheat, barley, oats, rye, and malt. Gliadin induces gastrointestinal mucosal injury, probably through an immune complex–mediated process. In patients with celiac disease, gliadin may cause growth failure without the classic signs of bulky, foul-smelling diarrhea, abdominal distention, and irritability. The diagnosis of celiac disease requires three small bowel biopsies: one showing intestinal injury while the patient is on a general diet, one showing normal mucosa while on a gluten-free diet, and one showing injury when gluten is reintroduced. These strict diagnostic criteria are necessary, since a gluten-free diet is difficult to adhere to and must be maintained throughout the patient's life.

Cystic Fibrosis

Cystic fibrosis (CF) is an inherited disease of unknown etiology. There is generalized dysfunction of exocrine glands. Patients may have chronic pulmonary disease or pancreatic insufficiency or both. CF may present in any number of ways from infancy through childhood. Eighty percent of children with CF have pancreatic insufficiency. Despite pancreatic enzyme replacement, steatorrhea persists. Along with the anorexia of chronic disease and the increased caloric needs of children with chronic respiratory distress and frequent infections, this steatorrhea leads to chronic energy deficiency. Textbooks often describe patients with CF as having voracious appetites. This may be true for infants, but older patients with CF usually have anorexia and depressed intakes.

Infants with CF should be given either breast milk plus MCT oil supplements or MCT-containing formulas (see Table 8–13). In older children, energy intake can be increased by encouraging frequent snacks. All food must be preceded by oral pancreatic enzymes. Diet supplements such as glucose polymers and MCT oil can be incorporated into recipes. (MCT oil does not need to be hydrolyzed by pancreatic lipase and is therefore a better-absorbed form of fat than long chain triglycerides [see Chapter 21].)

Despite reduced levels of pancreatic proteolytic enzymes, levels of serum proteins are often normal in patients with CF. Fat malabsorption can result in deficiencies of fat-soluble vitamins. Patients with cystic fibrosis are given supplements of vitamins A, E, and sometimes K. It is possible that deficiencies of vitamins A and E may contribute to the pathology of this disease. In experimental animals, vitamin A deficiency has resulted in flattening of ciliated cells in the lung, squamous metaplasia, and bronchiectasis. Vitamin E and linoleic acid are involved in prostaglandin metabolism (see Chapter 1). Prostaglandin $F_{2\alpha}$ ($PGF_{2\alpha}$) levels are elevated by deficiencies of these two nutrients. $PGF_{2\alpha}$ causes bronchoconstriction and pulmonary vasoconstriction. Vitamin D supplements are not usually prescribed. Clinical rickets is rarely seen except in those patients with liver involvement. Early and consistent vitamin supplementation may alter the course of CF. Water-miscible analogues of fat-soluble vitamins will be better absorbed.

Chronic Liver Disease

Bile acids are necessary for micelle formation, the mechanism through which long chain fats are transported across the intestinal mucosa. Inadequate secretion of bile acids, as seen in chronic cholestatic liver disease, leads to steatorrhea and consequent energy deficit and deficiency of fat-soluble vitamins (see Chapter 22). In infants, use of special MCT-containing formulas will increase net caloric balance. MCT oil can be used to supplement breast milk feedings, and can also be used in recipes for older children.

Deficiencies of vitamins D and E are more significant clinically than vitamin A deficiency. Some children with chronic liver disease manifest a neurologic syndrome consisting of areflexia and posterior column signs (loss of vibration sense, dysmetria, weakness). This syndrome can be reversed with parenteral vitamin E and may be prevented by supplementing patients starting early in the course of their disease.

The rickets of liver disease is usually refractory to normal doses of vitamin D; it is caused primarily by malabsorption of vitamin D and partly by faulty hepatic hydroxylation of vitamin D precursors (see Chapter 14). Use of phenobarbital to stimulate bile flow in patients with cholestasis may cause increased production of inactive vitamin D metabolites.

A coagulopathy due to decreased hepatic synthesis of clotting factors and vitamin K malabsorption results as liver failure progresses. The vitamin K malabsorption can be demonstrated early in the course of the disease and is manifested as a prolonged prothrombin time correctable with parenteral vitamin K.

All children with chronic liver disease should begin supplements of water-miscible analogues of fat-soluble vitamins early in the course of their disease.

Chronic Renal Disease

Children with chronic renal failure are subject to nutrient excesses and deficiencies as a result of altered kidney function (see Chapter 23). Uremia induces anorexia, and this exacerbates the deficiencies. There are three major imbalances, involving fluids and electrolytes, protein-energy, and calcium–phosphorus–vitamin D.

Fluid and Electrolyte Imbalance

Problems with fluids and electrolytes vary depending on the specific renal tubular involvement of the disease. The majority of patients with chronic renal disease will have some edema and will be overloaded with sodium. Laboratory evaluation will demonstrate increased BUN creatinine, increased serum phosphate, and metabolic alkalosis. Hyperkalemia occurs only when renal function is severely impaired. Because of their smaller size, children have a lower tolerance for extremes of sodium and potassium intake than adults.

Protein-Energy Imbalance

Almost all patients with chronic renal disease have inadequate caloric intake. This is due to uremia-induced anorexia, lack of interest in a restricted diet, depression, altered taste perception, and/or other factors. Adequate calories are needed to maintain body energy stores and positive nitrogen balance. These patients retain nonprotein nitrogen (particularly urea), but nitrogen as a body protein is depleted, and muscle wasting is common. A high calorie, moderately protein-restricted diet is recommended. Calories can be added by use of carbohydrate polymers (Polycose, Controlyte, Caloreen, and others) or by emphasizing use of gravies, cream, mayonnaise, butter, syrups, jam, and frosting. Protein of high biologic value (high essential-to-nonessential amino acid ratio) such as egg should be used (see Chapter 1). Use of oral essential amino acid or ketoanalogue amino acids as protein sources in children with renal disease has not been validated in practice.

Calcium-Phosphorus-Vitamin D Imbalance

Children develop renal osteodystrophy for several reasons. Their kidneys are unable to hydroxylate provitamin D to its active 1,25 form. Calcium absorption from the gut is diminished, but phosphorus absorption is normal. The phosphate load becomes exaggerated as glomerular filtration rate (GFR) declines. As phosphate rises and calcium decreases, parathormone (PTH) is stimulated. PTH causes bone resorption in a compensatory attempt to normalize serum calcium.

Another cause of bone resorption is the acidosis that accompanies renal failure. Calcium is lost from bone as it acts to buffer acid. Use of steroids will aggravate this osteodystrophy.

Bone demineralization and disturbed osteoid formation can be controlled and may be prevented by use of calcium supplements, a moderate restriction of dietary phosphorus, use of phosphorus-binding gels, and vitamin D. Recently, synthetic 1,25(OH) vitamin D_3 has been used to increase the usually dismal growth rate seen in children with chronic renal disease (see Chapters 14 and 23).

Supplementation With Other Vitamins and Minerals

In addition to supplementing patients with renal disease with calcium and vitamin D, other vitamins and minerals are required. Status of vitamins A, B_6, C, and folate is particularly tenuous; supplements are recommended because dietary restrictions may limit intake of foods rich in these nutrients.

In general, dietary restrictions become stricter as renal failure progresses. Use of dialysis may ease some of the restrictions (for example, PO_4, K) but may exacerbate other deficiencies (such as calories, vitamins, trace minerals). It is postulated that early restriction of phosphorus and dietary protein may lessen renal failure, but this has yet to be proved.

Cancer

Malnutrition in patients with cancer may result from tumor-host interaction, effects of anticancer therapy, and psychologic factors (see Chapter 24). The tumor may cause altered sense of taste or may compete with normal tissues for ingested nutrients.

- Certain tumors can cause malabsorption by increasing gut motility, by inducing a protein-losing enteropathy, or by anatomic destruction.
- Chemotherapeutic agents may prevent a child from eating. For example, methotrexate can cause ulcerative stomatitis, and vincristine can induce a peripheral neuropathy that may make mouth movement too painful to permit eating. Most chemotherapeutic agents cause anorexia, nausea, and vomiting.
- Radiation to the abdomen may cause enteritis and malabsorption.
- Anorexia is a common sign of psychologic depression.
- "Anticipatory emesis" is frequently seen in teenagers who may begin to vomit even before their chemotherapy is begun.

These factors often prompt physicians to begin nutritional augmentation. When nausea and vomiting are predominant factors, the parenteral route may be used. Some children have indwelling central lines (Broviac or Hickman catheters) for venous access, since this can become a major problem in children receiving chemotherapy. These lines may be used in a select group of patients for in-hospital or at-home parenteral nutrition. There is an increased risk of infection in these children when lines are broken and used for multiple purposes (such as blood drawing, medications, and nutrition). This is in addition to any therapy-induced immunosuppression which puts them at special risk for sepsis. **Total parenteral nutrition is not recommended for all patients with tumors.**

When diarrhea is a problem unassociated with vomiting, as with postradiation enteritis, elemental enteral feedings may be used. When anorexia is a problem, a dietary history may reveal types of foods that are well accepted or times of day when foods are taken more easily. Prepared, balanced supplements may be used. Formal nutritional counseling may give parents positive ways they can intervene in improving their child's intake.

Neurologic Disease

The quality of life for patients with meningomyelocele may be improved by controlling the obesity that is prevalent in these patients. Reaching ideal body weight can decrease the incidence of fractures and will facilitate ambulation. Fluids should be encouraged to minimize kidney infections. Their use, plus adding fiber to the diet, will help prevent constipation. These principles hold true for other patients who are not ambulatory due to other causes (such as spasticity with contractures or hypotonia).

Patients with impaired sucking and swallowing abilities may need nonoral routes of enteral feeding, including gastrostomy or nasogastric tube placement. Careful attention must be paid to the energy and fluid needs of these patients, whose intake is not self-regulated. If aspiration is not a hazard, some oral feeding will give the child experience with sensations and social interaction. On the other hand, use of nonoral routes to deliver the bulk of nutrients may relieve extreme tension associated with feeding that may have existed when parents tried to force feed a child who was failing to thrive.

Anticonvulsants increase the need for vitamin D, folate, and B vitamins. Suggested dosages for vitamin D supplementation range from 500 to 1200 IU per day. Folate supplementation may precipitate seizures in a minority of patients who are sensitive. In one small group, 5 mg per week of folate brought folate levels to normal and reversed phenytoin-induced gingival hyperplasia. Ideal vitamin supplementation for children on long-term anticonvulsant therapy has yet to be defined.

Congenital Heart Disease

Infants with congenital heart disease are generally term infants of normal weight. Many will suffer from malnutrition and growth failure, especially infants with cyanotic heart disease, although there is no linear correlation of growth with oxygen saturation. Infants with congestive heart failure (due to left-to-right shunting, pulmonary hypertension, and so on) are at high risk for growth failure, although infants with hemodynamically balanced lesions may also be small.

Children with congenital heart disease have an increased basal metabolic rate and require more calories to grow than the average child. Many of these children also will be on fluid restriction. During hospitalization, if these children are provided with parenteral nutrition, 20 percent intravenous fat is extremely useful as a concentrated calorie source. (This should be used with caution in babies with pulmonary hypertension.) Infants can be fed enterally with formulas that contain 24 to 30 kcal per ounce. This can be accomplished by adding less water to concentrated liquid, or by adding modular ingredients (easily absorbed glucose polymers or MCT oil or both). When concentrated formulas are used, the renal solute load is high. These infants are at risk for dehydration if their water losses are increased, such as through vomiting or diarrhea or in hot weather. Low sodium formulas such as SMA, PM 60/40, or Lonalac may be used.

When solids are added to the diet, sugar or oil may be added to increase caloric density. Low sodium foods are emphasized.

Folate and riboflavin deficiency has been reported in children with congenital heart disease. Folate and calcium intake may be below the recommended level in infants who are consuming a limited amount of formula.

Growth failure is most severe in infancy, and older children may show increases in growth, particularly if they undergo surgical repair. Caloric intake should be maintained. A "prudent diet" consisting of low fat foods is not appropriate for a child with congenital heart disease before growth is completed.

Diabetes Mellitus

Diabetes mellitus (see Chapter 17) is the most common endocrine disorder in children. In most cases, there is total inability to secrete insulin. A picture consistent with adult-onset diabetes is seen rarely, usually in obese, black teenage girls.

The management of diabetes involves use of insulin, dietary counseling, and exercise. The goals of treatment are

1. maintenance of normal growth and body weight
2. prevention of hypoglycemia
3. encouraging accurate regulation of serum glucose within a fairly narrow range
4. maintaining serum cholesterol less than 210 mg per dl and overnight serum triglycerides less than 130 mg per dl

These goals must be adjusted within the context of the patient's age, emotional maturity, and family system. For example, school-age children may have erratic eating habits, and tight glucose control may not be possible. Teenagers should be encouraged to use a multiple dose per day insulin regimen, but in practice, compliance in this age group can be extremely difficult to ensure. Family support for the child with a chronic disorder is a critical factor in optimal management.

In the past, patients with diabetes were told to weigh and measure all foods and to avoid all concentrated sweets, but such dietary management currently is changing. The exchange system published by the American Diabetic Association is still the mainstay in dietary teaching of diabetics. The suggested distribution of nutrients is a 50:35:15 ratio of carbohydrate-to-fat-to-protein. At least 60 percent of the carbohydrate should be in the form of complex carbohydrates. Fiber has been purported to cause a slower rise in serum glucose. New research has begun to challenge some previously held truths, and it is no longer held that all complex carbohydrates cause a slow glucose response. When we eat cooked white potatoes, the response of serum glucose is similar to that seen after ingestion of pure glucose. Although rice, bread, corn, and potatoes are all equivalent in the exchange system, they may induce very different glycemic responses, with potatoes causing the most rapid and rice the most gradual (Chapter 18, see p. 427). Food combinations may produce different responses than those of their individual components. The in vivo responses of serum glucose to most foods are unknown. In the meantime, diabetics should be encouraged to eat frequent, small meals in order to avoid wide swings in serum glucose. An alternative is multiple dosing of insulin, but this can be achieved only in some pediatric patients.

Inborn Errors of Metabolism

There are many inborn errors of metabolism, each requiring specialized therapy.

Phenylketonuria

The best studied and best known of these metabolic defects is phenylketonuria (PKU). Children with this disorder have decreased activity of phenylalanine hydroxylase, so that phenylalanine cannot be converted to tyrosine and rises to toxic levels. If patients with this disorder eat complete protein, mental retardation almost always occurs. This can be prevented by feeding the patient a low phenylalanine formula during infancy (such as Lofenalac), then using phenylalanine-free protein hydrolysates plus foods that are either low in protein or protein-free for older children. The principle behind this therapy is to give the patient enough phenylalanine to build body protein, but not enough to reach toxic serum levels. The child with PKU has the same basal requirement for phenylalanine as a normal child. Too severe restriction can result in failure to thrive and negative nitrogen balance. Dietary restrictions must be maintained for at least the first 5 years of life, and perhaps for the patient's entire lifetime.

Other Amino Acidopathies

Other, less well studied amino acidopathies which are responsive to a similar type of diet therapy include maple syrup urine disease, tyrosinemia, homocystinuria, and histidinemia. Specialized formulas exist for each of these conditions.

Vitamin-Responsive Inborn Errors

Some inborn errors are vitamin responsive. There are several disorders of propionic acid metabolism in which enzymes requiring cofactors are defective. In a subgroup of patients with one of these disorders (some, but not all patients with methylmalonic acidemia), daily administration of vitamin B_{12} causes striking improvement. In another disorder of propionic acid metabolism, daily doses of biotin along with diet therapy alleviate symptoms. In these instances, the defective enzymes have low affinity for the cofactor vitamin. High doses of the vitamin compensate for the defect.

Nonessential Nutrients

There are some inborn errors of metabolism that involve nonessential nutrients. Galactosemia and hereditary fructose intolerance are disorders in the metabolism of the respective hexoses and can be treated by totally removing the offending sugar from the diet. This may prevent mental retardation and liver disease.

Glycogen Storage Diseases

In some of the glycogen storage diseases, serum glucose falls due to various defects in glycogenolysis. These patients need to be treated with frequent feedings of glucose-containing formulas. Some must avoid all nonglucose sugars. Overnight enteral drips are being used to prevent hypoglycemia. However, the benefit of continuous overnight feedings awaits further study, since some of these patients may be at higher risk for hypoglycemic episodes when not receiving the feedings.

Familial Hyperlipidemias

Familial hyperlipidemias (see Chapter 18) are somewhat responsive to dietary control. Patients with hypercholesterolemia (type 2a) are treated by following a low cholesterol diet (less than 100 mg per day) and by increasing the ratio of polyunsaturated-to-saturated fats in their diet. Those with hypertriglyceridemia (type 4) are treated with a dietary regimen with less cholesterol restriction and with emphasis on control of obesity (excess calories). Sugars can cause hypertriglyceridemia even in normal individuals, so a carbohydrate-restricted diet low in simple sugars is emphasized. In patients with familial combined hyperlipidemia (type 2b), both cholesterol and triglycerides are elevated. For these individuals, the appropriate diet will improve the serum lipoprotein profile but may not correct it. Drug therapy may be an adjunct, however, to dietary management. A conservative approach to use of lipid-lowering drugs is warranted in growing prepubertal children.

CHRONIC PEDIATRIC NUTRITION PROBLEMS

Food Allergies/Food Intolerance

Food intolerance may be due to many mechanisms, not all of which are allergic, that is, immune mediated (see Chapter 5). Unfortunately, the term "food allergy" has been used to describe a wide range of adverse reactions to food.

It is more difficult to define food allergy than it is to describe inhalant allergy. Like inhalants, foods are complex substances; however, they are altered partially by digestion before they contact the intestinal mucosa. For example, a single milk protein may yield up to 10 new antigens after partial hydrolysis under experimental conditions mimicking the upper gastrointestinal tract. Foods may contribute haptenes that combine with host proteins before exerting immune stimulation. Skin testing to detect IgE antibodies may therefore be nonspecific, and controversy has arisen regarding its clinical value.

True Food Allergy

Reaginic Allergy. True food allergy may be reaginic (IgE-mediated) or nonreaginic. Immediate-onset, IgE-mediated food allergy may manifest itself as urticuria, rhinitis, vomiting, diarrhea, or even acute anaphylaxis. The most common foods that induce these reaginic responses are nuts and legumes, soy, cow's milk, and seafood. Corn and citrus may also cause reactions. Because of the immediate onset of symptoms, these food allergies are the most readily identifiable true allergic reactions.

Nonreaginic Allergy. Nonreaginic (IgG-, IgM-, or T cell–mediated) food allergies are being investigated currently. One example is celiac disease. In contrast to reaginic reactions, symptoms appear a long time after the ingestion of gluten. Although the etiology of celiac disease is not known, current evidence suggests that genetically predisposed patients become sensitized to gliadin, a component of gluten. According to this theory, immune complexes and T cells then cause small intestinal mucosal destruction. Other diseases that may also be caused by this mechanism include cow's milk– and soy-induced intestinal injury, eosinophilic gastroenteropathy, and Heiner's syndrome (iron deficiency, gastrointestinal symptoms, patchy pneumonitis, and occasionally pulmonary hemosiderosis).

Food Intolerance

Nonimmune mechanisms may cause food intolerance that is then interpreted as allergy. Certain pharmacologically active substances may cause neurologic or hypertensive reactions. Coffee, tea, cola, and chocolate contain methylxanthines. Licorice contains glycerrhizinic acid, which has a mineralocorticoid effect. Vasoactive amines are found in cheeses, red wine, tomato, and pineapple. Other chemicals may cause acute asthmatic attacks, such as the azo dye tartrazine and the preservative bisulfite.

Hyperactivity. Do foods cause other intolerances, such as the tension-fatigue syndrome or hyperactivity? The answer is unclear. The best explored case is that of the Feingold diet, which is based on the theory that artificial colors and preservatives and salicylate-containing foods cause hyperactivity. Because of the ubiquitous nature of these substances, adherence to this diet requires a major reorganization of the child's eating habits. This change, as well as the attendant increased attention and change in family dynamics, may be responsible for some of the reported success of this regimen. Diet crossover studies and specific blind challenge studies suggest that, at best, there may be a small group of individuals who are extremely sensitive to food additives; however, there is no objective evidence to support the Feingold theory for the majority of patients.

Megavitamin Supplementation. Of note concerning diet and hyperactivity: Some have suggested that megavitamin supplementation may aid children with this disorder. However, controlled, double-blind studies have not supported this theory. Megavitamin dosing may cause a deterioration in behavior and has been found to elevate transaminases.

Food Elimination Diets

The only absolute way to establish the diagnosis of food allergy or intolerance is through double-blind, placebo-controlled oral food challenge. In practice, this may be difficult to arrange. A sequence of food elimination and reintroduction is the more common method of diagnosis. Individual foods or food families (such as nuts and legumes) are eliminated for 2 to 4 weeks. Parents must be instructed to read the labels of prepared foods, since many products contain hidden potential allergens such as soy, milk solids, or corn syrup. If the child is old enough, he or she should be included in the dietary instruction. Elimination diets must be nutritionally adequate. Alternative supplements may be necessary if the food to be evaluated is the major source of some nutrients in the patient's diet (such as the protein and calcium in milk). If the symptoms recur when the food is reintroduced, other potentially instigating factors should be evaluated (for example, rhinitis may be due to a coincidental viral illness). Symptoms should then disappear when the food is again eliminated.

The biggest danger of elimination diets is lack of follow-up. If no conclusion is drawn as to whether a food actually is responsible for symptoms, the parents will continue to withhold it. If this is done for more than one food, a dangerously limited diet can result. Parents tend to suspect food allergy more often than it can be verified.

Failure to Thrive (FTT)

FTT is a complex biopsychosocial problem. It represents 1 to 5 percent of hospital admissions and up to 10 percent of visits to a rural outpatient clinic. It is usually defined as weight less than the 5th percentile or a deceleration in weight gain so that weight measurements cross two major percentile lines on standard growth grids.

Traditionally, FTT has been divided into organic and nonorganic FTT. It is now clear that this is a false division, and that many cases have both organic and nonorganic components. The work-up of all children with FTT should include evaluation of both physical and psychosocial risk factors (Table 8–15).

Although any disease may cause FTT, few do so without suggestive signs and symptoms. Laboratory tests should be ordered based on positive findings

Table 8–15. RISK FACTORS IN FAILURE TO THRIVE

Organic Risk Factors
  Prenatal
    Toxins
    Infections
    Malnutrition
  Perinatal
    Prematurity
    Difficult delivery
    Prolonged neonatal hospital stay
  Developmental delay
  Difficult temperament
  Positive review of systems (e.g., frequent infections, vomiting, diarrhea, and so on)
  Positive physical findings (e.g., wheezing, heart murmur, major or minor congenital anomalies, and so on)

Psychosocial Risk Factors
  Life stresses
    Financial
    Marital
    Disorganized lifestyle/mobile family
    Personal losses
    Chronic illness
    Social isolation
    Unplanned difficult pregnancy
    Maternal depression
    Child perceived as sick or bad

(From Bithoney, W.G., and Rathburn, J.: Failure to thrive. In Levine, M.D.: Developmental-Behavioral Pediatrics. W.B. Saunders, Philadelphia, 1983, p. 54, with permission.)

in the history and physical examination. A developmental assessment must be included. Delays in social, language, or motor milestones may be a cause or a result of malnutrition. In most studies based on hospitalized children with FTT, the most frequent organic diagnoses were gastrointestinal and neurologic disease (Table 8–16).

Psychosocial causes of FTT may be as simple as inadequate parental education and/or family resources, or include complex situations involving parental substance abuse, chaotic family structure or child neglect, or both.

Recently, researchers have attempted to define the biologic component of FTT by using standard measures of malnutrition, such as triceps skinfolds and mid-arm muscle circumference (see Chapter 3). Although in the majority of cases the FTT will result from family dysfunction or disturbed parent-child interactions, inadequate feeding and resultant malnutrition are the final common denominator. Children do not become well nourished on love alone, and a nutritional prescription should be part of the management of all cases of FTT. It is much easier to order a nutritional prescription and follow weights and anthropometrics than it is to design a psychosocial intervention and follow its success. However, the best treatment of FTT involves evaluation of the child's physical, developmental, nutritional, and psychosocial status, and coordinated therapy in each area of need.

Obesity

Obesity (see Chapter 16) is the most common nutritional disorder in the United States, with perhaps 5 to 30 percent of children and adolescents affected. Obesity commonly runs in families, although true genetic obesity syndromes are rare. No clearcut metabolic abnormality has been found in obese patients. Despite this, in some studies, obese children have been found not to consume excessive calories when compared with age-matched nonobese children. Energy expenditure may be somewhat less in obese children, although it is not clear whether this is a cause or an effect of obesity. However, as overweight persists, children are less likely to participate in peer activities.

Childhood obesity predisposes a patient to adult obesity, although spontaneous remissions do occur. Childhood obesity is highly correlated with childhood hypertension. Although some complications of obesity, such as slipped femoral epiphysis or Blount's disease (tibia vara), do occur early on, the most significant problems for obese children are psychologic. Isolation from peers and low self-esteem may thus begin at an early age.

Therapy

Therapy for obesity must be geared to the patient's age, and in all instances an assessment of the family's eating patterns and nutritional knowledge should be obtained.

Table 8–16. STUDIES OF ULTIMATE DIAGNOSES IN FAILURE TO THRIVE[*]

	English (1978)	Sills (1978)	Hannaway (1970)	Riley et al. (1968)	Shaheen et al. (1968)	Ambuel and Harris (1963)
No. of cases	77[†]	185[†]	100[†]	83[†]	287[‡]	100[‡]
Diagnoses (%)						
Organic	53%	18%	49%	48%	85%	68%
Gastrointestinal[§]	(19)	(8)	(12)	(14)	(15)	(9)
Neurologic	(14)	(4)	(18)	(12)	(18)	(10)
Genitourinary	(4)	(0)	(5)	(5)	(5)	(4)
Endocrine	(4)	(1)	(5)	(1)	(4)	(5)
Cardiac	(7)	(1)	(4)	(2)	(13)	(31)
Other	(5)	(5)	(5)	(13)	(29)	(9)
Environmental	38%	55%	39%	31%	15%	NR[‖]
No cause (or constitutional)	9%	26%	12%	20%	NR[‖]	32%

[*] From Berwick, D.: Nonorganic failure-to-thrive. Pediatr Rev 1:265, 1980, with permission.
[†] Children hospitalized to diagnose FTT.
[‡] Survey of all children in hospital who have FTT.
[§] Includes cystic fibrosis.
[‖] Not reported.

Infants. Although it has been theorized that fat babies become fat adults, this is not consistently true. Infants should not be put on reducing diets, regardless of their weight. Exceptional obesity or that accompanied by short stature, slow mentation, or other unusual physical findings should prompt consideration of the rare genetic causes of obesity (Table 8-17). If the weight is disproportionately greater than that expected for length, the physician should delve deeper into feeding practices. Is food being used as a pacifier or as proof of parental adequacy?

Toddlers and Young Children. Parents become more concerned about their children's obesity in the toddler to preteen years. In some cases, the child's obesity may become the focus of other unrelated family problems. In this age range, reducing diets are inappropriate and should not be used. Instead, emphasis should be placed on improving family patterns of eating and exercise and on nutrition education. Simple dietary manipulation, such as the use of 2 percent fat milk rather than whole milk and decreasing family use of prepackaged, easy-to-eat snacks, may be recommended. Every effort should be made to increase the family's level of activity. This may range from sports participation to measures such as walking upstairs to speak to a family member rather than yelling. The goal for these children is maintenance of body weight as opposed to weight loss.

Adolescents. True reducing diets may be used in teenagers, although young adolescents may lack the cognitive maturity and personal independence to put these into effect. As noted earlier, there is some evidence that weight loss should not be attempted prior to the completion of puberty. Teenagers and their parents should participate in planning their dietary and exercise regimen. Peer groups are useful in this age range. Emphasis must be placed on improving self- and body-image. The goals of therapy should be realistic and attainable, since success reinforces positive attitudes and actions.

Table 8-17. DIFFERENTIAL DIAGNOSIS OF OBESITY

A. Genetic syndromes
   1. Prader-Willi
   2. Laurence-Moon-Bardet-Biedl
   3. Frohlich's
   4. Alstrom's
B. Hormonal causes
   1. Cushing's disease (hyperadrenalcorticism)
   2. Hypothyroidism
   3. Pseudohypoparathyroidism
   4. Stein-Leventhal syndrome
C. Exogenous obesity

Extreme or fad diets are especially contraindicated in teenagers (see Chapter 6). Balanced reducing diets for teens should include enough protein to facilitate the normal adolescent increase in lean body mass and should take into account the greater-than-adult requirements for nutrients such as calcium. Morbidly obese teens should undergo surgery such as gastric stapling only after all medical therapy (including prolonged hospitalization) has failed.

CHAPTER 9

Geriatric Nutrition

Early in the 21st century it is expected that about 20 percent of the United States population will be over 65 years of age and that 11 percent will be over age 75. The proportion of the population represented by people over 65 will grow four times as fast as younger age groups. It is estimated that by 2050, half the United States population will be over age 50 and almost 10 percent of the population will be 80 years old or over (the aged "baby boomers"). Since the human lifespan has reached approximately 115 years, the elderly segment of the population, in numbers and in years of remaining life, has become important enough to warrant special consideration of its specific nutritional needs and problems.

Our present knowledge about the effects of aging on human nutritional needs is scant. However, specific changes in the body's physiology and particular social circumstances influence nutritional status and demand our attention. As the prevalence of illness increases with age, more attention must be paid to the interactions between drugs and nutrients and to the nutritional imbalances resulting from therapeutic diets.

Some lifetime dietary practices have been implicated as major risk factors for the "killer diseases" in the United States, principally cardiovascular disease, hypertension, and cancer. Lifelong nutritional inadequacies can contribute to diseases such as osteopenia (diminished bone mass). The elderly confined to hospitals often have minimal nutritional reserves and are therefore at increased risk of developing malnutrition.

However, lifelong habits cannot be changed quickly or radically, even when change is indicated; dietary recommendations thus must be appropriately designed for older people. Even simple nutrient requirements such as water intake, if not adequately met—especially with summer heat or fever—may prove disastrous. Nutritional counseling of the elderly must take their long-term habits into account and must also emphasize attention to general well-being and proper physical activity.

THEORIES OF AGING

Theories of the mechanism of aging focus on derangements during formation of cellular proteins or on changes in proteins after they are formed:

- accumulation of DNA and RNA errors
- increased cross-linking, especially in collagen (24 to 40 percent of the body's protein)
- formation of highly reactive products of free radical reaction with unsaturated fatty acids in cells, disrupting membranes and freeing enzymes to attack the cell
- reduction of immune function with abnormal cell proliferation and autoimmune reactions

- decline in endocrine function
- accumulation of toxins because of metabolic error
- reduced effectiveness of the nervous system

Nutrition may influence most of the nongenetic factors and perhaps some of the genetic factors as well, thereby playing possible preventive or therapeutic roles in aging.

MANIFESTATIONS OF AGING

The Cardiovascular System

Collagen rigidity and elastin degradation contribute to rigidity of arteries and increased blood pressure (Table 9–1). Systolic blood pressure increases from age 20 to the age of 70 or 80, while diastolic pressure tends to plateau by age 60. In addition, reduced cardiac output results in diminished capacity to adapt to increased physical exertion, so that heart rate and blood pressure are raised more than they would be in younger persons in similar circumstances. (See Chapter 19 for more information on the role of nutrition in cardiovascular disease.)

Table 9–1. MEAN NORMAL VALUES, EFFECTS OF AGE

		Age (years)		
		20–44	*45–59*	*60–74*
Blood pressure (mm Hg),	women	118/75	135/84	151/86
	men	125/81	137/88	145/86

		Age (years)		
		20–49	*50–75*	*76+*
Energy needs (kcal),	women	2100	1800	1600
	men	2900	2400	2050
Plasma cholesterol (mg/dl),	women	182	227	225
	men	192	212	205
Plasma triglycerides (mg/dl),	women	85	120	130
	men	127	143	130

The Respiratory System

Reduction of the lungs' elastic recoil and weakening of the respiratory muscles lead to a decrease in both oxygen diffusion and capacity for coughing and deep breathing.

Bone

Bone loss begins earlier in women than in men (age 35 versus age 50), accelerates at the menopause, and proceeds at a faster rate in women (8 percent versus 3 percent per decade). This demineralization may be lessened in part by increasing calcium intake to 1.5 g per day and also by participating in 1 hour of endurance exercise four times per week (see **Osteopenia**, p. 242).

Skin and Hair

The skin becomes wrinkled, with loss of elasticity, mottled pigmentation, dilatation of the capillaries, senile purpura, warts, skin tags, and cherry angiomata. It blisters more easily and has diminished water-holding capacity, thus becoming drier. The hair grays, with hair loss from scalp and body, while growth of hair on the ear increases. It is doubtful, however, that nutritional factors have a major role in any of these processes.

Memory

Short-term memory may be related to the synthesis of acetylcholine in the brain. While such synthesis can be increased by dietary supplements of choline (in the form of lecithin), there is no evidence to date that ingestion of lecithin improves memory in the elderly or is effective in the prevention or treatment of presenile or senile dementia (Alzheimer's disease). Significant memory loss, however, is not part of the normal aging process.

PHYSIOLOGY AND NUTRITION

Aging significantly affects digestion, absorption, utilization, storage, intracellular transformation, and excretion of nutrients. Body composition undergoes specific changes (Fig. 9–1). Metabolic processes affecting glucose metabolism and blood lipid levels are altered (see Table 9–1).

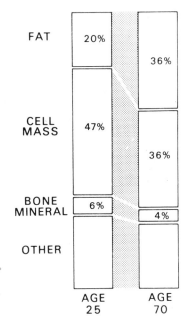

Figure 9-1. Idealized representation of the age-related change in body composition of male subjects. (Young females, age 25, have nearly twice as much body fat as do males but show a smaller increase of fat—and loss of cell mass—with age than do males.) (From Williams, R.H. (ed.): Textbook of Endocrinology, ed. 6. W.B. Saunders, Philadelphia, 1981, p. 1200, with permission.)

Sensory Changes

Numerous physiologic changes with aging may adversely affect food intake. Taste is altered, a change that may result from a decrease in the number of taste buds, among other more complex factors. Sensitivity to sweet taste diminishes, and some individuals report increasing perception of bitter and sour tastes. A 10-fold increase in the threshold for smell may also contribute to reduced enjoyment or appreciation of food. Vision and hearing are frequently impaired, possibly interfering with food shopping, preparation, and eating.

Mechanics of Eating

Fifty percent of Americans lose their teeth by age 65, and ill-fitting dentures usually are worse than none at all. Difficulties in biting and chewing that develop in edentulous patients affect the mechanics of eating. Malocclusion and missing or loose teeth are added problems for many. Individuals with dental problems may avoid such nutrient-rich foods as meats, nuts, raw fruits and vegetables, and hard-crusted bread. (See Chapter 20 for a further discussion of dental disease.)

With increasing age, osteoarthritis may reduce the mobility of the mandibular joint and impair chewing, or may bring problems in cutting food. Because the oral mucosa of the aging person is friable and easily bruised or injured, burning or soreness of the mouth is not uncommon. Oral candidiasis may inhibit proper food intake. A decrease in salivary secretion may make chewing and swallowing difficult and may contribute to increased dental caries and impaired immune response (IgA). There may also be difficulty in swallowing because of esophageal disease; some individuals cannot initiate swallowing because of oropharyngeal disease or neurologic disorders such as stroke or pseudobulbar palsy. Recurrent aspiration may be a problem with meals, liquid supplements, and tube feeding.

Digestion

Motility is decreased in amplitude and synchrony throughout the gastrointestinal tract, possibly contributing to constipation. Decreased secretion of mucus and digestive enzymes—amylase, lipase, trypsin, pepsin—occurs. However, there is no significant impairment in the ability to digest most foods, although some data suggest that protein digestion may be less efficient. There may be a decrease in the bioavailability of polyglutamate forms of folacin derived from foods, but synthetic sources of folic acid are well absorbed. Absorption—especially of calcium—diminishes, but this occurs primarily in very advanced age.

The prevalence of achlorhydria increases as the quantity of gastrointestinal secretions declines. This disorder may interfere with protein digestion and mineral absorption, may contribute to proliferation of bacteria in the intestinal tract, and has been thought to increase the potential for stomach cancer.

Gastrointestinal Tract Disorders

Dietary protein deficiency in the elderly is associated with structural and functional changes of the gastrointestinal tract, as it is in younger patients (see also Chapters 13 and 21). The variety of medications taken by many older persons alters the functions of the gastrointestinal tract. Constipation is a persistent problem, while pancreatic deficiency and jaundice in hepatic failure occur with increasing frequency.

Peptic Ulcer

Half of all patients hospitalized for bleeding peptic ulcer are over age 65, and mortality and the incidence of perforation are increased in the elderly. Chronic ingestion of aspirin increases susceptibility to peptic ulcer formation.

A gastric ulcer in an older person is more likely to be located in the juxtacardiac region, rather than in the antral region. About 10 percent of patients over age 60 with peptic ulcer disease develop gastric outlet obstruction. These patients are not allowed oral intake and must be maintained by intravenous feeding (Chapter 12). Bezoars from undigested plant fiber material may occur following vagotomy or gastrojejunostomy.

Ulcerative Colitis

About 7 percent of cases of ulcerative colitis occur after age 65, with rectosigmoid involvement common. Systemic manifestations are minimal. (See Chapter 21 for management.)

Diverticulosis

About one third of adults over age 60 have diverticulosis—a common cause of rectal bleeding—and one fourth of these individuals develop diverticulitis. An increase in fiber in the diet will bring improvement for 85 percent of these patients.

Constipation

Because constipation is a common complaint among the elderly, up to 50 percent of those over age 70 are regular users (and abusers) of laxatives. Drinking prune juice and a warm beverage on arising can be helpful in relieving this condition without laxative use, which tends to impair motility and perpetuate the disorder. Constipation of recent onset should be investigated.

Gallstones

About one third of people over the age of 70 have gallstones. Those who develop cholecystitis but cannot tolerate surgery may be treated with chenodeoxycholic or ursodeoxycholic acid.

Pancreatitis

The incidence of acute pancreatitis increases in elderly individuals. The disorder is related to gallstones, alcoholism, cancer chemotherapy, use of diuretics, trauma, administration of steroids, and complicating viral diseases.

BODY COMPOSITION AND METABOLISM

Changes in body composition with aging (see Fig. 9–1) include a marked increase in the proportion of fat and decreases in lean body mass and bone mass—changes that are closely associated with the decline in metabolic rate. The major loss of body mass is in muscle, which contributes importantly to both metabolic rate and physical strength. Glycolytic activity of cells increases while oxidative phosphorylation decreases, resulting in decreased basal metabolic rate, especially in the cells of the brain, skeletal muscle, and heart—all major contributors to resting energy expenditure. When combined with decreased activity, these changes generally bring a decline in energy consumption of approximately 5 percent per decade between the ages of 40 and 60 and of 10 percent per decade after age 60 (Fig. 9–2). (See Chapter 1 for further discussion of metabolic rates.)

NUTRITIONAL REQUIREMENTS

Lack of data has prevented agreement as to whether the elderly have increased needs for some nutrients. Dietary guidelines also are difficult to develop because of wide variation in the characteristics of the elderly. There are obvious differences between a person of age 70 who has remained active and healthy and one of the same age who is inactive and diseased. Rates of deterioration of renal, gastrointestinal, cardiovascular, muscular, skeletal, and mental function vary widely. Fifty percent of elderly people have some limitation of activity, however, and more than 15 percent are incapacitated for any major activity.

Caloric Intake

To compensate for diminished energy requirements and to prevent excessive weight gain, caloric intake of the elderly usually needs to be adjusted downward. Such reduction should be less for those who remain active. While food consumption should be adjusted to prevent the patient from being significantly overweight or underweight, there is no justification for creating anxiety about the need for weight loss among the elderly who are only moderately overweight.

In order to meet protein and micronutrient needs but limit caloric intake, elderly persons whose physical activity is reduced must consume foods of increased nutrient density. Good advice is to maintain their intake of nutrient-rich lean meat, fish, eggs, milk, and vegetables (provided they can be chewed and swallowed without difficulty) while curtailing their consumption of calorie-dense purified fats and carbohydrates. Of course, fat and cho-

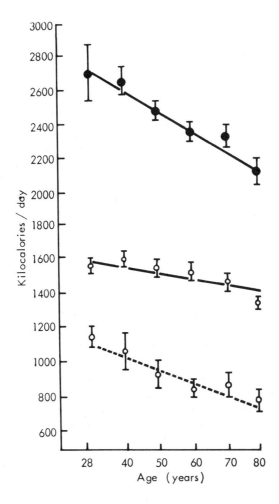

Figure 9-2. In a classic study of energy intake and expenditure in aging, McGandy and colleagues found that average daily calorie intake decreased about 600 kcal per day from age 30 to age 80 in men of high socioeconomic status. One third of the decline could be correlated with reduced basal metabolism; two thirds with reduced physical activity. ●————● total intake; ○————○ basal expenditure; ○---○ expenditure for activity. (Adapted from Munro, H.N.: Nutrition and aging. Br Med Bull 37:84, 1981.)

lesterol intake should be controlled whenever advisable (see Chapter 19 for indications).

Protein

The protein requirements of the elderly probably do not differ from those of younger persons. However, a high protein intake is not advisable, since renal function deteriorates with age. (Blood flow to the kidneys is halved between the ages of 35 and 80.) It has even been suggested that a high protein diet may accelerate aging of the kidneys (see Chapter 23 for a discussion of renal failure). The protein content of the diet should thus be maintained at approximately 12 percent of total calories consumed.

NUTRITIONAL DEFICIENCIES

Recent surveys indicate that over 10 percent of the aged have intakes lower than two thirds of the RDA for calcium, iron, vitamin A, and water-soluble vitamins. In addition, vitamin D and zinc intake may be inadequate in elderly women.

A 1968–1970 10-state nutrition survey of low income people (lowest quartile of income) revealed that in those over age 60 the most prevalent nutrient deficiencies were iron, vitamin A (Hispanic Americans), riboflavin (blacks and Hispanic Americans), and vitamin C (men only). Food consumption among these low income older individuals was too low to meet nutritional standards, although clinical signs of deficiencies other than iron were found only infrequently. More recent research, however, suggests that iron deficiency in the elderly is not as common as had been supposed.

Osteopenia

Osteopenia—a reduction in bone mass that is greater than that expected considering an individual's age, sex, and race—is a major problem in the elderly. If the decrease in skeletal mass leads to mechanical failure, spontaneous fracture (the principal clinical manifestation of osteopenia) may occur. Hip and wrist fractures occur most frequently. It is estimated that one third of postmenopausal women have osteoporosis, and that one in five suffers a hip or vertebral compression fracture. Up to the age of 80, women are affected four times more often than men; after this age, the incidence of osteoporosis is equal in both sexes. For an unknown reason, blacks are less susceptible to this condition than whites.

Etiology

In idiopathic osteopenia of the elderly, the primary mechanism of bone loss may be decreased bone formation or increased bone resorption. Osteomalacia (adult rickets) is less common than osteoporosis and is attributable to vitamin D deficiency. There is controversy concerning the role of adequate dietary calcium intake in the prevention of osteoporosis. Estimates are that the average daily intake of calcium in the United States, especially among women, is typically less than 500 mg per day, whereas the calcium requirement is set between 800 mg and 1 g per day (see Chapter 2 for further discussion of calcium requirements). Middle-aged and elderly persons may need even more dietary calcium to remain in positive calcium balance, because of decreased absorption of calcium, increased urinary leak, increased secretion of parathormone, and poor adaptation to changes in dietary content. Postmenopausal women's decreased estrogen activity further contributes to bone demineralization.

Calcium absorption is decreased by oxalates (green vegetables) and phytates (unleavened wheat bread) in food. In addition, a dietary increase in the phosphate-to-calcium ratio or in the phosphate load (soft drinks, animal protein) may accentuate the decrease in bone mass.

Prevention and Treatment

A good lifelong calcium intake, especially in women of slight build and northern European extraction, may prevent osteopenia. Since it is difficult to maintain a high calcium intake (1 to 1½ g daily) from food sources alone, a supplement in the form of calcium carbonate, calcium lactate, or other salts in tablet or liquid form is recommended. The need for vitamin D and/or fluoride supplements or for estrogen administration is controversial, although adequate dosage of the latter has been recommended for menopausal women. A sustained program of 3 to 4 hours weekly of aerobic endurance exercise has also been shown to have a beneficial effect on bone mass.

If an increase in calcium intake is delayed until fractures occur or overt bone demineralization is observed on radiograph, the best result is likely to be an arrest of the process rather than repletion of bone. That is, a high level of calcium intake does appear to reduce bone resorption, but to date it has not been shown that demineralized bone is remineralized by the use of calcium supplements. It has been shown, however, that fracture frequency can be decreased under such a regimen, as well as with the administration of estrogens.

Anemia

Another problem common in the elderly that may represent nutritional deficiency is iron deficiency anemia. Although this condition may be related to inadequate dietary intake, it is more often caused by blood loss from the gastrointestinal tract, and this likelihood should be fully investigated. (See Chapter 15 for a discussion of nutritional anemias.)

OVERNUTRITION

Problems that can be caused or exacerbated by excessive intake of nutrients include obesity (calories), cardiovascular disease (calories, total fat, saturated fat, cholesterol, sodium), diabetes mellitus (calories, refined carbohydrates), and perhaps cancer (calories, fat, protein). These topics are discussed in detail in later chapters.

Obesity

Obesity is common in middle age and may persist in persons age 65 or older. Usual causes of obesity include failure to reduce food intake as physical activity decreases, overeating because of boredom or depression, and, rarely, intake of drugs that increase appetite. Food intake patterns of older persons often are more firmly set than those of younger people, and there may be less concern about the cosmetic problems of obesity. Weight reduction should be imposed when indicated for management of current health problems (not prevention of disease) and should stress slow weight loss on a balanced diet with vitamin and mineral supplements if daily caloric intake is less than 1300 to 1500 kcal. A diet high in fiber and low in refined sugars may be helpful in controlling not only obesity but also diabetes mellitus and constipation. Weight loss may lead to dramatic improvements in diabetes mellitus, hypertension, osteoarthritis, hyperlipidemia, low back pain, and exercise tolerance.

Cardiovascular Disease

Interestingly, the increase in blood pressure with age is absent in populations that do not have high sodium intake (see Chapter 19 for a complete discussion of the role of nutrition in cardiovascular disease).

Cancer

Cancer is primarily a disease of older people. It has been estimated that 50 percent of human cancer may be related to the diet, with deterioration in immune function also implicated in cancer causation. As discussed in Chapter 24, dietary practices particularly have been associated with cancers of the colon, breast, stomach, and prostate.

- Colon cancer may be related to dietary mutagens, effects of diet on bacterial flora, a deficiency in fiber, an increase in animal fat, and limited consumption of vegetables in the cruciferous family.
- The risk of breast cancer may be greater in the obese and may be correlated with dietary fat intake.
- The incidence of gastric cancer is correlated with intake of dried and salted fish, pickled and smoked foods, high levels of carbohydrates, and limited consumption of fresh fruits and vegetables.
- Prostate cancer is correlated with dietary meat and fat consumption.
- A link between low intake of retinoids (vitamin A and its analogues) and certain cancers has been reported.
- Skin cancer may be related to low selenium intake.

Malnutrition is a leading cause of death in cancer patients. Treatment of the tumor often exacerbates weight loss, while response to anticancer therapy may be compromised by poor nutritional status. Exuberant feeding of the patient, however, could stimulate tumor growth and may have no beneficial effect on survival. Problems in patient feeding may include anorexia, nausea, vomiting, diarrhea, maldigestion, malabsorption, alterations in taste and smell, protein loss, metabolic changes, and mechanical problems because of obstructions. (See Chapter 24 for recommendations for feeding cancer patients, which apply generally to elderly patients as well.)

NUTRITIONAL RISKS

Psychosocial Factors

Factors that may interfere with the pleasurable aspects of eating or the consumption of appropriate foods include

- social isolation
- the inferior status associated with aging
- loss of mobility
- effects of low income
- food beliefs and practices
- depression
- attitudes toward illness and death

Dissatisfaction with one's social role or with life in general, or a sense of dependence or changing body image may adversely affect appetite or eating patterns.

Isolation—whether the result of living alone, cultural isolation, or loss of mobility—is an important issue. Many aged individuals live alone and may not be motivated to shop, cook, and eat by themselves, while loneliness itself may diminish appetite. Cultural isolation occurs when customary foods are no longer available because of neighborhood changes, or when there are differences between the values of old-world elderly people and those of their assimilated children and grandchildren, who now prepare their meals. Loss of mobility may include the inability to operate an automobile, to use public transportation, or even to walk because of physical limitations or concerns about safety or cost.

Loss of income or reliance on a fixed income may be a critical factor. Poverty often means consumption of filling foods with minimal nutritional value and erratic scheduling of daily meals. Increased expenditures for health care may result in diminished spending for food and other essentials. Reliance on spoiled or rancid food may be an additional problem.

Depression may result from the aforementioned factors. For example, many elderly individuals, especially men and blacks age 75 and older, are chronically depressed by living alone. On the other hand, depression may be a reaction to illness. It often leads to anorexia, weight loss, and undernutrition, or it may result in overeating. Decreased food intake may further exacerbate the depression.

Fad Diets

Popular fad diets for weight loss are especially dangerous for the aged because of such diets' nutrient—particularly protein—deficiency. The elderly often are attracted by claims that adherence to a particular diet will prevent some acute or chronic illness, increase vitality, improve appearance or prolong life. Older persons with diminished hepatic, pancreatic, or renal function face special health risks from high protein–high fat diets. It is essential to provide rational alternative diets and discourage patients from ingesting potentially hazardous (and costly) megadoses of vitamins, minerals, or trace elements. (Chapter 6 discusses fad diets in greater detail.)

Therapeutic Diets

Therapeutic diets often are prescribed to treat medical problems of elderly patients. Such diets (discussed more fully in Chapter 10) may result in some nutrient deficiencies requiring supplementation:

- A fat-restricted diet has deficient amounts of fat-soluble vitamins.
- A diet that severely restricts sodium may also be low in protein.
- A high fiber diet may tend to decrease intestinal absorption of calcium, zinc, or other trace elements.

• Low calorie diet often will result in low intake of iron and many vitamins.

Food-Drug Interactions

The elderly consume 25 percent of all prescription drugs sold in the United States. Nutritional depletion (especially of minerals) or diet-related side effects are risks for those taking medications to treat hypertension, heart disease, peripheral vascular disease, chronic obstructive pulmonary disease, Parkinson's disease, dementia, cerebrovascular disease, diabetes mellitus, arthritis, and cancer. In addition, laxative abuse increases with age, possibly interfering with absorption of glucose or fat-soluble vitamins. (See Chapter 6 for more specific discussions of food-drug interactions.)

Alcoholism

Alcoholism is relatively common in individuals over 65, with a prevalence ranging up to 10 percent. Since their borderline diets and marginal digestive function may have already caused precarious nutritional balance, alcoholism in the elderly is likely to promote further deterioration. (Chapter 17 discusses the general nutritional effects of alcoholism.)

As reviewed in Chapters 14 and 17, alcoholic patients have increased need for B vitamins, including riboflavin, folacin, vitamins B_6 and B_{12}, and thiamin. Alcoholism is now believed to be the major cause of thiamin and folate deficiencies among the elderly in the United States. Both active and reformed alcoholics should be encouraged to consume foods high in essential nutrients, although milk may not be tolerated because of acquired lactose intolerance.

Medications prescribed for illness may interact with alcohol. In addition, disulfuram (Antabuse) may be hazardous for elderly patients with severely impaired liver function.

Caffeine

Ingestion of 200 mg of caffeine activates the cerebral cortex, reducing drowsiness and fatigue. The morning cup of coffee may energize, eliminate fatigue, slow the development of boredom, and increase motor and mental efficiency. On the other hand, caffeine taken in the evening may alter sleep patterns. Elderly persons with any type of cardiac arrhythmia or cerebrovascular disease should limit their consumption of caffeine.

Chronic Illness

Chronic diseases that lead to malnutrition in the elderly include heart failure, cancer, chronic neurologic disease with paralysis, alcoholic cirrhosis, chronic bronchitis and emphysema, arthritis, organic brain syndromes and psychosis, depression, end-stage renal disease, maldigestion, and malabsorption syndromes.

THE HOSPITALIZED PATIENT

All elderly hospitalized patients should have their nutritional status promptly assessed. (Chapter 3 contains a full discussion of nutritional assessment.) Briefly, risk factors to watch for include

- a history of inadequate food intake
- anthropometric measurements (percent ideal body weight, triceps skinfold, or mid-arm muscle circumference) that show depletion
- serum albumin below 3.5 g per dl (however, serum albumin in the aged may not fall even with serious malnutrition)

Acute illness commonly brings a marked reduction, or even cessation, in food intake. At the same time, the catabolic effects of diseases such as pneumonia and cholecystitis may increase nutrient requirements. Nutrient needs similarly increase with injury, surgery, or fractures. (Chapter 25 describes in greater detail the increased requirements of the stressed patient.) Vomiting as well as lack of food intake during preoperative periods when no food is permitted by mouth present additional nutritional problems. Resection of the stomach or intestine with lack of nutritional support has a negative impact on postoperative nutritional status.

Owing to their lack of nutritional reserves, most elderly individuals are unable to withstand starvation for more than 5 days. It is especially important to begin immediate adequate feeding of those patients at risk of malnutrition because of antecedent weight loss, alcoholism, and/or catabolic disease. Adequate nutritional support may increase resistance to infection and improve wound healing and general well-being. Physical activity should also be encouraged.

Feeding may be accomplished by enteral or parenteral routes, or by some combination of both. (Chapters 11 and 12 discuss these methods.) Nutritional supplements can also be helpful. Enteral nutrition by supplement or tube is useful in nursing homes and can also be used in the outpatient at home. If the enteral route is contraindicated, total parenteral nutrition should be used.

Patient acceptance can be facilitated by avoiding radical or rapid changes in the customary diet. Frequent feeding is often helpful. It is imperative that foods with high nutrient density be provided. Meals should include high quality protein, low amounts of fat, and an increased intake of complex carbohydrates relative to simple sugars. Each meal should provide a source of vitamin C, and it is vital to ensure an adequate intake of water. An example of a well-balanced main meal with foods of high nutrient density might include roast chicken, enriched steamed rice, broccoli, whole wheat enriched bread, orange slices, and low fat milk.

FEEDING REGIMENS IN NURSING HOMES

In the United States, more than one million elderly are in nursing homes. These patients commonly have very low calcium intake and low intakes of vitamin A, thiamin, riboflavin, and iron. In some instances vitamin C intake is also deficient. These deficiencies can be rectified by using more milk and milk products in meal preparation and by serving green and yellow vegetables and citrus fruit more often. Social interaction—encouraging the elderly to take their meals together with other patients in a communal dining room—as well as spacing meals about 5 hours apart may help to improve appetite.

NUTRITIONAL COUNSELING

Information about locally available meals and food distribution systems including government, local agencies, and "Meals on Wheels" should be provided for older persons. Congregate feeding programs offer the older person socialization and some nutrition education, often together with appropriate transportation to meal sites.

Additionally, nutritional counseling should be offered to

- elderly persons who live alone and are responsible for their own shopping and meal preparation
- those who purchase or prepare food for the elderly
- food service managers at domiciliary care facilities and nursing homes
- attendants responsible for feeding, or helping to feed, the elderly

SECTION III

Modalities for Nutritional Support

He had had much experience of physicians, and said "the only way to keep your health is to eat what you don't want, drink what you don't like, and do what you'd druther not."

Mark Twain (Samuel L. Clemens), 1835–1910, *Following the Equator,* Vol. 11, Ch. 13, "Pudd'nhead Wilson's New Calendar."

While the previous sections focused on the basic principles of nutrition and the special considerations appropriate throughout the life cycle, this section concentrates specifically on how to provide support for patients whose illnesses require special nutritional attention.

Chapter 10—**Diets as Therapy**—begins by explaining the role of the dietitian, and then discusses the regular hospital diet and modified diets, providing sample menus. The chapter concludes with a complete description of the diet order, including a clear exposition of the physician's role in formulating the therapeutic diet.

Chapter 11—**Enteral Nutritional Support**—explores all types of enteral formulas, then moves on to tube feeding, with a discussion of delivery systems, indications and contraindications, monitoring, and complications. Finally, we present guidelines for feeding via tube enterostomies.

In Chapter 12—**Parenteral Nutritional Support**—we consider all aspects of parenteral alimentation, including indications, determining the formulation, routes of administration, nutritional requirements, orders for specific disease states, monitoring, and complications.

CHAPTER 10

Diets as Therapy

Jane M. Greene, M.S., R.D., L.D.
Sandra B. Leonard, M.S., R.D., L.D.

As physicians become more aware of nutritional principles and the influence of nutritional status on the disease process, consultations between physicians and dietitians are becoming more common. Communication—verbal and/or written in the medical record—among all health care staff is essential to optimize the patient's nutritional care.

THE DIETITIAN

The term "dietitian" has been used since 1899 to describe persons working in a hospital to provide nutritious meals to patients. Home economists

253

performed these duties until 1917, when the American Dietetic Association was founded. By 1926 the group had established educational standards for membership, requiring a Bachelor of Science (B.S.) degree. By 1930 dietetic internships were initiated. Currently, most hospitals require that one be a Registered Dietitian (R.D.) in order to practice.

Registration Requirements/Licensure

To be eligible to take the registration exam, a dietitian must have completed a B.S. degree and satisfactorily served an internship. The 4-year curriculum usually involves courses in biology, chemistry (general, organic, biochemistry), human physiology, microbiology, food science, food preparation, and nutrition (basic, advanced, and diet therapy). Courses in statistics and computer science are included. The internship includes training in food service systems management, clinical dietetics, and community nutrition. This work experience ranges from 9 to 12 months.

Other routes to eligibility are coordinated undergraduate programs in which work experience is included with academic study during the 4-year undergraduate program or completion of a Master's degree in nutrition. Upon earning an advanced degree in nutrition, one works for 6 months under an experienced Registered Dietitian. After review and approval of the experience, these persons may take the registration examination. Once a dietitian becomes registered, a minimum of 75 hours of continuing education credits must be earned every 5 years to remain registered.

Many states are in the process of initiating or have recently passed legislation for licensure of dietitians in addition to the existing requirement of registration. Like registration, licensure is another sign of professionalism, and licensed dietitians are recognized as the nutrition authorities.

Administrative Dietitians

Over 50 percent of the dietitians in the United States work in hospitals as administrative or clinical dietitians. Administrative dietitians work primarily with hospital administrators and have little direct contact with the medical staff. They function as part of the hospital management team concerned with the standardization of food services in order to provide the best food for patients and, in some cases, staff.

Clinical Dietitians

The clinical dietitian has direct contact with the medical and paramedical staff concerned with the delivery of care to the patients. Traditionally, dietitians have been responsible for translating diet orders into meal plans and teaching patients about therapeutic diets prior to discharge. Today dietitians are prepared to take an active role in patient care.

Nutritionists

The term "nutritionist" is often used interchangeably with "dietitian." Although there is no official definition of "nutritionist," among professionals a nutritionist is thought of as one with advanced training, that is, Master's level, Ph.D., or fellowship, in nutrition. Unfortunately, since there is no official definition for nutritionist, persons often refer to themselves as nutritionists without having proper credentials (see Chapter 6).

Specific Responsibilities of the Dietitian

Responsibilities of the dietitian may include

1. Monitoring the dietary, physical, and biochemical parameters of the patient's nutritional status. In many hospitals the dietitian performs significant portions of the nutritional assessment. The medical record must be reviewed for pertinent findings. Additional information is gathered during an interview with the patient when possible (see Chapter 3).
2. Assessment and reporting the adequacy of the patient's intake of kilocalories, protein, and other essential nutrients. This is accomplished by doing calorie counts of the actual food eaten in the hospital. The nursing staff is instructed to record what the patient eats. The dietitian then calculates the total intake and the adequacy of that intake. Previous intake can also be assessed by 24-hour dietary recalls or food frequencies.
3. Evaluation and reporting of the patient's progress and ability to tolerate the present (or more advanced) diet. When feeding problems are documented, it is the dietitian's responsibility to visit the patient frequently to encourage maximal intake and to evaluate progress. Accurate reporting of this information is helpful to the physician in knowing when changes are indicated in the diet orders.
4. Consideration and recommendations about specifically defined diets or pharmaceutical products that the physician may order to optimize nutritional adequacy. With the wide variety of products available for use in either total or supplemental nutrition, the dietitian may assist the physician in pointing out products that have the properties best

suited to the patient's medical problems. Factors considered include caloric density, type and amount of fat and protein, osmolarity, palatability, and electrolyte content (see Chapter 11).

Dietitians also are involved in other areas including research, public health programs, and specialty areas such as diabetes mellitus, renal disease, cardiology, nutrition support, and pediatrics.

THE REGULAR HOSPITAL DIET

The regular hospital diet is designed for the patient who has no indication for therapeutic modifications in food intake. The specific nutrient content may vary widely from hospital to hospital, but all regular diets are aimed at providing appropriate amounts of protein, calories, and other nutrients for practically all healthy persons. The Recommended Dietary Allowances (see Chapters 1 and 2) are translated into basic food groups (Chapter 4) to provide a foundation for the regular diet. Table 10–1 indicates the number of servings and serving sizes of each food group to be supplied in the daily diet.

Some hospitals offer selective menus for patients on regular diets so that each individual patient may choose foods from a limited menu. There are two schools of thought regarding the composition of regular diets. Some believe that hospitals should teach by example so that the food is planned and prepared with only good nutrition principles in mind. Others think that it is more important to provide foods the patient is willing and able to eat. Generally, there is a compromise between these two viewpoints, with emphasis placed on meeting the needs of the individual patient. It is generally not appropriate to impose unnecessary restrictions on hospitalized patients. This

Table 10–1. BASIC FOOD GROUPS—REQUIREMENTS
THROUGH THE LIFE CYCLE

Food Group	Adult	Child	Adolescent	Pregnant	Lactating
Milk	2 cups	2–3 cups	4 cups	3–4 cups	4 cups
Meat	2 2-oz servings	2 1¹/₂-oz servings	2 2¹/₂-oz servings	2 2¹/₂-oz servings	2 2¹/₂-oz servings
Fruits/Vegetables	4 ¹/₂-cup servings	Same	Same	Same	Same
Bread/Cereals	4 or more servings	Same	Same	Same	Same
Fat/Sweets	Adjust according to individual needs				

The American diet as recommended should contain approximately 55% carbohydrate, 15% protein, and 30% fat.

Table 10-2. NUTRIENT COMPOSITION OF A TYPICAL
REGULAR HOSPITAL DIET

Nutrient	Amount/day
Kcalories	2000–2500
Protein	60 g
Sodium	2.5–3.5 g
Potassium	3.5–4.5 g
Calcium	1.0–1.3 g
Phosphorus	1.1–1.5 g
Magnesium	300–400 mg
Iron	7–9 mg
Zinc	13–14 mg

is especially true if the modifications keep the patient from receiving adequate protein and calories to meet the needs of convalescence from illness, injury, or surgery.

The regular hospital diet provides specific nutrients each day (Table 10-2). It does not take into account special needs arising from infections, metabolic disorders, chronic diseases, or other abnormal conditions that require therapeutic modifications of the diet.

MODIFIED DIETS

A modified or therapeutic diet may differ from the regular diet in

- consistency (liquid, soft)
- levels of individual nutrients
- energy level
- fluid content
- number of meals (three meals, three snacks)
- elimination of certain foods or nutrients

The Diet Manual

In general, diet manuals contain information regarding foods allowed and not allowed on each diet, the indications for use, sample menus (Table 10–3), and the nutritional adequacy of the diets. Examples of modified diets are listed in Table 10–4. The exact composition of specific therapeutic diets may vary among hospitals. It is therefore important that physicians familiarize themselves with a particular hospital's diets by reviewing the hospital diet manual. In larger hospitals, diet manuals are prepared by the dietary staff

Table 10–3. SAMPLE MENUS

	Clear Liquid Diet	Soft Diet	Diabetic
Approximate daily intake:	Kcalories, 1100 Protein, 42 g Fat, 1 g Carbohydrate, 227 g	Kcalories, 1650 Protein, 75 g Fat, 62 g Carbohydrate, 200 g	Kcalories, 1200 Protein, 85 g Fat, 44 g Carbohydrate, 126 g
Breakfast:	Grape Juice, 8 oz Orange Frostee, 6 oz (Citrotein Slush) Coffee Sugar	Orange juice, 8 oz Grits, 4 oz Plain scrambled egg, 1 Toast, 1 slice Margarine, 1 tsp Blackberry jelly Coffee, cream Milk 2%, 8 oz	Orange juice, 4 oz Grits, 4 oz Scrambled egg, 1 Margarine, 1 tsp Skim milk, 8 oz Coffee
Lunch:	Chicken broth, 6 oz Pineapple juice, 8 oz Raspberry gelatin with grape Citrotein, 5 oz Tea Sugar	Plain roast turkey, gravy, 3 oz Cranberry sauce Plain rice, 4 oz Roll, 1 Margarine, 1 tsp Peeled apricots, 4 Tea	Plain roast turkey, 3 oz Plain green beans, 4 oz Tomato wedge salad, 4 oz Roll, 1 Margarine, 1 tsp Unsweetened purple plums, 2 Skim milk, 8 oz
Dinner:	Beef broth, 6 oz Lemonade, 8 oz Punch Frostee, 6 oz (Citrotein Slush) Tea Sugar	Plain roast beef, 3 oz Plain whipped potatoes, 4 oz Plain green peas, 4 oz 1 peach with cottage cheese, 1 oz Roll, 1 Margarine, 2 tsp Plain gelatin cubes, 4 oz Tea	Lean roast beef, 3 oz Plain diced potatoes, 4 oz Sliced beets/onions, vinegar, 4 oz Unsweetened pear halves, 2 Margarine, 2 tsp Skim milk, 8 oz

Table 10-4. EXAMPLES OF MODIFIED DIETS

Consistency Modified Diets	Nutrient Modified Diets	Diets Excluding Certain Foods
Clear liquid*	Reduced kcal	Allergy
Full liquid*	High kcal	Gluten restricted
Soft	Low protein	Purine restricted
Low residue*	High protein	Tyramine restricted
High fiber	Low fat	Lactose restricted
	Low cholesterol	
	Low potassium	
	High potassium	
	Low sodium	
	Fluid restricted†	
	Force fluids	

*May be offered either orally or via feeding tube.
†When fluid restriction is indicated (hyponatremia, renal failure, congestive heart failure, and so on), specify degree of restriction (e.g., ≤ 1000 cc/day). This includes water and any other fluids (juice, milk), plus water content in solid foods.

with approval of hospital administrators, physicians, and other key personnel. A hospital diet manual generally is designed to be specific for the hospital using it and includes directions for the physician regarding ordering diets.

THE DIET ORDER

The physician is responsible for ordering a diet for every patient admitted. The purpose of a diet order, or diet prescription, is to let the dietitian (or food service) know the intention of the physician regarding a patient's diet. In formulating a diet prescription, the physician must consider the nature of the disease, what can be accomplished by the diet, and whether or not the patient will accept the diet. The characteristics of good diet orders are:

1. The diet prescription should be brief but specific. It should state in a few words or sentences what is intended.
2. The diet should be clear and contain only one meaning. If the dietitian can interpret the diet to be other than that intended, it is poorly written.
3. The diet order must be complete. Any changes that you wish to be continued must be repeated each time the diet is ordered. One cannot assume that the dietitian will automatically continue other modifications when a new diet is ordered.

4. The orders for individual patients should be consistent. That is, one modification in diet should not conflict with another.
5. If the diet prescription includes several therapeutic modifications, the most important modification should be listed first to give it priority.
6. Be sure that the patient actually needs all of the restrictions you are including. Many disease states require very restrictive diets; often, less stringent restrictions may accomplish what is necessary with less dissatisfaction on the part of the patient.
7. Avoid frequent changes in diet orders. As the patient's hospital course progresses, changes in the diet may be indicated. Once a diet is selected, it is important that the dietary staff be advised so that patient instructions can be started promptly. By having several days to work with the patient regarding discharge diet planning, the dietitian is better able to instruct the patient to understand and follow the diet at home.

The order is written in the medical record and should be consistent with the names given to various diets in the hospital manual. If the physician desires a diet different from that listed in the diet manual, this must be specified. Table 10-5 gives examples of problems that may result from inappropriate diet orders.

Table 10-5. SOME EXAMPLES OF PROBLEMS THAT CAN OCCUR FROM INAPPROPRIATE DIET ORDERS

1. A patient is ordered to receive no food (NPO) by the physician, who wants a laboratory test performed. According to hospital policy, the physician must indicate when the diet is to be resumed. The doctor assumed the diet would resume after the test. The patient is needlessly starved for several days.
2. A patient is having poor tolerance to regular food even after several modifications have been tried. The physician decides to stop regular food and try an enteral supplement. Although the doctor orders the supplement, he or she neglects to stop the other diet. The patient continues to receive a tray and also gets the supplement. Food intolerance continues as the patient eats the regular food rather than try the supplement.
3. A patient has severe edema and congestive heart failure and a low sodium diet is ordered. The dietary department interprets "low sodium" to be 2000 to 3500 mg sodium per day, whereas the physician thought the patient was receiving 1000 mg sodium. The patient's fluid retention persists.

In ordering a therapeutic diet, the physician must consider the patient's age, sex, level of activity, and cultural, economic, and family situation in relation to the patient's specific medical and nutritional needs. Table 10–6 provides indications for using some of the most frequently requested diets, how the diet should be ordered by physicians, and additional comments. It is important to recognize that some diet regimens are based on traditional dietary practices rather than on documented evidence, such as

- Routine restriction of caffeine, black pepper, chili powder, and so forth, may not be warranted for all patients with peptic ulcer disease.
- In patients with Crohn's disease, unless in the acute phase, elemental formulas or total parenteral nutrition are generally not necessary.
- Many lactose-intolerant patients can tolerate cultured dairy products (e.g., buttermilk, yogurt) and small amounts of cheese and butter, especially when ingested with other foods that delay gastric emptying.
- Severe fat restriction may not be necessary for patients with steatorrhea—a low fat diet (40 to 50 g fat) plus medium chain triglyceride (MCT) oil may be tolerated.

Table 10–6. INDICATIONS FOR USE
OF SOME COMMON DIETS

Type of Diet	Indications	Comments
Regular	All adult patients who do not need any specific dietary modifications	Calorie (2000–2500) and protein (70–100 g) contents vary in different hospitals.
Diabetic (Chapter 18)	For the management of patients with either insulin-dependent (type I) or non–insulin-dependent (type II) diabetes mellitus. The primary goal is to attain as nearly normal state of blood glucose as possible without undue inconvenience or risk of hypoglycemia.	Weight control may be one of the primary goals in early management of the diabetic. Diet should be ordered in the following manner: _____ kcal, _____ g PRO, _____ g CHO, _____ g FAT, _____ meals, _____ snack(s).

(Continued)

**Table 10–6. INDICATIONS FOR USE
OF SOME COMMON DIETS**—Continued

Type of Diet	Indications	Comments
		As persons with diabetes are especially vulnerable to premature or accelerated atherosclerosis, the diet should also be directed at reducing this risk, and modified in fat content/composition and cholesterol intake.
Weight control (Chapter 16)	For management of persons who need to gain or lose weight	Weight control diets should be tailored to the individual patient and ordered by calorie level.
		If calories are restricted to < 1300 kcal, vitamin and mineral supplements may be indicated.
Low sodium (Chapters 19 and 23)	Control of edema and hypertension.	There is no indication for *routine* restriction of sodium in hospitalized patients.
	500 mg—severe restriction; difficult to provide and rarely indicated—congestive heart failure; cirrhosis with massive ascites.	The diet should be ordered as _____ mg sodium, *not* sodium chloride. 1 tsp table salt (5 g) contains 2 g sodium.
	1000 mg—moderate restriction—congestive heart failure.	The sodium content of drugs taken by patient must be considered (see Chapter 19, Cardiovascular Disease).
	2000 mg—mild restriction—hypertension; cirrhosis with ascites.	
Consistency Modifications		
Clear liquid	First phase of postoperative dietary progression.	Inadequate in all nutrients; should only be used for 24–48 hr.

Table 10–6. INDICATIONS FOR USE
OF SOME COMMON DIETS—Continued

Type of Diet	Indications	Comments
	Dietary preparation for colon surgery. Decreased function of GI tract, such as recovery from ileus or surgery.	Examples: coffee, tea, Koolaid, carbonated beverages, strained lemonade and juices, fruit drinks, clear broth, plain or flavored gelatin, hard candy. Consider low residue enteral supplements in place of clear liquid diet—especially if patient is malnourished.
Full liquid	Second phase of postoperative dietary progression. Difficulty chewing and swallowing.	Inadequate in most nutrients. High in lactose: many patients who have not eaten for a while develop lactose intolerance. Examples: eggnog, custard, plain ice cream or yogurt, well-cooked refined cereals, cream soups with pureed vegetables, butter, margarine, cream, half-and-half, unstrained juices. Consider enteral supplement instead.
Soft	May be indicated for some postoperative and convalescing patients. Transition from full liquid to a regular diet.	Modifies the regular diet by changing its consistency to soft. May need to restrict gas-forming, highly seasoned, or fried foods. (Continued)

Table 10-6. INDICATIONS FOR USE
OF SOME COMMON DIETS—Continued

Type of Diet	Indications	Comments
	Patient who has difficulty swallowing.	Examples: See Table 10–3 for sample menu.
		Patients may prefer commercially prepared supplements.
		Some patients with difficulty chewing or swallowing can handle a "soft mechanical" diet (i.e., regular diet, ground).
Fat modified		
A. Low fat (Fat restricted) (Chapter 21)	Improves symptoms of steatorrhea in: Crohn's disease Gallbladder disease Gastrectomy Short gut syndrome Sprue Whipple's disease Pancreatic insufficiency Cystic fibrosis Cirrhosis and other liver diseases	All forms of fat are restricted; no attempt is made to differentiate among various forms.
		Substitution of dietary medium chain triglycerides for long chain triglycerides may improve fat absorption, palatability and caloric intake.
		Diet order should indicate low fat diet or low fat diet with MCT and the level of fat (e.g., 35 g of fat).
		Dietary fat can be liberalized as control with supplemental enzymes is achieved, when appropriate.
		To promote weight gain and maximize nutrient intake, patient should be given the greatest amount of fat tolerated.

Table 10-6. INDICATIONS FOR USE
OF SOME COMMON DIETS—Continued

Type of Diet	Indications	Comments
B. Hyper-lipidemia Diet (Chapter 19)	Reduce elevated levels of serum cholesterol and triglycerides to reduce risk of heart disease.	Fat (amount and type), cholesterol, carbohydrate, and alcohol restriction is determined by which lipids (lipoproteins) are elevated in blood.
		When possible, determine levels of all serum lipoproteins so that nutritional management may be tailored to the specific lipoprotein abnormality.
		Weight control emphasized.

INFORMING THE PATIENT ABOUT DIETARY MODIFICATIONS

When modifications are indicated, it is the physician's responsibility to explain the need for dietary changes to the patient. It can be upsetting to a hospitalized patient to receive a tray with significant modifications and not know why. By making the patient aware of the importance of the dietary modifications, the patient is more likely to accept this change in his or her normal dietary pattern. Once the physician has explained the importance of the diet in relation to this specific disease state, the dietitian and other health personnel can further emphasize the importance of the diet in treating the patient's condition and, in selected patients, in long-term management of the disease.

CHAPTER 11

Enteral Nutritional Support

When the gut works, use it.

Nutritional support via the enteral route involves the delivery of nutrients into the alimentary canal at any point from the mouth to the small intestine. Nutrients may be provided by voluntary ingestion (drinking, sipping) or delivered by a tube placed into the stomach or small intestine, or through surgically created "ostomies" leading into either one of these organs. The products consumed or introduced are usually liquid and may consist of blenderized food or commercially prepared nutritional supplements or formulas. Constituents range from modular products of fat, carbohydrate, and protein, together with vitamins and minerals, to complete mixtures of nutrients, or some combination thereof. Macronutrients may be in the form of complete

266

proteins, complex carbohydrates and triglycerides of long-chain fat, from foods or chemically defined—or they may be partially digested or in the form of end products of digestion (elemental, chemically defined). Products may be ready-prepared, usually canned, or may require dissolving and mixing. Enteral feedings may be delivered continuously by pump or introduced as a bolus.

Formulations may be used as supplements to the usual dietary intake when it is judged to be inadequate. However, in some circumstances it may be both convenient and economic to ingest the entire diet as a formula. Patients may be given their diet via tube feeding both in and out of the hospital. Whenever possible, the enteral route should be used for nutritional support, and is preferable to intravenous alimentation. Enteral feeding generally is cheaper, safer, and more physiologic. It may not be simpler, however, especially because of the proliferation of enteral formulas, tubes, and delivery systems constantly changing in a highly competitive setting. With increasing awareness of the importance of nutritional support over the past decade, the process of enteral feeding has been made easier and more acceptable to patients and health care professionals. Obviously, the enteral route can be used only if the gastrointestinal tract is both accessible and functional.

This chapter discusses types of formulas, sites of feeding, tubes and pumps; classifies products; and reviews indications for, complications of, procedures for, and monitoring of enteral feeding. Details may be found in the references provided and in current product information.

TYPES OF FORMULAS

Formulas may be classified as complete, modular, or special. Commercial formulas generally are low residue, and therefore can be consumed by patients prior to various radiographic and other diagnostic procedures involving the gastrointestinal tract. Some products make visualizing the bowel for endoscopy difficult, while consumption of others may yield intestinal gas, a hazard for some electrocoagulation procedures (polypectomy). Complications may be avoided by consulting with physicians who carry out these procedures concerning the enteral products their patients are permitted to ingest prior to study.

Most nutritionally complete products provide between 1 and 2 kcal per ml. More concentrated formulas do not provide sufficient water, especially when accompanied by a high nitrogen load. Adequate water supplements (dilute fluids) should be administered. A sample formulary for enteral feeding, and other products of therapeutic equivalence, is presented in Table 11–1.

**Table 11-1. SAMPLE ENTERAL NUTRITION FORMULARY
AND THERAPEUTIC EQUIVALENTS**

Classification	Sample Product	Equivalent
I. POLYMERIC		
A. Hypertonic		
1. Containing lactose	Instant breakfast	Compleat b
		Meritene
		Blenderized tube feeding
2. lactose free		
a. Low residue	Sustacal	Ensure
		Precision HN
		Travasorb
	Ensure Plus	Ensure Plus HN
		Isocal HCN
		Sustacal HC
		Magnacal
		Two Cal HN
b. High fiber	Enrich	
B. Isotonic	Osmolite	Compleat Modified
lactose free		Isocal
		Osmolite HN
	Travasorb MCT	Isotein HN
II. MONOMERIC		
A. Standard amino	Vital High Nitrogen	Vivonex
acid formula		High Nitrogen Vivonex
		Criticare HN
		Travasorb MCT
B. High branched chain	Stresstein	Traumacal
amino acid formula	Vivonex T.E.N.	Traum-Aid HBC
III. MODULAR		
A. Carbohydrate source	Polycose Powder	Moducal
		Sumacal
B. Fat source	MCT oil	
	Microlipid	
C. Protein source	Pro-mix	Pro Mod
		Propac
		Casec
D. Protein supplement	Citrotein	SLD
with carbohydrate		Gevral
		High protein gelatin
IV. DISEASE-SPECIFIC		
FORMULATIONS		
A. Hepatic	Travasorb hepatic	Hepatic Aid
B. Renal	Travasorb renal	Amin Aid
C. Pulmonary	Pulmocare	

Table 11–1. SAMPLE ENTERAL NUTRITION FORMULARY
AND THERAPEUTIC EQUIVALENTS—Continued

Classification	Sample Product	Equivalent
V. SEMISOLID NUTRITIONAL SUPPLEMENT	Forta pudding	Sustacal pudding Commercial pudding

Complete

Complete formulas provide all essential nutrients (carbohydrate, protein, fat, vitamins, minerals) and either contain lactose or are lactose-free.

- They may be hypertonic, with osmolality exceeding that of the extracellular fluid, or be isotonic.
- Protein, carbohydrate, and fat may be derived from various dietary sources (Table 11–2), ranging from extracted dietary nutrients (cereal, cornstarch, meat, eggs, milk, soy, vegetable oils) to end products of digestion (elemental).
- Products may be powder, liquid, or in pudding form.
- They may be flavored, or flavor packages may be added.
- Elementary diets generally have higher osmolality and are less palatable, and therefore are better suited to tube feeding than to voluntary oral ingestion.

Indications for Specific Formulas

- Lactose-free formulas are indicated in cases of lactose intolerance or lactase deficiency (see Chapter 21), which is common in patients with moderate or severe celiac or tropical sprue, kwashiorkor, and severe forms of gastroenteritis, and in alcoholics. Other disaccharidases may also be abnormal in these disease states.
- Formulas with intact protein may be used in patients with normal pancreatic exocrine and small bowel absorptive functions.
- Formulas with hydrolyzed protein are indicated when absorptive surface is reduced and with exocrine pancreatic insufficiency.
- Crystalline amino acids are used in patients with hepatic or renal failure.
- Medium chain triglycerides (MCT) often are used in combination with long chain triglycerides (LCT) to provide easy digestibility and absorption (MCT) along with essential fatty acids (LCT).

**Table 11–2. SOURCES OF NUTRIENTS
IN ENTERAL FORMULAS**

Carbohydrate	
Starch (polysaccharides)	Hydrolyzed cereal solids
	Pureed green beans
	Modified corn starch
	Tapioca
	Soy polysaccharide
Glucose polymers (partially hydrolyzed cornstarch)	Glucose polysaccharides $\Big\}$ ($>$10 units)
	Glucose polymers
	Glucose oligosaccharides (2–10 units)
	Maltodextrins
	Corn syrup
	Corn syrup solids
Disaccharides	Sucrose
	Lactose
	Maltose
Monosaccharides	Glucose
	Fructose
Protein	
Intact	Pureed beef
	Egg white solids
	Nonfat and whole dry milk
	Whey
	Soy protein isolate
	Casein isolates
	Egg albumin
	Lactalbumin
	Na^+, Ca^{++}, and K^+ caseinates
Hydrolyzed protein (polypeptides, peptides)	Casein
	Whey, soy, meat protein
	Lactalbumin
	Collagen
Crystalline amino acids	L-amino acids
Fat	
Long chain triglycerides	Corn oil
	Sesame oil
	Partially hydrogenated soybean oil
	Soybean oil
	Sunflower oil
	Safflower oil
Medium chain triglycerides	Fractionated coconut oil
Mono- and diglycerides	

Modular

Modular products provide
- sources of protein with or without carbohydrate
- carbohydrate as powder or liquid
- sources of long or medium chain fatty acids alone or with carbohydrate

Modular products may be mixed together or added to food or other formulas and may also be used to prepare gelatin, sodas, floats, or freezes. However, these products alone are insufficient to meet RDAs for all nutrients.

Special

Special formulas are designed to meet the needs of patients with hepatic, renal, or pulmonary failure. Their electrolyte content generally is limited. Mineral content of complete formulas may vary by 50 to 100 percent; thus, if mineral content—calcium, sodium, potassium—is an important factor in the diet, the specific composition of the product to be used should be known.

Patients with renal failure should be given formulas limiting intake of protein, potassium, phosphorus, and magnesium and avoiding excessive intake of some vitamins and trace minerals. Enteral formulas composed of the essential amino acids are specifically designed for patients with renal failure. A low protein intake enriched in branched chain amino acids is provided by some specific enteral formulas and may be desirable in patients with hepatic failure. Both renal and hepatic formulas contain minimal amounts of electrolytes, vitamins, and minerals, which must be supplemented according to individual patient needs. Pulmonary formulas are designed for patients with hypercapnia. They contain an increased proportion of calories from fat and less from carbohydrate so that the respiratory quotient (RQ) is lower, thereby decreasing the ventilatory load and the work of breathing. A "stress" formula has increased branched chain amino acids and is calorie dense. Since most enteral products are equivalent to a 2 g sodium diet, they are generally tolerated by patients with cardiac failure. Patients who require severe fluid restriction may be managed with a formula providing 2 kcal per ml.

TUBE FEEDING

Tube feedings can be provided through the nasogastric portal, or via cervical esophagostomy, gastrostomy, duodenostomy, the nasoduodenal, nasojejunal, or jejunostomy route. The tip of the tube is placed in the stomach or small intestine.

The physical characteristics of the formula will affect the patient's tolerance of the feeding (e.g., gastric retention, diarrhea), which also is influenced by administrative techniques. Osmolality will influence gastric emptying, which is slowed by solutions with osmotic pressures more than or less than 200 mOsm. Hypertonic solutions may cause severe diarrhea, electrolyte depletion, and dehydration. Bolus administration of hypertonic solutions may delay gastric emptying, causing nausea and vomiting.

Complete formulas, whether hypertonic or isotonic, meet the needs of most tube-fed patients. Modular or special formulas may be indicated in patients with hepatic, renal, pulmonary, or cardiac failure and in those with diabetes mellitus, malabsorption, or disorders of acid-base balance. These formulas may be two to 15 times the cost of conventional complete hypertonic or isotonic formulas. Nevertheless, when they obviate the need for even more expensive parenteral alimentation, they may be cost effective, although they are difficult to prepare, administer, and monitor. Recently developed formulas contain a high proportion of branched chain amino acids for use following surgical procedures and in patients with nonsurgical trauma and sepsis (see Chapter 25). Tube-fed patients are more comfortable when they are permitted to drink additional water, breathe through the nose, have good oral hygiene, and gargle. Patients also should be encouraged to be active.

Delivery System

Tubes

A major advance in tube feeding was the introduction of the soft, small-bore feeding tubes that minimize complications of long-term feeding and patient discomfort from the size and stiffness of the tube. The small-bore, soft tube permits the patient to continue to swallow. Early tubes were made of rubber; later came progressive changes to polyethylene, polyvinyl, and finally polyurethane or silicone, weighted with mercury or beads. Silicone and polyurethane tubes may require added stiffening in order to be passed. Various devices have been employed, including an accompanying larger, stiffer tube with or without gelatin embedding or coating, guide wires, stylets, or weights. Length and diameters of tubes vary, ranging from 36 to 45 inches and from 5 to 18 French. There are various devices to hold the tubes in place.

Containers and Pumps

Feeding containers may be glass or semirigid or nonrigid plastic bottles or bags holding 250 to 1600 ml. Some are prefilled. It is essential that the enteral delivery system—bottle, tubing, and contents—not be confused with intravenous delivery systems to avoid possible lethal infusion of enteral formulas intravenously.

Enteral feeding pumps are designed for continuous slow-drip infusion of hyperosmolar formulas, ensuring a constant delivery rate and reducing gastric pooling of solution with retention leading to aspiration and osmotic diarrhea. A number of inexpensive, portable pumps designed for enteral feeding are available, making it unnecessary to use intravenous pumps.

Continuous Feeding

Delivery of continuous enteral feeding into the jejunum may be advantageous in reducing the potential for aspiration. Continuous feedings are usually necessary to deliver formulas directly into the small intestine. A recommended infusion rate into the stomach or jejunum is 50 ml per hour, increasing daily by 25 ml per hour to the rate necessary to provide energy needs. Dilution to isotonicity also is recommended, followed by gradual increase to full strength.

Four or 5 days may be required to reach the calorie goal determined by the usual process of nutritional assessment in developing the nutritional prescription. It is likely that vitamin and mineral requirements will not be met until the patient is receiving full-strength formula, possibly necessitating specific supplementation. Tube-fed patients generally do not receive the calories prescribed and suffer from a calorie deficit; patients whose requirements—especially for repletion—cannot be met by enteral feeding may need added peripheral intravenous alimentation (see Chapter 12).

Chronic nasogastric feedings may be carried out at home or in the hospital by passing a tube each evening and administering continuous-drip feedings at night while the patient sleeps. This regimen has been used with success in children with Crohn's or glycogen storage disease.

Indications

Indications for nasoenteric tube feeding (Table 11–3) include patients with

- neurologic or psychiatric disorders preventing satisfactory oral intake
- disorders of the oropharynx, esophagus, or upper gastrointestinal tract who cannot eat
- burns or various diseases of the gastrointestinal tract, including short bowel syndrome
- treatment regimens of chemotherapy or radiotherapy

In patients with fistulas, an elemental diet can be infused distal to the fistulous tract.

Table 11–3. INDICATIONS FOR NASOENTERIC
TUBE FEEDING

1. Severe protein and/or calorie malnutrition
2. Anorexia
3. Fractures or neoplasms of head and neck, preventing oral intake
4. Neurologic or psychiatric disorders, preventing oral intake
5. Coma or depressed mental state
6. Serious illness with very high metabolic requirements (burns)
7. Enterocutaneous fistulas
8. Short bowel syndrome
9. Bowel preparation for surgery in seriously ill or malnourished patients
10. Crohn's disease
11. Type I glycogen storage disease
12. Chemotherapy or radiotherapy
13. Renal or hepatic failure

Contraindications

Patients in whom there are contraindications to nasoenteric tube feedings include those with

- complete or incomplete gastric or intestinal obstruction
- severe gastroesophageal reflux (especially nasogastric feeding)
- ileus

In patients needing long-term enteral feedings, esophagostomy, gastrostomy,
or jejunostomy is the preferable procedure, although nasoenteric tube feedings have been used with success for periods up to 18 months. Alert patients
with intact gag reflexes and no pulmonary disease generally do well with
nasogastric feeding. Those with gastroparesis or delayed gastric emptying
and those who are at increased risk for aspiration or have just had surgery
should be fed into the duodenum or jejunum.

Implementation

The procedure for inserting nasoenteric tubes is detailed in Table 11–4.
Required supplies include the tube, 10- and 50-ml syringes, lubricant, emesis
basin, stethoscope, towel, tissues, alcohol sponges, cup of water with straw,
benzoin, and nonallergenic tape. Metoclopramide (10 mg every 6 hours) may
be given to stimulate gastric emptying if the tube does not pass spontaneously
into the duodenum after 8 to 24 hours. The patient's head must be elevated to
prevent regurgitation while tube feeding is being carried out. Gastric residuals should be checked and must not exceed 150 ml. If the patient develops

**Table 11-4. PROCEDURE FOR INSERTING
NASOENTERIC TUBE**

1. Provide privacy.
2. Explain procedure and purpose.
3. Place patient in sitting position or elevate head of bed to 45 degrees. Flex patient's neck slightly.
4. Stiffen tube by cooling in ice water.
5. Lubricate stylet and insert into feeding tube.
6. Determine nostril with optimal patency.
7. Estimate distance to stomach—measure from tip of nose to earlobe, earlobe to xiphoid, +50 cm.
8. Lubricate end of tube. Pass it with patient swallowing water using a straw.
9. Advance tube with patient's neck flexed and while patient swallows.
10. Patient may rest when tube is past nasopharynx.
11. If patient coughs, withdraw tube into nasopharynx and repass.
12. Confirm position in stomach by aspiration of gastric contents and abdominal radiogram.
13. Place patient in right lateral decubitus position if tube is to enter the duodenum. Confirm location of tube by radiogram.
14. Remove stylet.
15. Secure tube with tape to forehead, cheek, nose, or upper lip.
16. Begin feeding.
17. Document in chart.

severe diarrhea that is unresponsive to antidiarrheal agents, tube feedings may be temporarily discontinued and usually restarted in 48 hours.

Monitoring and Complications

Monitoring of metabolic status and fluid and electrolyte balance comparable to that recommended for those receiving parenteral nutrition (Table 12-6) is necessary in tube-fed patients. The complications of enteral alimentation may be gastrointestinal, metabolic, infectious, mechanical, and/or psychologic. They can be treated easily and should be prevented with appropriate monitoring. Nausea, vomiting, and diarrhea are the most common gastrointestinal complications, said to occur in 10 to 20 percent of patients.

Nausea and Vomiting

Potential causes of nausea and vomiting include

- smell of the formula, especially the elemental products
- high osmolality leading to gastric retention

- rapid rate of infusion
- lactose intolerance
- excessive fat (exceeding 30 to 40 percent of total calories)

Nausea and vomiting may be prevented or managed by

- adding flavorings and using polymeric formulas whenever possible
- diluting hyperosmolar formulas to isotonic strength, then slowly increasing the concentration over several days, or using isotonic formulas
- infusing into the stomach at 40 to 50 ml per hour and into the small intestine at 20 to 25 ml per hour, and advancing by 25 ml per hour every 12 to 24 hours if tolerated
- using lower-lactose or non–lactose-containing formulas, especially in patients predisposed to lactose intolerance (see Chapter 21)

Diarrhea

Factors that may cause diarrhea include

- hyperosmolality
- lactase deficiency
- fat malabsorption
- cold feedings
- protein malnutrition

Diarrhea may be treated or prevented by

- using isotonic or hypertonic solutions diluted to isotonic strength, with controlled slow infusion and gradual increments
- using low lactose or low fat products in situations of lactose intolerance or fat malabsorption
- infusing refrigerated formulas initially at a slow rate until formula has warmed to room temperature (however, some clinicians advocate keeping formula chilled while hanging)
- slowing infusion rate to 20 to 25 ml per hour
- using antidiarrheal agents

Factors independent of the enteral formula that may cause diarrhea should be investigated and appropriate treatment administered. If no cause can be identified, tube feedings should be discontinued, slowed, or diluted for 24 to 48 hours and slowly advanced. Peripheral parenteral nutrition may be used in the interval (see Chapter 12).

Constipation

Constipation may be caused by dehydration, impaction, or obstruction. Fluid intake must be greater than output by 500 to 1000 ml, or more in the febrile patient.

Metabolic Complications

Metabolic complications encountered in tube feeding include excess or lack of water, sugar, potassium, phosphorus, sodium, or magnesium and lack of vitamin K or essential fatty acid. In order of decreasing frequency, the most common (more than 10 percent of patients) are

- hyperkalemia
- hyponatremia
- hypophosphatemia
- overhydration
- hyperglycemia
- hyperphosphatemia
- zinc deficiency

These complications may be prevented or treated by

- controlling the infusion rate
- switching to another type of formula
- providing supplements
- restricting water
- monitoring intake, output, and clinical status
- checking electrolytes daily as feedings are initiated, and at least weekly when flow rate is established
- using formulas with a higher percentage of fat, if not contraindicated

Metabolic complications are common in patients with renal failure, especially when associated with metabolic acidosis.

Aspiration and Infection

Aspiration pneumonia and contamination of the formula are the most common infectious complications. Aspiration of stomach contents in patients who are obtunded or who have decreased ability to close the glottis (patients with tracheostomy or endotracheal tube) may be subtle. Any combination of tachypnea, tachycardia, fever, hypoxemia, and pulmonary infiltrate should be considered evidence of aspiration. Aspiration of a large volume may produce acute pulmonary edema. Aspiration is less likely when the head of the bed is elevated 30 degrees at all times. More dilute, nasojejunal feedings may be preferable to minimize aspiration and its adverse consequences. Vigorous coughing or vomiting may dislodge a tube placed beyond the pylorus, increasing the risk of aspiration. A residual that is 10 to 20 percent greater than the hourly flow is an indication to stop feeding in patients who are continuously fed.

Treatment of aspiration includes correction of hypotension or sequestration of fluids within the alveoli, as well as mechanical ventilation using positive pressure early on. The role of steroids and prophylactic antibiotics is controversial. Appropriate cultures and institution of antibiotics are warranted when purulent sputum is observed.

Formulas are easily contaminated by personnel who place them in the delivery system, but the potential for contamination can be minimized by use of proper sterile technique and prefilled pouches or canned rather than mixed formulas. Enteral formulas can probably hang for 8 to 12 hours at room temperature without clinically significant contamination, although cultures are positive from 40 to 60 percent of the time and a 4-hour hang time is preferable. The delivery system—with the exception of the feeding tube—should be changed every 24 hours.

Mechanical Complications

Mechnical complications of tube feeding are reduced considerably with use of fine-bore, soft, mercury-weighted tubes. The tube may be inadvertently inserted into the trachea. Perforations are rare with silicone tubes but may occur with polyvinyl and polypropylene tubes. Clogging is more likely when the internal diameter of the tube is less than 2 mm. Blenderized diets or those with fibers are not recommended for use with such small tubes. Tubes should be irrigated either after bolus feeding or once or twice daily when the infusion is continuous.

ENTEROSTOMIES

Tube enterostomy delivers nutrient formulas via the stomach, jejunum, pharynx, or cervical esophagus. This route is indicated when the nasoenteric route is unavailable or when enteral alimentation is prolonged. Tubes are usually placed surgically as a primary procedure, or in conjunction with gastrointestinal surgery. Percutaneous endoscopic gastrostomy and jejunostomy procedures have become available more recently and obviate the need for surgery.

Gastrostomy is the most common method of feeding by tube enterostomy and is used in patients who have normal gastric and duodenal function and intact gag reflexes, but who do not have significant esophageal reflux. Gastrostomy is contraindicated in patients at high risk of aspiration.

Jejunostomy is commonly used for feeding in conjunction with other abdominal surgical procedures and when gastrostomy is contraindicated. Feeding by jejunostomy can be instituted 1 day following major abdominal surgery. A tube can be inserted into the pharynx or cervical esophagus and passed into the stomach for feeding patients undergoing head and neck surgery.

Bolus feedings into the stomach can be carried out at home in enterostomy patients, with a low complication rate. Bolus feedings may begin by introducing 50 to 100 ml of isotonic or slightly hypotonic formula every 3 hours. The formula should be increased by 50 ml every one or two feedings up to a maximum of 250 to 300 ml every 3 to 4 hours, followed by an increase to full strength. Patients should not recline for at least 2 hours following a bolus feeding.

CHAPTER 12

Parenteral Nutritional Support

Advances in technology over the past two decades have made it possible to provide all the nutrients needed daily by the parenteral route, so-called total parenteral nutrition (TPN). Access is via a central vein that permits introduction of hypertonic nutrient solutions, hence the term hyperalimentation. TPN may be continued over long periods, usually at home. Alternatively, nutritional needs may be only partially provided by the intravenous route, complementing oral or enteral intake. This form of parenteral feeding usually is provided through a peripheral vein.

INDICATIONS

The indication for TPN is unavailability of the enteral route for either voluntary eating or involuntary delivery of nutrients via enteral tube feeding (see Chapter 11). Candidates for parenteral nutrition include previously adequately nourished, minimally stressed patients expected not to resume adequate enteral intake for 7 to 14 days. Elderly patients should be considered for intravenous nutrition support if the anticipated period of limited nutrient is 5 days or longer (see Chapter 9).

- The gastrointestinal tract may be obstructed, diseased, excised, or otherwise nonfunctional or inaccessible for handling nutrients.
- Nutritional needs for repletion or treatment of severe malnutrition or a catabolic state (e.g., burns) may exceed the capability of the oral or enteral route.
- Oral intake may be contraindicated in treating a diseased gastrointestinal tract, as in Crohn's disease (see Chapter 21), or bowel rest may be prescribed in the healing of a pancreatic pseudocyst (see Chapter 22).

The oral/enteral route is preferable to the intravenous for a number of reasons, including safety and cost: TPN costs 4 to 10 times as much as tube feeding, apart from the hospitalization required to initiate, and/or special supervision for long-term at-home TPN. Nonetheless, administration of TPN permits better treatment of some diseases, allows some patients to survive who would otherwise die, permits patients who otherwise would not be candidates for surgery to undergo surgical procedures with healing of wounds and recovery, and provides a form of high level nutritional support that may reduce morbidity and mortality in the hospital and shorten the hospital stay. Safe, appropriate use of TPN requires coordination and application of the skills of a team consisting of physician, pharmacist, nurse, and dietitian, with compulsive attention to detail through the entire process. Procedures and policies should be known and strictly followed not only by this team but also by the hospital staff.

THE PRESCRIPTION

The usual procedures of nutritional assessment must be followed (see Chapter 3) to arrive at a nutritional prescription, specifically of calories and protein (and fluid), that also provides for any specific increased nutrient needs, special requirements, or contraindications.

Determining the Formulation

The tolerated or required daily fluid level must be determined, permitting derivation of the formulation to provide this therapy. Solutions of dextrose (to provide calories) and amino acids (for nitrogen/protein) are mixed, and appropriate electrolytes, vitamins, and trace minerals are added. A solution of lipid emulsion also provides a source of calories and essential fatty acids.

The central intravenous route will permit infusion of hypertonic solutions, such as 35 percent glucose. However, feeding cannot be initiated with 3 liters of such a solution—providing 1050 g glucose—owing to the adverse metabolic effect of the sudden introduction of such a high glucose load. The TPN regimen is therefore ordered with stepwise increment of nutrients until the goal is reached. This approach assumes that the patient is relatively stable. Unfortunately, many patients given TPN are severely, acutely ill, often in intensive care units, with multiple organ failure influencing their nutritional needs. The art of TPN thus requires tailoring the nutritional prescription to the medical, as well as the nutritional, needs of the patient.

ROUTES OF ADMINISTRATION

The site of parenteral infusion of nutrients (central or peripheral) depends on the calorie level and source, fluid tolerance, and vascular access.

- Central TPN should not be carried out without experienced personnel and appropriate facilities.
- Peripheral parenteral nutrition (PPN) is of limited value as the sole source of nutritional support, since in usual circumstances, calories are limited to a maximum of 1500 to 2000 daily.

Central

Parenteral hyperalimentation through a central vein can deliver greater nutrient loads via hypertonic solutions because blood flow in the superior vena cava rapidly dilutes these solutions more than 1000-fold. Central infusion usually is mandatory when the use of lipid emulsions as a source of calories is contraindicated or when fluid volume must be limited.

Peripheral

Solutions infused through a peripheral vein must be of appropriate osmolarity to avoid sclerosing the vein and stimulating development of thrombophlebitis. Osmolarity is determined by the sum of the concentrations of glucose, amino acids, and electrolytes. Lipid solutions are relatively isotonic; their infusion simultaneously with the glucose–amino acid–electrolyte solution reduces the osmolarity. We do not recommend use of heparin or corticosteroids specifically for the purpose of preventing thrombophlebitis from infusing higher concentrations of glucose (exceeding 10 percent) into a peripheral vein. The intravenous site should be changed every 48 hours.

INITIATING TPN

Central vein access requires placement of a catheter, a surgical procedure that must be carried out using aseptic technique. Meticulous attention must be given to skin preparation at the insertion site to prevent sepsis. The TPN line ideally should not be used for other purposes. The procedure initiating TPN is carried out in a surgical suite or clean treatment room. In long-term infusion, catheters are placed at distant sites and tunneled, as for home TPN or when using Hickman catheters. Central vein access may involve either the subclavian or external or internal jugular vein, with the subclavian vein preferred to facilitate dressing changes. Subclavian vein catheterization also permits the patient free movement of the arm and neck. The procedure for central vein catheterization is detailed in Table 12–1.

Institution of TPN is never an emergency procedure. Depending on institutional rules, orders for nutrient solutions may not be processed around the clock. Once the central line is in place, 10 percent glucose can be infused until orders for TPN are filled.

The specific parenteral nutrition solution is prepared in the pharmacy, with additions and mixing done under a laminar flow hood. Solution bottles not in use are stored refrigerated and protected from light. The intravenous tubing is fitted with an in-line filter to stop air, particulate matter, and most microorganisms; this line is used for the glucose–amino acid solution. Intravenous fat emulsions should not be filtered. The administration set should be changed every 24 hours. Extension tubing is changed at the time of dressing change (usually thrice weekly). To avoid air embolism, the patient should perform the Valsalva maneuver when either the administration set or extension tubing is changed. In the patient who cannot cooperate, tubing should

Table 12-1. PROCEDURE FOR CATHETERIZATION OF
SUBCLAVIAN VEIN FOR TOTAL PARENTERAL NUTRITION

1. Equipment:
   TPN solutions
   Normal saline
   IV tubing
   Administration set with in-line filter for glucose-amino acid solution
   Extension set
   Fat emulsion administration set
   Catheter
   Venesection tray: syringes, needles, sponges, scissors, medicine glasses,
      drapes/towels, skin needles, needle holder, silk
   Skin preparation: tincture of benzoin, 70% isopropanol, iodophor solution,
      razor, soap
   Xylocaine, 0.5% without epinephrine
   Sterile surgical supplies: gloves, masks (gown, head cover optional)
   Adhesive
   IVAC pump
2. Adequate lighting.
3. Instruct patient in Valsalva maneuver; practice.
4. Shave, if necessary.
5. Place in Trendelenberg position, head down 15 degrees.
   Position patient supine with small roll of towels medial to scapula.
   Turn head away from side of catheterization.
6. Use aseptic technique. Mask patient.
7. Establish sterile field, provide solutions, catheters, IV fluids, tubing (flushed).
8. Cleanse skin.
9. Drape area.
10. Anesthetize skin, periosteum of clavicle, and first rib.
11. Insert catheter using syringe with negative pressure attached to needle directed
    beneath clavicle aiming toward sternal notch.
12. When venous blood is obtained, instruct patient to perform Valsalva
    maneuver, detach syringe, insert catheter through introducer needle (tell
    patient to breathe). Advance catheter several centimeters. Place patient
    head up, with head tilted toward catheter.
13. Connect catheter to IV tubing, check blood flow.
14. Suture catheter.
15. Cover site, hub/extension tubing connection with air occlusive dressing using
    tincture of benzoin, gauze.
16. Tape all connections not secured with Luer lock.

be changed at the beginning of expiration. Connections should be taped if there is no Luer lock.

A closed system of infusion of parenteral nutrition solutions through the central venous catheter is mandatory to reduce the potential for sepsis. The central line must not be used for obtaining blood samples, for measurements of central venous pressure, or for administration of medications, blood, albumin, or other substances. Any violation of the line should be justified by written order on the patient's chart.

Nutrient solutions are infused by pump at a constant rate. Delays in delivery should not be compensated for; that is, there is no catch-up. Glucose–amino acid solution bottles should be changed at least every 24 hours. The 500 ml bottle of lipid emulsion should be infused for no longer than 12 hours.

When TPN is terminated—or if the infusion solution is interrupted for any reason—10 percent glucose should be administered at the same infusion rate for at least 3 or 4 hours. A blood culture should be obtained through the catheter before it is removed, and the catheter then removed aseptically and portions of the tip sent for culture.

Nutrient solutions infused through a peripheral vein should be prepared in a manner similar to those for central TPN. Maintenance and care of intravenous tubing and dressings also are similar, except that dressings are changed when the site is changed. Administration of peripheral infusions by pump at a constant rate also is preferred.

REQUIREMENTS

All essential nutrients—water, energy, protein (essential amino acids), essential fatty acids, minerals (electrolytes, trace minerals), vitamins—must be provided in TPN (see Chapters 1, 2, and 14).

Energy

Energy requirements are influenced by body size, gender, age, level of activity, and underlying disease and nutritional state. The resting energy expenditure is increased by the stress factor of the specific illness (see Chapter 3). The calorie level is increased if the goal is to replete the underweight or marasmic patient.

The bulk of the calories (60 to 80 percent) is supplied by the dextrose solution. Because the glucose is hydrated, dextrose in intravenous solutions provides 3.4 kcal per g (instead of the usual 4). The caloric value and osmolality of dextrose concentrations commonly used for mixing or delivery in TPN are listed in Table 12-2. The optimum ratio of carbohydrate to fat calories in

Table 12-2. DEXTROSE SOLUTIONS

Concentration, %	Kcal/l	mOsm/l
5	170	252
10	340	505
20	680	1010
25	850	1267
30	1020	1515
35	1190	1764
40	1360	2020
50	1700	2520
60	2040	3030
70	2380	3530

TPN has not been determined. In the severely stressed patient, however, glucose should provide at least 80 percent of basal energy requirements.

Lipid

Lipid emulsions provide 1.1 (10 percent concentration) or 2 kcal per ml (20 percent concentration) because of their lipid (9 kcal per g) and glycerol content. Lipid emulsions in concentrations of 10 and 20 percent are derived from soybean oil or safflower oil or both; the emulsions also contain egg phospholipids and varying amounts of cholesterol. The composition of some products is shown in Table 12-3. While the requirement for essential fatty acid may be met by weekly provision of 500 ml of a 10 percent fat emulsion, it is recommended that at least 20 percent of daily energy requirements be provided as lipid. The FDA allows up to 60 percent of calories to be provided as lipid administered intravenously (see Chapter 14 for a description of the symptoms and signs of essential fatty acid deficiency).

Fat emulsions are contraindicated in patients with allergy to eggs or with hypertriglyceridemia, especially chylomicronemia. Plasma lipids should be measured prior to the administration of any fat emulsion, or at minimum the standing plasma test should be performed. Lipid emulsions must be used with caution in patients with severe pulmonary disease (adult respiratory distress syndrome), coagulopathy, or severe thrombocytopenia. After a test dose of 50 ml of a 10 percent fat emulsion is infused over 1 hour, the lipid emulsion can be infused at maximum rates of 125 ml per hour for the 10 percent solution, and 60 ml per hour for the 20 percent solution (central). Lipid emulsions usually are infused at slower rates in peripheral veins (500 ml per 12 hours). Some TPN regimens require that lipid solutions be infused only via peripheral vein. It now is possible to add the lipid to the 3 liter bags now

Table 12-3. SOME INTRAVENOUS FAT EMULSIONS

Fat	PL*	Glycerol	Concentration, % Kcal/l	Osmolality, mOsm
10	1.2	2.4	1100	280–300
20			2000	330–340

		Composition				
			Fatty Acid, %			
Fat Source	Cholesterol	Palmitic 16:0	Stearic 18:0	Oleic 18:1	Linoleic 18:2	Linolenic 18:3
Soybean oil	19–31 mg/dl	9	3	26	54	8
Safflower oil/ soybean oil	5–12 mg/dl	9	3	18	66	4

*PL = phospholipid

available for delivering the TPN mixture (3 in 1 total nutrient admixture, or TNA system).

Protein

Protein requirements are determined in the course of nutritional assessment, with protein status indicated by anthropometric measurements (mid-arm muscle circumference) and appropriate blood or urine tests, or nitrogen balance (see Chapters 1 and 3). Nitrogen for parenteral nutrition is usually supplied in the form of solutions of L–amino acids (except glycine) in which essential and nonessential amino acids are mixed. Solutions are usually packaged in 500 ml bottles, with the amino acid concentration varying between 5 and 15 percent. The composition of some amino acid solutions is detailed in Table 12–4. The nutritional benefit of administering albumin as a protein source is questionable, and the product is expensive. The usual glucose–amino acid solution is prepared by mixing the amino acid solution with a stock solution of dextrose, usually 50 to 70 percent. Orders are usually written in terms of the final concentration to be administered. The most economic preparation of 1 liter solutions mixes an entire bottle of glucose solution with a full bottle of amino acid solution. The day's infusion also can be made up in a plastic bag holding up to 3 liters and mixing the required amount from stock solutions.

Varying amounts of the individual amino acids are offered in commercial solutions. Special solutions enriched in branched chain amino acids or containing only essential amino acids (Table 12–4) are used in nutritional support of stressed patients and in patients with hepatic or renal failure.

TABLE 12–4. COMPOSITION OF SOME AMINO ACID FORMULATIONS

Amino acids, % of total content	Formulation								
	Aminosyn (Abbott)	FreAmine III (McGaw)	Travasol (Travenol)	Travasol (Travenol)	NephrAmine (McGaw)	RenAmin (Travenol)	Aminosyn-RF (Abbott)	HepatAmine (McGaw)	FreAmine HBC (McGaw)
Essential									
Branched chain { Isoleucine	7.3	7.0	4.8	6.0	10.4	7.7	8.9	11.2	11.0
Leucine	9.5	9.2	6.2	7.3	16.3	9.2	14.0	13.8	19.9
Valine	8.1	6.7	4.6	5.8	11.9	12.6	10.2	10.6	12.8
Lysine (salt)	7.3	10.3	5.8	5.8	16.7	6.9	10.3	7.6	5.9
Methionine	4.0	5.4	5.8	4.0	16.3	11.2	14.0	1.2	3.6
Phenylalanine	4.4	5.7	6.2	5.6	16.3	7.5	14.0	1.2	4.6
Threonine	5.3	4.0	4.2	4.2	7.4	5.8	6.3	5.6	2.9
Tryptophan	1.6	1.5	1.8	1.8	3.7	2.5	3.2	0.8	1.3
Nonessential									
Alanine	12.9	7.2	20.7	20.7	—	8.6	—	9.6	5.8
Arginine*	9.9	9.6	10.4	11.5	—	9.7	11.5	7.5	8.4
Histidine*	3.0	2.8	4.4	4.8	4.6	6.5	8.3	3.0	2.3
Proline	8.7	11.3	4.2	6.8	—	5.4	—	10.0	9.1
Serine	4.3	6.0	—	5.0	—	4.6	—	6.2	4.8
Tyrosine	0.7	—	0.4	0.4	—	0.6	—	—	—
Glycine	12.9	14.2	20.7	10.3	—	4.6	—	11.2	4.8
Cysteine	—	0.2	—	—	0.4	—	—	0.2	—
Available concentrations, %	5, 7, 8.5, 10	8.5, 10	†5.5, 8.5	10	5.4	6.5	5.2	8.0	6.9
Aliquot size, ml	500	500	500	250	250	300	500	750	—

*Considered essential in renal failure.
†Available without or with electrolytes.
Travenol also makes a solution (Aminess) for patients with renal failure that contains essential amino acids with histidine (5.2%, 400 ml).
Abbott also makes a high-branched chain formulation (Aminosyn-HBC 7%).

Amino acids provide 4 kcal per g. The usual parenteral nutrition solutions provide 1 to 2 g protein per kg ideal body weight daily. The solutions are usually administered in final concentrations of 4.25 to 5 percent for central TPN and in final concentration of 2.125 percent for peripheral infusion.

Fluid

The fluid requirement must provide for adequate urine excretion and must replace insensible losses (see Chapter 1). The renal solute load, which determines urine volume, is itself determined by the nitrogen and electrolyte load. The usual renal solute load is approximately 600 mOsm. Since the healthy kidney can concentrate urine to 1200 mOsm per liter, 500 ml of urine should be a sufficient volume. The patient receiving TPN may excrete a larger volume of urine because of a higher solute load resulting from catabolism of protein, provision of high protein levels in the TPN solutions to provide for anabolism, or because of impaired renal concentrating ability.

Insensible fluid losses in patients with burns, tachypnea, or fever may also be higher than the usual 500 to 1000 ml daily. An additional 360 ml of fluid is lost daily for each degree centigrade of fever. Extra fluid losses from diarrhea, nasogastric suction, and fistula and wound drainage must be considered in calculating fluid requirements. These losses also add to electrolyte requirements. (See also Chapters 2 and 21, and Tables 2-4 and 2-6.)

Daily body weights and intake and output volumes are needed to calculate fluid requirements. Fluid shifts that result when muscle tissue is broken down or replaced, or when glucose or fat is oxidized, must also be considered. Edema is observed when there is an excess of interstitial fluid of 3 to 5 kg or more. Retained fluid will be excreted with correction of hypoproteinemia; thus, the patient may experience weight loss despite increase in lean body mass or adipose tissue. Edema may occur also as a result of refeeding (see Chapter 13).

Minerals

Usual daily requirements for trace minerals and electrolytes are shown in Table 2-4, and electrolyte content of body fluids in Table 2-6. Needed trace minerals and electrolytes may be provided by incorporating them into the TPN glucose–amino acid solution or by infusing them through a peripheral site. The basic solutions have some electrolyte and mineral content, which varies with the product. In addition, electrolyte packs that contain mixtures of varying amounts of some minerals are available.

Sodium, Chloride, and Potassium

The sodium requirements (approximately 100 mEq per day) is usually met in the form of sodium chloride plus sodium lactate, sodium phosphate, or sodium acetate. Edema may be a sign of excessive body sodium, while sodium depletion may be manifested by unexplained weight loss. Serum sodium levels are not always reliable indicators of body sodium status; serum sodium levels also indicate the status of body water. Chloride is provided as sodium chloride and potassium chloride. Requirements for potassium provided as chloride, phosphate, or acetate, average about 100 mEq daily when an anabolic regimen is being administered. Provision of glucose solutions with resultant entry into cells also drives potassium intracellularly. The requirements for potassium are increased in the first few days of provision of hypertonic, high concentrations of glucose. Potassium is also used in protein synthesis, along with nitrogen. Severe hypokalemia is averted in part by a gradual increase over several days to the full calorie-protein regimen. Serum potassium levels should be closely monitored, especially in patients with impaired renal function (see Chapter 23).

Phosphorus

Phosphorus also shifts into the cell during anabolism because of incorporation into tissue protein. Adequate phosphorus should therefore be provided in anticipation of such shifts. Hypophosphatemia is the most common acute mineral complication of the TPN regimen and may be life-threatening (see also Chapter 14). Phosphorus may be provided in the form of a monobasic or dibasic salt; for this reason, phosphorus orders should be written in quantities of milligrams or millimoles, rather than milliequivalents. The initial TPN regimen in patients with normal renal function should prescribe 1200 to 1500 mg (40 to 50 millimoles) phosphorus daily; 20 to 40 millimoles daily should suffice for maintenance.

Calcium

Even if calcium is not provided in the daily TPN regimen, hypocalcemia is rare because calcium can be mobilized from bone. Provision of 10 to 20 mEq calcium per day (as gluceptate) will minimize bone resorption. Hypocalcemia can result from hyperphosphatemia, magnesium deficiency, or bicarbonate infusion (see Chapter 14). Hypercalcemia and bone disease in TPN resulting from vitamin D administration are discussed under the section on Complications, p. 299.

Magnesium

Magnesium should be provided daily (20 mEq), as the sulfate, for patients with normal renal function.

Acidosis and Alkalosis

Metabolic acidosis should be managed by adding acetate rather than bicarbonate to the TPN solution, as bicarbonate may precipitate with any added calcium, and its buffering capacity may be decreased by formation of CO_2. Metabolic alkalosis may be managed with addition of sodium, potassium, or ammonium chloride, or 0.1 N hydrochloric acid.

Trace Minerals

Trace mineral status is not easily evaluated (see Chapters 2 and 14). The precise requirements for trace minerals when administered by the intravenous route are unknown; they are estimated at less than the RDA, or the safe, adequate intakes for the oral route. Trace element deficiency will develop in patients receiving TPN for prolonged periods without supplementation. Since most patients receiving TPN are either stressed or malnourished and presumably depleted of micronutrients, it is appropriate from the beginning to include some or all of the required trace minerals in the TPN regimen.

Zinc. The daily maintenance requirement for zinc administered intravenously is estimated at 2.5 to 4 mg. The catabolic patient requires 2 mg more than that amount daily; zinc losses from small bowel fistulas or suction are about 12 mg per liter, while stool losses amount to 17 mg per kg. These losses, seen most commonly in the clinical setting in patients with Crohn's disease—almost half of whom have low zinc levels—should be anticipated and repleted. (Crohn's disease is discussed in Chapter 21.)

Copper. Copper should also be provided daily but should be administered with caution in patients with extrahepatic biliary obstruction, prolonged intrahepatic cholestasis, or cirrhosis. Requirements in premature infants are especially high (see Chapter 8).

Additional Trace Minerals. Manganese, chromium, molybdenum, and selenium supplements are also included as part of the daily TPN regimen in additive preparations that provide amounts considered adequate for maintenance. Specific supplementation of iodine usually is not necessary, although some trace mineral combinations contain iodine.

Iron

Iron is not routinely added to TPN solutions, since iron overload or sequestration is a common accompaniment of chronic disease (see Chapter 15), and its administration may worsen disease processes as well as be contraindicated in the presence of some infections. Nonetheless, some patients receiving TPN may be iron deficient and require supplementation; these patients are best identified by measurement of serum ferritin levels (see Chapter 15).

Vitamins

All vitamins except vitamin K can be provided in a mixture for intravenous use that meets daily requirements in patients with no contraindications (Table 2–4). Vitamin K (10 mg) can be provided weekly in parenteral form. Mixtures containing only water-soluble vitamins for intravenous use at levels that meet or exceed daily requirements are not readily available. The malnourished, nutritionally depleted patient—especially the alcoholic—may require increased amounts of B vitamins for repletion and should be presumed deficient in these nutrients. These patients may be prescribed multivitamins and specific water-soluble vitamins daily. Vitamins A and D may be contraindicated in patients with renal failure, so that only water-soluble vitamins should be administered. Micronutrients—trace minerals and vitamins—usually are added to the day's first bottle of glucose–amino acid solution if liter bottles are used in the regimen.

Insulin

Insulin may be added to the glucose–amino acid solution for continuous infusion. Supplementary insulin may be provided by subcutaneous or intramuscular injection, or infused continuously through a peripheral vein.

ORDERS

TPN orders are written daily, using a particular form (Fig. 12–1A and B) for TPN or TNA. Table 12–5 details the procedure for writing orders for a hypothetical patient prescribed total intravenous feeding because of an episode of recurrent acute pancreatitis. A 50-year-old afebrile male, his height is 170 cm (68 in) and his body weight of 56 kg is 80 percent of ideal. Triceps skinfold measurement is 9 mm (70 percent of standard), and mid-arm muscle circumference measures 22.2 cm (87 percent of standard). Bowel sounds are absent and the abdomen is tender. Nasogastric suction yields 700 ml bile-tinged secretion daily. Urine output is "adequate." Serum albumin is 2.5 g per dl. The regimen prescribed in Table 12–5 meets fluid, protein, and energy needs. Catheter care is prescribed to meet requirements to avoid infection.

A

DAILY PARENTERAL NUTRITION ORDER SHEET FOR ADULTS

Please prescribe enough TPN to last for 24 hours.

REPEAT YESTERDAYS TPN FLUID & RATE (absolutely no changes): ☐

ADMINISTRATION ROUTE: ☐ Central ☐ Peripheral   PN DAY#_____

AMINO ACID SOURCE: ☐ Regular ☐ Other_____

SUPPLY AMINO ACIDS: (final concentration) _____% or total _____Gm

SUPPLY DEXTROSE: (final concentration) _____% or total _____Gm
(Note: 3.4Kcal/Gm x Grams of Dextrose = Kcal total)

FINAL VOLUME: _____ml   RUN AT A RATE OF: _____ml/hr

ADDITIVES:

    ELECTROLYTE PACK I _____ml (The average anabolic dose is 1ml/kg/day.)
       Each 25ml contains Sodium 25mEq, Potassium 20mEq, Magnesium 5mEq, Calcium
       5mEq, Chloride 30mEq, Acetate 25mEq.

    ELECTROLYTE PACK II_____ml (The average anabolic dose is 1ml/kg/day.)
       Each 25ml contains Sodium 25mEq, Potassium 40mEq, Magnesium 8mEq, Calcium
       5mEq, Chloride 33mEq, Gluconate 5mEq, Acetate 41mEq.

☐ SODIUM AS: Chloride_____mEq   Acetate_____mEq   Phosphate_____mEq

☐ POTASSIUM AS: Chloride_____mEq   Acetate_____mEq   Phosphate_____mEq

☐ CALCIUM AS: Chloride_____mEq   Gluconate_____mEq

☐ MAGNESIUM AS: Sulfate_____mEq

☐ TRACE ELEMENT PACKAGE (Contains Zinc 3mg and Copper 1.2mg)

☐ MULTIPLE VITAMIN INFUSION (MVI-12) 10ml

OTHER: _____   _____

      _____   _____

      _____   _____

      _____   _____

IV FAT EMULSION __ 10% __ 20% _____ml over _____hrs at _____ml/hr _____Kcal total
(Lipid 10% = 1.1Kcal/ml; Lipid 20% = 2Kcal/ml -- Run 10% over 6-12 hrs & 20% over
8-12 hrs)

See reverse side for additional information and other available products.

	For Nurse's Use	
	Time Needed:	Signature:

_____ _____ _____
Physician's Signature   Beeper#   Date/Time

For Pharmacy Use Only		
Calculations By:_____ Date & Time Prepared:_____	Prepared By:_____	
Base Solution:_____ Additives:_____R.Ph. Label:_____R.Ph. Lipids:_____R.Ph.		

PS 960 Rev. 12/87

Figure 12–1. *A* and *B,* Sample hospital forms for parenteral nutrition.

B   RECOMMENDED DAILY REQUIREMENTS FOR ELECTROLYTES

```
Sodium......................60-180mEq
Potassium...................60-180mEq
Calcium......................5-30mEq
Magnesium....................8-24mEq
Phosphate...................10-20mM
```

MULTIVITAMIN MIX-12 (Abbott or USV) 10ml PROVIDES:

```
Vitamin A...................3300 I.U.(1mg)
Vitamin D....................200 I.U.(5mcg)
Vitamin E.....................10 I.U.(10mg)
Vitamin C....................100mg
Niacin........................40mg
Vitamin B2.................3.6-4.93mg
Vitamin B1...................3-3.35mg
Vitamin B6...................4-4.86mg
Dexpanthenol.................15mg
Folic Acid..................400mcg
Vitamin B12...................5mcg
Biotin.......................60mcg
```

TRACE ELEMENTS

Consult your hospital formulary for other trace elements
which may be needed in cases of severe malnutrition or long
term TPN.

PHOSPHATE

Phosphate is available as sodium or potassium salts. When
ordering sodium (as phosphate) for each 4mEq of sodium, 3mM
of phosphate are supplied. When ordering potassium (as
phosphate) for each 4.4mEq of potassium, 3mM of phosphate
are supplied.

CONSULT YOUR PHARMACIST TO DETERMINE WHICH ANIONS AND
CATIONS ARE CONTAINED IN THE AMINO ACID SOLUTION CURRENTLY
BEI.G STOCKED IN THE PHARMACY

*The ADULT PARENTERAL NUTRITION ORDER SHEET was prepared
under the direction of the Nutrition Committee by authority
of the Executive Committee of the Medical Staff.*

Figure 12–1. *Continued.*

Physical therapy should be added to the regimen of all patients who are able to be physically active.

Because specific alterations in this regimen are required in differing disease states, all orders must be written to meet individual patient's daily needs. Requirements and provisions in renal failure (Chapter 23), hepatic failure (Chapter 22), trauma and sepsis, and in patients with cardiac or pulmonary disease (Chapter 25), are detailed elsewhere.

Renal Failure

Briefly, the patient with renal failure may require

- fluid restriction with use of the most concentrated solutions of dextrose (70 percent) and lipid (20 percent)
- a formula of essential amino acids

**Table 12–5. DEVELOP PRESCRIPTION
FOR TOTAL INTRAVENOUS FEEDING**

TASKS	EXAMPLES—How To; What
1. Determine IBW.	106 + 8 × 6 = 48 154 lb = 70 kg
2. Determine fluid requirements and tolerances.	*2000–3000* ml = "maintenance" if normal kidneys *700* ml = gastrointestinal replacement *500* ml = increased insensible losses (tachypnea) 360 ml/°C = *3200–4200* ml

3. Determine protein requirement.
    0.8 g/kg for maintenance
    1.5+ for anabolism
        extra for stress
	2 g/kg IBW × *70* kg (maintenance, anabolism, stress)
	
	= *140* g

4. Determine energy requirements.	*20* kcal/kg IBW for maintenance/activity *15* kcal/kg IBW for anabolism—for max N balance 25–50% above BEE = 5 kcal/kg IBW for stress = *40–45* kcal/kg × *70* kg = *2800*–3150 kcal/day
5. Determine desired percentage fat calories (usual 20%).	*500* ml 10% lipid emulsion provides *550* kcal (~20% of caloric needs) 12 hr = 40 ml/hr

6. Determine glucose calories.
    IV = 3.4 kcal/g
	2800 kcal total required
	550 kcal from lipid
	= *2250* kcal from glucose
	    divide by 3.4 kcal/g IV glucose
	= *662* g glucose

7. Order amino acid–glucose solution.	2700–3700 ml 662 g dextrose, 140 g amino acids/24 hr = *110*–150 ml/hr

(Continued)

Table 12-5. DEVELOP PRESCRIPTION
FOR TOTAL INTRAVENOUS FEEDING—Continued

TASKS		EXAMPLES—How To; What				
8. Add electrolytes based on preexisting deficiencies or excesses.	**Electrolyte**	**Needs (anabolic + NG replacement)*/day**				
	100 { Na, mEq	60–200	+	~60	=	120–260
	K, mEq	60–200	+	~6	=	66–206
	Cl, mEq	80–120	+	~70	=	150–190
	20 { Mg, mEq	8–20	+	—	=	8–20
	P, mMoles	13–26	+	—	=	13–26
	Ca, mEq	10–20	+	—	=	10–20
9. Add vitamins.		10 ml MVI-12 added each day. Suspect deficiency water soluble vitamins, add extra vitamins B and C.				
10. Add trace elements.	**Mineral**	**Needs (anabolic + GI replacement)/day**				
	Zn, mg	2.5–4.0	+	8.4	=	11–12
	Cu, mg	0.5–1.5	+	—	=	0.5-1.5
	Mn, mg	1-2	+	—	=	1-2
	Cr, µg	10–20	+	—	=	10–20
	Add each day.					
13. Order monitoring (see Table 25–6).						
14. Order catheter care.						
15. Order physical therapy—needed to replete somatic muscle.						

*Mixture of bile and gastric juice.

- varying amounts of protein, depending on treatment with hemodialysis or peritoneal dialysis
- possibly increased amounts of pyridoxine, folate, and vitamin C, avoidance of vitamin A, and intake of specific forms of vitamin D

The patient may also exhibit varying problems with dextrose (glucose intolerance) or lipid (hyperlipidemia), as well as specific electrolyte needs and acid-base problems.

Liver Disease

The patient with liver disease may require

- fluid and/or sodium restriction if hyponatremia or ascites is present
- protein restriction and use of an amino acid formula consisting of or enriched in branched chain amino acids, in the presence of encephalopathy
- increased amounts of fat- and/or water-soluble vitamins

Other Disease States

Fluid restriction may also be necessary in the cardiac patient, while fluid requirements in the ventilator-dependent patient may be increased. In the latter case the ratio of fat to glucose calories may need to be increased maximally to decrease metabolic rate, CO_2 production, and the respiratory quotient (RQ). Caloric needs may require revision in the patient with cardiac cachexia, while the ventilator-dependent patient needs adequate calories, with emphasis on fat as an energy source. Cardiac arrhythmias may be worsened with electrolyte imbalance. Hypophosphatemia increases the tendency to hypoxia in the presence of apparently adequate arterial blood gas values.

Monitoring

The patient receiving parenteral nutrition must be monitored daily. A schedule for blood chemistries, blood count, specific nutritional assessment parameters, intake, output, body weight, urine sugar and acetone, and prothrombin time is presented in Table 12–6. Appropriate adjustments must be

Table 12–6. MONITORING OF PATIENT RECEIVING PARENTERAL NUTRITION*

1. *Baseline* SMA-6, SMA-12, magnesium, triglycerides, prothrombin time, CBC with differential and platelet count (transferrin, prealbumin, nitrogen balance, vitamins, trace minerals in malnourished).
2. Strict intake and output throughout.
3. Weigh daily.
4. Urine for sugar and acetone q 6 h throughout (blood glucose if positive or in patient with renal failure).
5. SMA-6 daily until stable, then three times weekly.
6. SMA-12 daily until stable, then weekly.
7. Magnesium twice weekly until stable, then weekly.
8. CBC with differential and prothrombin time weekly.
9. Repeat triglyceride determination 3 to 4 hr after initial dose of lipids and weekly.
10. Nitrogen balance—24 hr urine for creatinine and urea nitrogen—biweekly if initial is negative or patient's condition is unstable; otherwise weekly.
11. Biweekly prealbumin.
12. Repeat vitamin/mineral tests and anthropometrics q 3 wk.

*In patients with acute metabolic problems, add serum lactate.

promptly made to prevent or treat complications. Parameters relating to blood sugar, lipids, and electrolytes need close attention in the early phase, and as the patient stabilizes, these measurements may be needed only weekly. Body weight must be obtained daily, but the other anthropometric measurements of calorie and protein stores change slowly and should be repeated only after several weeks (Fig. 12–2). While serum albumin changes slowly, except in response to fluid shifts, serum prealbumin levels rapidly reflect protein anabolism and therefore should be obtained twice weekly in severely stressed patients (see Chapters 13 and 25).

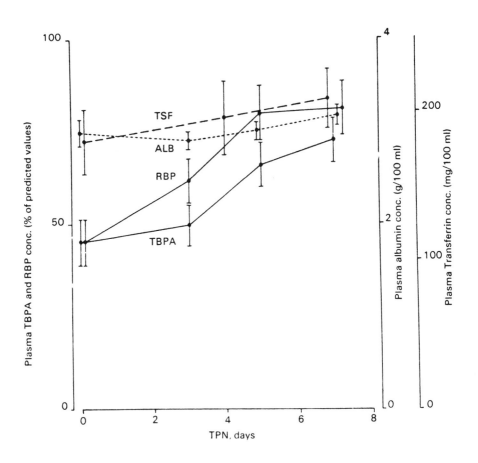

Figure 12–2. Response of nutritional assessment parameters in 10 patients to an effective TPN regimen. TSF = transferrin; ALB = albumin; RBP = retinol-binding protein; TBPA = thyroxine-binding prealbumin. (From Carpentier, Y.A., Barthel, G., and Bruyns, J: Assessment of nutritional status in man. Proc Nutr Soc 41:410, 1982, with permission of Cambridge University Press.)

COMPLICATIONS

Metabolic

Complications relating to provision of large amounts of dextrose intravenously include

- glucose intolerance
- hyperglycemia and glycosuria
- hyperosmolarity

Insulin secretion may be depressed or insulin resistance may be present even in the nondiabetic patient, especially in those with trauma or sepsis (see Chapter 25). Glucose intolerance is less likely when insulin secretion is gradually stimulated over a period of several days by progressive increments of glucose delivery. This is best accomplished by infusing lower concentrations of glucose initially. However, some regimens use concentrated solutions administered at lower flow rates. Such regimens may result in suboptimal delivery of amino acids and may not meet fluid needs unless these are provided by other routes.

Hyperglycemia with glycosuria is treated with insulin. If the patient continues to require a fixed amount of insulin, this should be prescribed as an addition to the TPN solution and added by the pharmacist. Most patients with mild hyperglycemia are controlled with the addition of 5 to 10 units of insulin per liter of TPN solution.

Electrolytes, Glucose, Calories, and Fat

Rapid shifts of potassium, phosphorus, and magnesium intracellularly with resultant lowering of their concentrations in serum are observed unless adequate or increased amounts of these electrolytes are included in the TPN regimen.

Provision of glucose in amounts that exceed caloric needs produces excessive amounts of CO_2 in the process of fat synthesis over and above glucose oxidation, thereby increasing the ventilatory load. This makes patients acidotic and increases difficulties in weaning them from respirators. Excess glucose (and calories generally) also increase the metabolic rate, and may precipitate cardiac as well as pulmonary failure. In addition, prolonged excess glucose increases hepatic steatosis, since fat is stored not only in adipose tissue but also in the liver. This may result in abnormal liver function tests and, in infants, leads to intrahepatic cholestasis, jaundice and biliary cirrhosis, and hepatic failure.

Excessive carbohydrate calories may produce hyperlipidemia from excessive release of very low density lipoproteins from the liver into the plasma.

**Table 12-7. COMPLICATIONS OF CENTRAL
VEIN CATHETERS, PLACEMENT,
INDWELLING, AND REMOVAL**

Air embolus
Arterial puncture
Arteriovenous fistulas
Brachial plexus injury
Cardiac perforation
Catheter embolus
Chylothorax
Hemothorax
Hemorrhage
Hydrothorax
Misplaced catheter
Pneumothorax
Sepsis
Shearing of catheter
Subcutaneous emphysema
Thoracic duct injury
Thrombophlebitis

These complications are decreased by providing only an appropriate, not an excessive, amount of calories, and by reducing glucose concentrations in maintenance TPN regimens from 25 percent to 20 or even 15 percent.

Contraindications to fat emulsions were discussed earlier in this chapter. Manifestations of deficiency or excess in vitamins and minerals are reviewed in Chapter 14.

Mechanical

Mechanical complications of TPN include thrombosis or embolism (Table 12-7). Air embolism is a rapidly fatal complication of central vein catheterization. Patients should be instructed that if TPN infusion connections are accidentally broken, they should immediately occlude the lumen of the catheter or tubing and seek assistance. The infusion system may be flushed with heparin and appropriate measures taken to resume the infusion if the central line has not been contaminated. A contaminated line should be clamped and a peripheral infusion of 10 percent dextrose introduced; the central venous catheter should then be removed.

Signs of air embolism include

- dyspnea
- tachypnea

- cyanosis
- chest pain
- tachycardia
- disorientation
- coma
- cardiac arrest

If air embolism is suspected, place the patient in the left lateral decubitus position with the head dependent (Trendelenberg) and administer oxygen. Aspiration of air through the central line may be attempted.

Septic

The incidence of septic complications of TPN is inversely related to the quality of care afforded the patient's infusion site, with particular attention to the skin, infusion system, and TPN solutions. In experienced hands the rate of infection is minimal but may rise as high as 50 percent when care is negligent. TPN should be carried out only in a hospital with trained personnel assigned the responsibility of the procedure.

Fever in a patient receiving TPN may be a sign of catheter sepsis or may be due to other causes. The source of infection should be sought by culture of urine, blood, sputum, wounds, and nutrient solutions for bacteria and fungi. The catheter must be removed if the patient is in unexplained septic shock.

If fever persists and the source has not been identified within 24 hours, remove and culture the central line, obtaining blood cultures through the catheter just prior to removal. A new catheter should **not** be introduced via guidewire into the same site. Antibiotics should be administered for 24 to 48 hours prior to insertion of a new catheter and line if bacteremia is present. Peripheral parenteral infusion of nutrient solutions can be used in the interim.

SECTION IV

Disorders of Undernutrition and Overnutrition

Famish'd people must be slowly nurst,
And fed by spoonfuls, else they always burst.

George Gordon, Lord Byron, 1788–1824, "Don Juan,"
Canto II, Stanza 158.

Having generally examined nutritional support in Section III, we now turn to some specific disorders relating to undernutrition and overnutrition.

Chapter 13—**Starvation and Protein-Energy Malnutrition (PEM)**— deals with the biology of starvation and protein-energy malnutrition, discussing the acute phase of semistarvation and the body's adaptation to the condition. The chapter then focuses on immune function and clinical syndromes of malnutrition, concluding with a section on the causes and results of hospital malnutrition.

In Chapter 14—**Nutrient Deficiency Diseases and Toxicities**—we build upon the basic information presented in Chapters 1 and 2, turning our attention toward the causes, symptoms, diagnosis, and treatment of vitamin and mineral deficiencies and toxicities and of essential fatty acid deficiency.

Chapter 15—**Nutritional Anemias**—delineates the function of specific nutrients involved in hematopoiesis by presenting causes, symptoms, diagnosis, and treatment of anemias stemming from deficiencies of iron, folate, and vitamin B_{12}.

Chapter 16—**Obesity, Anorexia Nervosa, and Bulimia**—first presents background information on energy needs and fat stores, as well as on the etiology of obesity. The chapter then focuses on theories, complications, and treatment of obesity, followed by a discussion of anorexia nervosa and bulimia.

In Chapter 17—**Alcoholism**—we discuss the metabolism of alcohol, alcohol intoxication and withdrawal syndromes, nutritional deficiencies and metabolic disorders related to alcohol use, and alcohol's effect on the digestive, cardiovascular, and nervous systems.

CHAPTER 13

Starvation and Protein-Energy Malnutrition (PEM)

THE BIOLOGY OF STARVATION

Fasting and Semistarvation

Starvation in the healthy human subject has a predictable course that has been vividly described in a number of studies.

IRA Hunger Strikers

Descriptions of the signs and symptoms of the IRA hunger strikers in Northern Ireland have recently provided a rare look at the effects of acute starvation in previously well-nourished, healthy young men. The mean time of death was 62 days after food was first refused. At 42 days of fasting, nystagmus appeared, together with severe spells of nausea, vomiting, and dizziness. These symptoms lasted 4 or 5 days, followed by a week of *physical and psychologic revival*. Speech then became slurred, hearing failed, and the starving men slowly went blind, even losing the sense of smell. Their minds, however, remained intact, with the men awake and memory of recent and past events persisting. Unconsciousness occurred only terminally, quickly followed by death.

Classic Studies

Descriptions of behavior and metabolic factors associated with starvation are found in two classic studies: F. G. Benedict's 1915 study of a professional faster who was observed for 30 days of fasting; and Ancel Keys and colleagues' *The Biology of Human Starvation* (1950), which describes "The Minnesota Experiment" in which 32 healthy young conscientious objectors underwent semistarvation with provision of 50 percent of their caloric requirements for a period of 24 weeks. The latter two-volume publication reviews many earlier reports of fasting and starvation, in addition to describing numerous psychologic, physical, and biologic parameters in the subjects. Refeeding of the subjects at four levels of increased calories also is described.

A further source of information concerning the effects of semistarvation is the observations of 28 physicians confined to the Warsaw ghetto between 1940 and 1942, where their ration was restricted to 1800 kcal per day.

Acute (Early) Phase

Both fasting and semistarvation have (1) acute effects, and (2) metabolic adaptation. The first phase lasts a few days to a few weeks (typically 5 to 10 days); adaptation, especially to semistarvation, is achieved after 3 to 6 weeks. The adaptation permits individuals to survive more prolonged periods of energy deprivation than otherwise might be possible.

The Body's Caloric Stores. The caloric stores of the healthy human body could provide sufficient fuel for more than 80 days.

Fat. Eighty-five percent of available calories are in fat, the most energy-dense tissue. Fat tissue contains very little intracellular water and has the greatest number of calories per unit weight (see Chapters 1 and 3).

Protein. Since protein, which could provide about 14 percent of the potentially available calories, has vital cell and structural functions, the adaptation over time allows the body to avoid using protein as fuel in order to minimize its consumption during starvation.

Carbohydrate/Glucose. The small amount of carbohydrate in the body directly available for energy is in liver glycogen (muscle glycogen is not available for direct glucose production because of the absence of glucose-6-phosphatase in muscle). RQ measurements indicate that carbohydrate is a significant energy source only in the first few days of fasting, with rapid depletion of liver glycogen. Glucose must nonetheless be provided, especially to the brain and to other tissues (erythrocytes, bone marrow, renal medulla, and peripheral nerves).

Gluconeogenesis. Provision of glucose via gluconeogenesis is thus essential for survival in starvation. Substrates for glucose synthesis include the end product of glycolysis, lactate, which is resynthesized to glucose in the liver and kidney (Cori cycle; Fig. 13–1). Protein-derived amino acids form the second substrate for glucose synthesis (alanine cycle; Fig. 13–2). Since animals lack the ability to reverse pyruvate decarboxylation to acetyl coenzyme A, new glucose cannot be synthesized directly from fatty acids under usual circumstances.

Hormonal Changes. A small decline of 10 to 15 mg per dl in blood glucose concentration with brief starvation results in a decline in circulating insulin and an increase in circulating glucagon. The hormonal milieu results

Figure 13–1. Major substrates in gluconeogenesis. In the Cori cycle, glucose is synthesized from lactate with the energy derived from free fatty acid oxidation. The glycerol moiety of triglyceride enters into gluconeogenesis directly. In the alanine cycle glucose is synthesized directly from amino acid. (From Saudek, C.D., and Felig, P.: The metabolic events of starvation. Am J Med 60:118, 1976, with permission.)

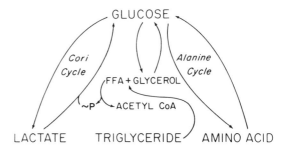

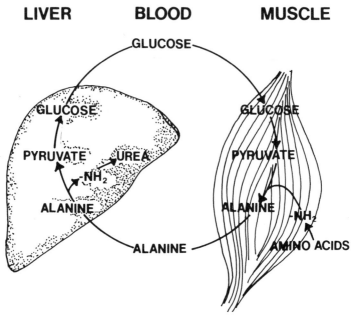

Figure 13-2. The glucose-alanine cycle. Alanine, synthesized in muscle from trans-amination of glucose-derived pyruvate, is taken up by the liver and reconverted to glucose. (From Saudek, C.D., and Felig, P.: The metabolic events of starvation. Am J Med 60:121, 1976, with permission.)

in stimulation of lipolysis, and fatty acids are provided to meet the energy requirements of muscle and liver with stimulation of hepatic ketogenesis. In addition, there is a decrease in extracerebral glucose utilization with a shift to fatty acids and ketones.

Amino Acid Utilization. Although all essential amino acids other than leucine are potentially glucogenic (see Table 1–8), there is a pattern of amino acid utilization by muscle that results in the output of alanine (representing 30 to 40 percent of the total amino acid output from muscle) and glutamine exceeding all others. Uptake of alanine and glutamine is specific, in that the gut utilizes glutamine, and alanine is taken up solely by the liver for use in gluconeogenesis.

Glucose-Alanine Cycle. There appears to be a glucose-alanine cycle (see Fig. 13–2) in which alanine is synthesized in muscle by transamination of pyruvate derived from glucose metabolism. The alanine is released by muscle, taken up by the liver, and reconverted to glucose after deamination. In the meantime the branched chain amino acids (leucine, isoleucine, and valine) are preferentially utilized by muscle, providing the major source of nitrogen for alanine synthesis. In the initial days of starvation, the output of alanine from muscle increases as does the fractional extraction of alanine by

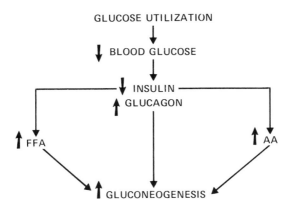

Figure 13–3. Metabolic adaptation during early starvation leading to increased gluconeogenesis. (From Saudek, C.D., and Felig, P.: The metabolic events of starvation. Am J Med 60:122, 1976, with permission.)

the liver. Glucose production by means of this mechanism provides glucose primarily for the brain.

Meeting the Body's Energy Needs. Metabolic adaptation to early starvation is summarized in Figure 13–3. Most of the energy requirements are provided by fatty acid oxidation. Release of amino acids and free fatty acids is enhanced by decreasing levels of insulin, while glucagon stimulates hepatic glycogenolysis and gluconeogenesis. This initial adaptation provides glucose at the expense of rapid proteolysis.

Fat and Protein. In the initial phase of starvation, energy needs are met from breakdown of adipose tissue triglyceride, providing five sixths of calories; protein breakdown, primarily from muscle, yields the rest of calories (Fig. 13–4).

Glucose. The liver provides adequate amounts of glucose through gluconeogenesis and glycogenolysis; 80 percent of the glucose is used by the nervous system, mainly the brain, and is completely oxidized to carbon dioxide and water. The remaining glucose is taken up by other tissues, which metabolize it to lactate and pyruvate. This glucose enters the Cori cycle and shuttles energy internally, sparing gluconeogenesis from protein.

Fat Preferred to Glucose. The heart, renal cortex, and skeletal muscle utilize the free fatty acids released from adipose tissue or the ketone bodies produced by the liver. These tissues preferentially use fat rather than glucose during starvation, minimizing the need for gluconeogenesis from protein. Energy for the liver's metabolic activity is provided by fatty acid oxidation to acetyl-CoA, which is then preferentially incorporated into ketone bodies in fasting humans, rather than undergoing terminal combustion in the tricarboxylic acid cycle.

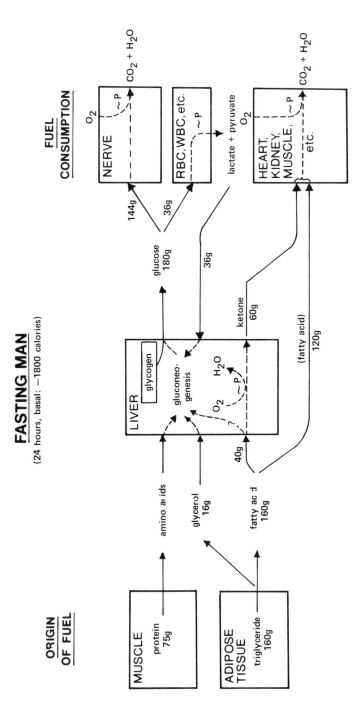

Figure 13–4. Fuel metabolism in man fasted 24 hours. (From Cahill, G.F., Jr.: Starvation in man. New Engl J Med 282:669, 1970, with permission.)

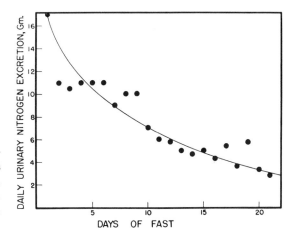

Figure 13-5. Decline in urinary nitrogen excretion in fasting man. (From Cahill, G.F., Jr.: Starvation in man. New Engl J Med 282:671, 1970, with permission.)

Nitrogen Excretion. Nitrogen excretion begins to decline rapidly after 1 to 2 days of starvation, plateauing at 2 weeks (Fig. 13-5). As urinary nitrogen excretion declines, the percent excreted as urine urea nitrogen decreases, conserving water required for urea nitrogen excretion, with a gradual increase in the amount of ammonia excreted (Fig. 13-6). Water needs are thus minimal in starved persons in a temperate, humid climate. At an estimated loss of 75 g per day, one third of the total body protein would be depleted in several weeks. Therefore, to prolong survival, a major reduction in nitrogen catabolism must occur.

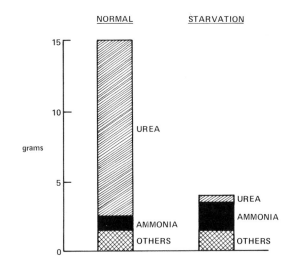

Figure 13-6. Urinary nitrogen secretion in normal man ingesting adequate energy and protein and after 5 to 6 weeks of starvation. (From Cahill, G.F., Jr.: Starvation in man. New Engl J Med 282:671, 1970, with permission.)

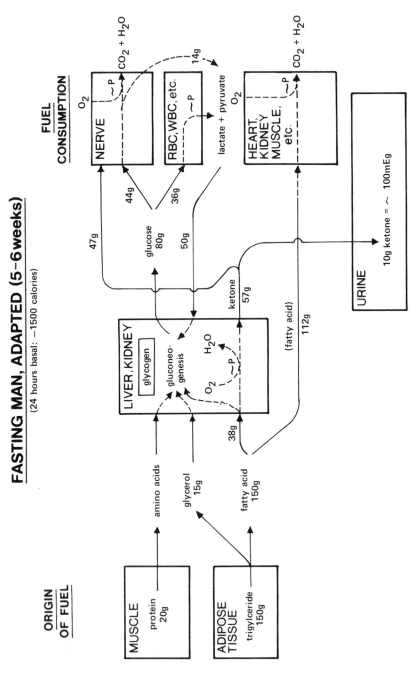

Figure 13-7. Altered fuel metabolism in man starved 5 to 6 weeks. (From Cahill, G.F., Jr.: Starvation in man. New Engl J Med 282:672, 1970, with permission.)

Adaptation (Prolonged)

Protein Catabolism. The late phase of starvation is characterized by alterations in protein catabolism that are manifestations of adaptation. Ninety percent of calories are provided by fat in prolonged starvation, and protein is conserved. Protein catabolism decreases from 75 to 20 g per day, and the ratio of fat to protein calories utilized increases from 4.8 to 17 (Fig. 13–7). In prolonged fasting, ketone bodies provide 50 to 60 percent of the brain's fuel requirements.

Gluconeogenesis. As the brain adapts to utilize ketone bodies, liver gluconeogenesis decreases, derived mainly from lactate, pyruvate, and glycerol, rather than from alanine and other amino acids. In prolonged starvation, the kidney synthesizes approximately the same amount of glucose as the liver, increasing from an initial 10 percent of gluconeogenesis. Renal gluconeogenesis parallels ammoniagenesis, with deaminated residues incorporated into glucose after donating the amino groups for ammonia formation.

Alanine and Ketones. The level of circulating alanine and the output of alanine from muscle are markedly and disproportionately reduced in prolonged starvation. This may be a response to hyperketonemia, which can inhibit the preferential oxidation of branched chain amino acids in muscle. Ketones are thus central in metabolic adaptation in late starvation. They replace glucose as a substrate for the brain and signal a reduction in protein catabolism and alanine output from muscle, thereby conserving protein and maintaining blood glucose homeostasis (Fig. 13–8).

Metabolic Rate and Physiologic Changes. The basal metabolic rate has a rapid decline of 20 percent in the first 3 weeks of prolonged semistarvation, followed by a slower decline of another 20 percent over the next 3 months

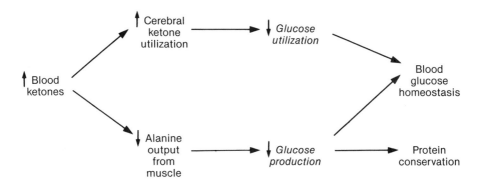

Figure 13–8. Metabolic adaptation in late starvation leading to protein conservation. (From Saudek, C.D., and Felig, P.: The metabolic events of starvation. Am J Med 60:124, 1976, with permission.)

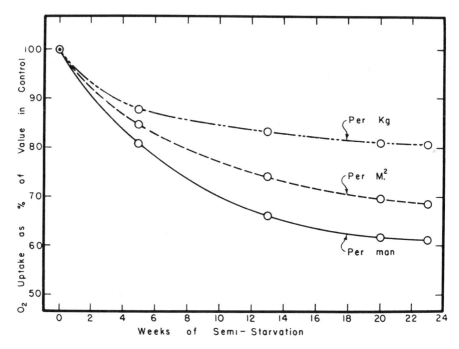

Figure 13-9. Mean basal metabolism of young man before and during 24 weeks of semistarvation expressed as percent of control values of oxygen uptake for man, per square meter of body surface and per kg body weight. (From Keys, A., et al.: The Biology of Human Starvation, Vol. 1. University of Minnesota Press, Minneapolis, 1950, p. 329, with permission.)

(Fig. 13-9). This exceeds the loss of body weight and lean body mass and represents an adaptation of decreased caloric expenditure, thus decreasing the body's rate of deterioration. There is also a corresponding decrease in the physical work performed by starving persons. Among the physiologic changes noted in starved men are decreases in cardiac work, muscle tone (especially of red muscle fibers), and the level of T_3.

Loss of Body Weight. Although there have been reports of survival with 50 percent weight loss, humans generally do not survive a loss of body weight that exceeds 40 percent. Weight loss is a function of both caloric deprivation and time (Table 13-1). The healthy young adult can withstand a weight loss of 5 to 10 percent below ideal, and can starve 14 days with little impairment of mental acuity or physical work. Death from malnutrition is unlikely until more than 25 percent of body weight is lost. At only 30 percent of maintenance caloric requirements, this level of weight loss is reached in 3 months; with half of caloric requirements, in 6 months; and at 60 percent of maintenance requirements, a 25 percent weight loss occurs within a year. Weight

Table 13-1. WEIGHT LOSS AS A FUNCTION OF
DECREASED CALORIC INTAKE AND TIME

Caloric Intake (% of Maintenance Requirements)	Weight Loss (% of Initial)		
	3 Mo	6 Mo	12 Mo+
90	5	8	10
80	8	12	15
70	10	15	20
60	12	20	25
50	15	25	30
40	20	30	35
30	25	35	40
20	30	45	—

(Adapted from Keys, A., et al.: The Biology of Human Starvation. Vol. 1. University of Minnesota Press, Minneapolis, 1950, p. 129.)

loss of 10 lb per month over several months in the nonobese is associated with symptoms and signs of PEM.

Summary of Metabolic Changes. Adaptation to prolonged starvation may be summarized as follows:

1. Modest initial fall in blood sugar, which plateaus until the end stages and then drops sharply.
2. Gradual increase in levels of free fatty acids, keto acids, and ketone bodies, leading to acidosis and ketonuria.
3. Decrease in protein breakdown.
4. Marked decrease in protein synthesis.
5. Decreased muscle uptake of glucose, with lowered levels of circulating insulin.
6. Decrease in gluconeogenesis.
7. Maintenance of increased carnitine for fatty acid transport.
8. Increase in hepatic ketogenesis equivalent to 100 percent fatty acid uptake.
9. Decreased release of glucogenic amino acids by muscle.
10. Inhibition of alanine extraction by liver.

Changes in Body Composition. Finally, changes in body composition with prolonged starvation result in

- decrease of 80 percent in body fat, most occurring late
- 22 percent decrease in lean body mass, most occurring early

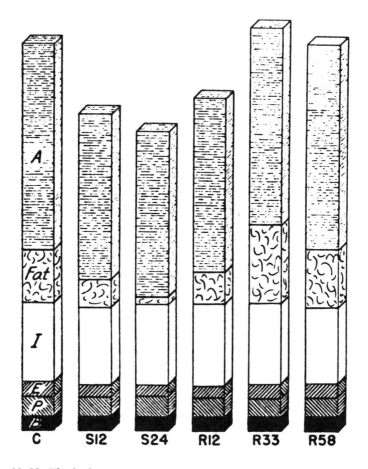

Figure 13–10. The body composition of young man before and during 24 weeks of semistarvation and after refeeding. C = control; S = semi-starvation weeks; R = refeeding weeks; B = bone mineral; P = plasma; E = erythrocytes; I = interstitial fluid; A = lean body mass. (From Keys, A., et al.: The Biology of Human Starvation, Vol. 1. University of Minnesota Press, Minneapolis, 1950, p. 329, with permission.)

- little change in the interstitial extracellular fluid compartment, which assumes a relatively larger proportion of the total body and may lead to manifest edema (Fig. 13–10)

Death. In the natural history of starvation, it is usually assumed that death occurs when there is a critical depletion of lean body mass (Fig. 13–11). However, physicians who observed the IRA hunger strikers concluded that death occurred when there was a critical depletion of body fat.

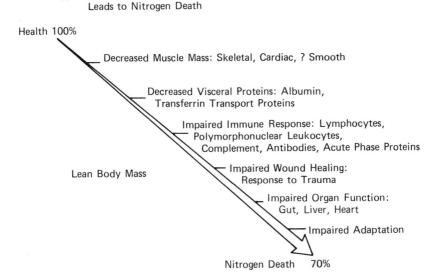

Figure 13–11. Loss of lean body mass leads to clinical signs and symptoms and eventually to death. (From Steffee, W.P.: Malnutrition in hospitalized patients. JAMA 244:2633, 1980, with permission.)

THE BIOLOGY OF PROTEIN-ENERGY MALNUTRITION

Anthropometric Indicators

There are other anthropometric indicators of calorie depletion in addition to body weight, and various indicators of protein status in PEM. These include measurements of triceps skinfold thickness and mid-arm muscle circumference, serum albumin, total lymphocyte count, and serum prealbumin (see Chapter 3). The degree to which these measurements equate with standard measurements is used to classify individuals with PEM as mildly, moderately, or severely depleted in calories stores (triceps skinfold), somatic protein stores (mid-arm muscle circumference), or visceral protein (albumin, total lymphocyte count). These measurements are used to determine the degrees of nutritional depletion and weight loss (Table 13–2).

Prealbumin Levels

The need for adequate intake of protein and calories to achieve nitrogen balance (see Chapter 1) is evident also in the maintenance of normal plasma

Table 13-2. DEGREES OF NUTRITIONAL DEPLETION

Parameter	Mild	Moderate (Significant)	Severe
Triceps skinfold, % standard*	>50	50–25	<25
Mid-arm muscle circumference, % standard†	>80	80–65	<65
Serum albumin, g/dl	>3.0	3.0–2.1	<2.1
Total lymphocyte count/cm	>1200	1200–800	<800
Weight loss, % initial (usual)			
Time			
1 wk	<1	1–2	>2
1 mo	<2	2–5	>5
3 mo	<5	5–7.5	>7.5
6 mo	<7.5	7.5–10	>10

*Standard = 12.5 mm (men), 16.5 mm (women).
†Standard = 25.3 cm (men), 23.2 cm (women).
(Ranges of normal are provided in Tables 3–3, 3–4, and 3–8.)

prealbumin values (Table 13–3). Normal levels of prealbumin were maintained on a high energy diet even when protein was decreased to half. However, on a low energy diet, even a high protein intake could not maintain normal prealbumin levels in the obese subjects studied. Prealbumin responds rapidly to refeeding, with a significant increase noted within 4 days (see Fig. 12–2). Plasma prealbumin decreased in these underfed subjects when no change was observed in plasma albumin or transferrin. Retinol-binding protein may be even more sensitive to protein status than prealbumin. With more severe malnutrition, plasma transferrin and albumin concentrations also fall.

Immune Function

Immune Deficits

Nutritional imbalance must be recognized as a significant, frequent cause of immunodeficiency that should be diagnosed and treated. A nutritional etiology of immunocompetence must be included in the evaluation of the anergic, malnourished person, especially children and the elderly.

Protein deficiency impairs a variety of immune mechanisms, the deficits correlating with the degree of malnutrition. Atrophy of thymic and lymphoid tissues is prominent; tonsil size is diminished, with a marked decrease in the number of thymus-dependent lymphocytes (T cells). An absolute decrease in the number of T cells is seen, together with a decrease in killer and helper

Table 13-3. EFFECTS OF ENERGY AND PROTEIN
RESTRICTION ON SERUM PREALBUMIN

Protein intake/day	Prealbumin mg/dl			
Energy intake/day	80 g	60 g	40 g	20 g
40 kcal/kg IBW*	30	30	29	24
9 kcal/kg IBW				
Day 6	28	17	21	15
Day 12	21	20	17	15
Day 24	19	17	15	13
Refeeding (day 4)	—	24	—	—

(Adapted from Shetty, P.S., et al.: Rapid-turnover transport proteins: an index of subclinical protein-energy malnutrition. Lancet 2:231, 1979.)
*IBW = ideal body weight.

cells and an increase in suppressor cell number. The number of null cells, possibly representing immature cells, may increase. Despite the atrophy of lymphoid tissues, B cell number may or may not be affected. Immunoglobulin levels may thus be normal, although secretory IgA is diminished. Antibody formation to specific antigens is variable, lymphocyte response to mitogens is poor, and delayed cutaneous hypersensitivity to a variety of skin cell antigens decreases. Inflammatory reactions and leukocyte phagocytic functions are defective, especially bactericidal activity, and there also is decreased chemotaxis, which may be a result rather than a cause of infection. Levels of serum complement components are low, especially C3 and factor B, while C4 is normal. Opsonins are decreased.

Functional Tests

Functional tests of immune response are altered with protein malnutrition in that delayed cutaneous hypersensitivity is diminished. Antibody titer may be increased, reflecting previous exposure to antigens, but response to a specific antigen may be decreased and blast transformation is diminished.

Infection

Not only do these changes result in increased susceptibility to infection, but the infection is masked. For example, patients with PEM commonly have infections such as measles, herpes simplex, tuberculosis, or gram-negative septicemia. However, they manifest gangrene rather than suppuration, fever and leukocytosis are absent, measles is characterized by scant rash and giant cell pneumonia, and herpes simplex may be disseminated. The prevalence of tuberculosis increases fourfold in starved individuals as weight drops below 85 percent of ideal. Diarrhea is not only more prevalent in PEM patients, but associated fatality also increases. Similarly, fatality from measles is markedly higher. Malnourished patients with amebic infections show an increase in hepatic infection.

Alterations in immune function respond rapidly—within days—to repletion with adequate protein and calories. Thus, when treating infection in PEM patients it is important to provide a high level of nutritional supplementation along with appropriate antibiotic or other specific therapy.

Severe protein-energy malnutrition also can be precipitated by common infections, including

- measles
- pertussis
- repeated acute diarrheal episodes
- chronic malaria
- schistosomiasis
- massive infestations of hookworm, Trichiuris, or Strongyloides.

Micronutrient Deficiencies

Severe protein-energy malnutrition usually is accompanied by deficiency of micronutrients. Some of these significantly affect the immune system, but the extent of their contribution and their importance in dietary rehabilitation remain unclear. Iron, zinc, and vitamin A and their effects on the immune system and the development of immunodeficiency are especially important. Impaired immunity has also been attributed to deficiencies of magnesium, selenium, folate, pyridoxine, and vitamins C and E. Excess intake of vitamins C and A, on the other hand, may impair immune responses.

CLINICAL SYNDROMES

The clinical syndromes of protein-energy malnutrition are distinguished by differences in body weight, expressed as percentages of standard weight for age norms (see Fig. 8–1). These syndromes are

1. Underweight: Persons who are 60 to 80 percent of standard, without edema.
2. Kwashiorkor: Body weight of 60 to 80 percent of standard, with edema.
3. Marasmus: Body weight less than 60 percent of standard, no edema.
4. Marasmic kwashiorkor: Body weight less than 60 percent of standard, with edema.

While these classic syndromes have typically been associated with infants and children in Third World countries, it has become customary to apply the term also to adult "sick" patients, often with less severe deficiencies.

Kwashiorkor

Causes

Kwashiorkor was first described in Ghana, where it afflicted children from 1 to 3 years of age (Fig. 13–12). The term relates to the weaning from the breast of the first child because of a new pregnancy. Sickness follows 3 to 4 months after the child has been weaned to dilute gruel, as a result of chronic deficiency of protein and energy.

Kwashiorkor is specifically caused by lack of protein in the diet relative to the energy content. Intake of starchy foods such as banana, cassaba, and other roots and tubers is excessive—a diet that stems from poverty, lack of knowledge, taboos, and family disorganization.

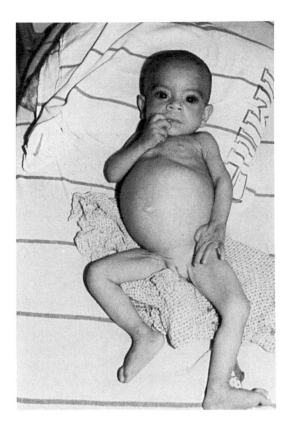

Figure 13–12. Child with kwashiorkor. (From Dr. T. Kuske)

General Symptoms

Children are apathetic, sad and irritable, weak, inactive, and anorexic. The body temperature may be subnormal, and there may be intermittent diarrhea and vomiting following meals. Motor development is retarded and infection is common.

Clinical Signs of Protein Deficiency

In addition to edema, about 30 percent have a fatty liver, and there may be weight deficit and failure to thrive (see Chapter 8). Subcutaneous edema may mask the muscle wasting. Children may exhibit a moon face, enlarged liver, and edema, with puffy eyes, swollen hands and feet, and finally generalized edema. There are variable changes in the chest-to-head ratio, mid-arm muscle circumference, and weight for length. Serum albumin ranges from 0.7 to 2 g per dl.

Among the factors affected by the clinical signs of protein deficiency are the hair, skin, facies, anthropometrics, and serum albumin. The hair has been described variously as light colored, straight, and dyspigmented, with dark hair turning first brown, then red, then blond and gray. The hair is dry, thin, silky, brittle, and pluckable, falling out easily, and leaving patches of baldness. The pigment changes start at the hair line (flag sign) and reflect the duration of the deficiency state.

Both changes of hyperpigmentation and hypopigmentation of the skin occur, with desquamation leading to the so-called flaky paint dermatosis, in which the flaking skin has the appearance of flaking enamel paint. This lesion can progress to skin ulcerations and fissures, which can involve the lower limbs, buttocks, and perineal regions.

Treatment

Prevention of protein malnutrition is the primary goal. Treatment is dietary, with provision of adequate protein, commonly in the form of milk, for 1 week, progressing to a mixed diet including added potassium and magnesium for 2 weeks, with hospitalization lasting a total of 2 to 3 weeks.

CASE 13a: KWASHIORKOR/ETHANOL

A 35-year-old black woman was hospitalized with a 2-week history of progressive dyspnea on exertion, orthopnea, and paroxysmal nocturnal dyspnea. Over the past 6 months her hair had began to change color from black to red, and about 3 weeks before admission her hair had begun to fall out. She developed upper respiratory symptoms and became progressively weaker. About 2 weeks before admission, because of shortness of breath, she had begun to sleep on two pillows and had progressed to three. On the day of admission she drank a half-pint of liquor and two beers and became progressively weaker and could not walk. She also noticed a worsening of her chronic lower extremity edema. She reported dry, scaly skin, chronic abdominal pain, and 10 to 15 episodes of greasy, orange, watery diarrhea for 4 months; her stools were floating.

The patient had been hospitalized 8 months earlier for acute pancreatitis; serum albumin was 2.5 g/dl. She gave a history of heavy alcohol abuse, claiming to have decreased about 2 years before to one beer per day. (Her family disputed this.) She was hospitalized 6 years earlier with chronic pancreatitis thought secondary to alcohol abuse. She had two pseudocysts and was placed on TPN for 6 weeks and underwent surgical drainage. She had smoked one to two packs of cigarettes per day for 23 years.

On examination, the woman was cachectic, appeared much older than her stated age, and had alcohol on her breath. Blood pressure was 105/80, pulse 92, respirations 18, weight 43.8 kg, height 5 feet 3 inches (about 80 percent of IBW). Hair was sparse and reddish. Eyebrows were sparse, and there was bitemporal wasting. Sclerae were muddy and the cornea were normal. The tongue was slightly reddened. There were bilateral basilar rales. The heart rate was occasionally irregular and S3 and S4 were audible. There was mild, right upper quadrant abdominal tenderness. There was 4+ pitting edema of the lower extremities from the hip inferiorly but no jugular vein distention. Desquamative changes were present over both palms, and the skin was dry and hyperkeratotic. The neurologic examination was normal.

Laboratory tests (abnormal values): white blood count and platelet count were normal, with MCV 106.6 fl. Serum sodium, potassium, chloride, bicarbonate, glucose, BUN, creatinine, magnesium, and phosphate were normal, with calcium 7.1 (mg/dl). Albumin was 1.6 g/dl, and total protein 5.4 g/dl. Other tests (IU): LDH 678, SGOT 1321, alkaline phosphatase 138, total bilirubin was normal; prothrombin time 13.2/12.0 seconds control, PTT 37.6/31.0 control. The chest radiograph showed cardiomegaly, fullness of the central hilar vasculature, and increased interstitial densities consistent with interstitial pulmonary edema. There was blunting of the right costophrenic angle suggestive of a right pleural effusion. ECG showed a normal sinus rhythm, rate 92, with left axis deviation, and low voltage in the frontal leads.

The initial diagnosis was congestive heart failure and severe malnutrition with probable kwashiorkor, secondary to her severe alcoholism, plus a possible malabsorption syndrome related to pancreatitis and pancreatic insufficiency. Serum and RBC folate and vitamin B_{12} were normal. Decreased T_3 with normal TSH was consistent with the euthyroid sick syndrome. A qualitative stool for fat was positive for neutral and split fats. A sonogram of the abdomen showed liver changes consistent with fatty infiltration without evidence of biliary obstruction. There was definite cholelithiasis and no ascites. The pancreatic area was grossly normal.

The nutrition service confirmed the diagnosis of kwashiorkor. Prealbumin 9.6 mg/dl, retinol binding protein 1.8 mg/dl, and transferrin 152 mg/dl were all deficient. Plasma retinol was deficient at 11 μg/dl, and vitamin E was extremely low at 80 μg/dl. Zinc was deficient at 52 μg/dl, and copper normal. Ionized calcium was low at 4.61 mg/dl. The patient was initially given lasix with diuresis and improvement in her shortness of breath. She was started on a low fat diet with supplementation with Vital and later with Osmolite HN and supplemental vitamins. She was started on Pancrease, 3 tablets with meals. Her stools became less frequent, decreasing to five per day. Her strength improved. She was discharged 2 weeks later to the Nutrition Clinic but did not keep her appointment. She was readmitted 1 month later with rhabdomyolysis following an acute drinking episode. Her hair and skin were improved, edema had cleared, and serum proteins were improved but were still at deficient levels.

LESSON:

This patient's protein deficiency resulted from poor intake, ethanol, and malabsorption. Skin and hair changes, infection, and heart failure resulted.

Marasmus

Marasmus is the most frequently encountered nutritional problem in developing countries, occurring at an earlier age than kwashiorkor. Children 6 to 18 months old exhibit gross wasting of muscle and subcutaneous tissue and marked stunting leading to growth failure. Infants appear emaciated, with large heads, redundant skin, and an "old" look (Fig. 13–13). Although irritable and fretful, children often have good appetites. There is hypothermia, motor retardation, and weakness. There are fewer hair and skin changes found in marasmus than in kwashiorkor, but the skin may be dry, hypopigmented, and scaling, with the hair at times dry, sparse, and light colored. Muscle atrophy leads to abdominal protrusion.

Conditions predisposing to marasmus are prolonged, markedly deficient dietary intake plus infection, resulting in lack of both protein and energy with their usual ratio maintained. Infection is usually of the lower respiratory tract. Fluid and electrolyte disturbance with dehydration are often present. Mortality exceeds 20 percent within a few days of hospitalization. Serum albumin approximates 2.5 g per dl.

Prevention of marasmus is achieved by adequate intake of breast milk supplemented at 3 months by appropriate foods. As with kwashiorkor, envi-

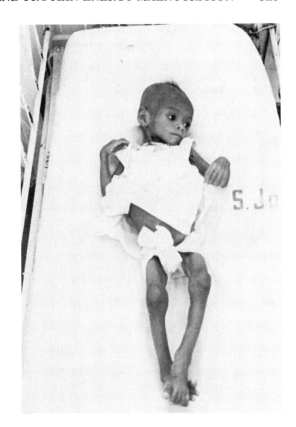

Figure 13-13. Marasmic infant. (From Dr. T. Kuske.)

ronmental factors predisposing to this disorder are frequent pregnancies, especially in teenage mothers, food taboos, poverty, wars, civil unrest, and natural disasters.

FEATURES OF PROTEIN-ENERGY MALNUTRITION

Autopsy studies of PEM reveal atrophy of the small intestine mucosa with a decrease in brush border enzymes, resulting in decreased absorption of nutrients. In addition, there is atrophy of the exocrine pancreas and fatty liver. With treatment and survival, the colonic mucosa returns to normal in 1 month and the small intestine has been reported to be normal in about 9 months. The fatty liver also resolves with treatment. Additional changes include a marked decrease in the size of the thymus—one-third to one-tenth normal size—with a decrease in T lymphocytes and in cell-mediated immunity.

PEM infants are especially susceptible to infections such as measles, gram-negative sepsis, Candida, histoplasmosis, and herpes. Other features are delayed wound healing with inadequate polymorphonuclear leukocytes, pus formation, an increase in necrosis, loss of bone mass, and a decrease in muscle mass and noncollagen protein.

Famine Edema

So-called famine edema is due to a relative increase in extracellular fluid with retention of sodium and water. The condition may result from hypoalbuminemia, a decrease in renal excretion of water and an increase in water reabsorption, a decrease in tissue tension, an increased fluid intake with increased thirst, or a decreased venous return. There is also low serum potassium and metabolic alkalosis.

Pneumonia

The most common cause of death in PEM is pneumonia. This is attributable in part to complicating abnormalities in the mechanics of ventilation: decreases in vital capacity and respiration rate, strength of respiratory muscles, minute volume, and tidal volume.

Protein Levels

Concentrations of plasma retinol binding protein (RBP) and prealbumin are greatly reduced in malnourished children and rapidly return to normal with refeeding. However, it is not clear whether there are significant differences in the levels of these proteins in kwashiorkor versus marasmus. It has been suggested that kwashiorkor results from a failure of the usual adaptation to protein deficiency, in which the liver is protected at the expense of muscle. The usual adaptation to starvation is seen in marasmus.

Amino Acid Levels

In kwashiorkor, the plasma free amino acid pattern exhibits a lowered concentration of the branched chain amino acids leucine, isoleucine, and valine, and also very low tyrosine. The ratio of branched chain essential to nonessential amino acids is low. An additional characteristic finding is a low tyrosine:phenylaline ratio (Fig. 13–14).

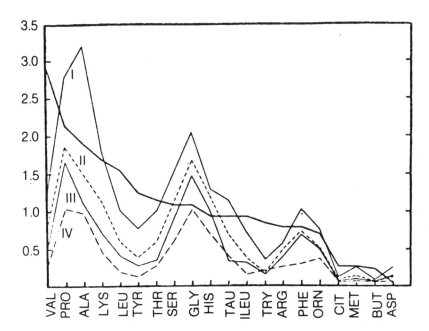

Figure 13–14. The average plasma amino acid patterns in children with kwashiorkor divided into four categories (I, II, III, IV), according to degree of deviation from the normal of seven amino acids plus tyrosine and the normal pattern. VAL = valine; PRO = proline; ALA = alanine; LYS = lysine; LEU = leucine; TYR = tyrosine; THR = threonine; SER = serine; GLY = glycine; HIS = histidine; TAU = taurine; ILEU = isoleucine; TRY = trytophan; ARG = arginine; PHE = phenylalanine; ORN = ornithine; CIT = citrulline; MET = methionine; BUT = amino butyric acid; ASP = aspartic acid. (From Holt, L.E., Jr., Snyderman, S.E., Norton, P.M., et al.: The plasma aminogram in kwashiorkor. Lancet 2:1345, 1963, with permission.)

Other Nutrient Deficiencies

In protein-energy malnutrition the intakes of other essential nutrients such as vitamins and minerals are also generally low. Specific clinical deficiencies, however, are less common because the requirements for other nutrients diminish when calorie and protein intake is limited. They may become manifest on refeeding.

Energy Versus Protein Deficiency

Most cases of severe malnutrition in children and adults fall between the extremes of pure energy and pure protein deficiency. More usual is a moderate to severe protein deficit superimposed on a severe calorie deficiency, or vice versa.

THERAPY

Nutritional therapy should be handled cautiously in the initial phases of treatment for PEM. Mortality in these children results from the complications, not from malnutrition per se. A high protein or calorie load initially may precipitate death by challenging physiologic functions that have maximally adapted to starvation. For children the initial dietary approach should provide about 1 g protein and 80 to 100 kcal per kg per day, with 20 percent of calories derived from fat. After 2 to 4 days the protein content of the diet should be gradually increased to 2, 3, and 4 g per kg, and the energy content increased in steps to as high as 200 kcal per kg per day. It is important to provide high levels of vitamins to replace those depleted and to meet the greater physiologic demand for vitamins and their mobilization (vitamin A) when a high calorie, high protein diet is ingested. Similarly, adequate amounts of minerals must be provided in the repletion.

HOSPITAL MALNUTRITION

Illness as a Precipitating Factor in Protein-Energy Malnutrition

The primary manifestation of protein-energy malnutrition in the United States adult population is a secondary decrease in energy intake below that needed to maintain body weight, coupled with an illness-related increase in energy expenditure. Significant causative factors include

- psychologic
- neurologic
- difficulty in ingesting and swallowing food
- problems with malabsorption and gastrointestinal disease
- sepsis
- malignancy
- postoperative problems of ileus, peritonitis, obstruction
- increased needs from trauma or infection
- metabolic alterations such as diabetic mellitus, or liver disease and liver failure
- renal insufficiency, acute or chronic

These problems are described in greater detail in the chapters that follow.

Incidence of Nutritional Deficiency in Hospitalized Patients

The incidence of nutritional deficiency, especially protein-energy malnutrition, is high in hospitalized patients. A number of studies beginning in the late 1960s and early 1970s brought these nutritional disorders to the attention of physicians. For example, 25 to 50 percent of medical and surgical patients hospitalized for 2 or more weeks may develop protein-energy malnutrition. For this reason, it is essential to recognize those factors adversely affecting patients' nutritional status and the parameters that identify patients at risk for significant malnutrition. This information should be used in the patient's initial nutritional assessment, and appropriate nutritional intervention prescribed. Unfortunately, extensive and complex diagnostic battery and treatment regimens add to patients' stress. Such adverse influences may worsen an already compromised nutritional status when a patient is hospitalized—the "skeleton in the hospital closet," a form of iatrogenic malnutrition. Studies have shown that nutritional parameters worsened in more than 75 percent of patients admitted with normal values.

Causes of Nutritional Deficiency

A number of omissions and oversights contribute to nutritional neglect. Many hospitals fail to measure and record patients' height and weight. For example, a recent chart review showed that 40 percent of patients on a medicine service did not have height recorded, and 21 percent were missing body weight measurement. Patients' food intake often is not observed or noted. Meals may be withheld frequently because of diagnostic tests. Prolonged use of intravenous feedings of 5 percent glucose and isotonic saline—the equivalent of quarter-strength Kool-Aid—are common.

All members of the health care team need to recognize that because nutritional requirements are altered due to injury or illness, it is especially important to assess patients' nutritional status throughout their hospitalization. Appropriate laboratory tests, particularly the hemogram and serum albumin, are universally available. Dietitians and nurses are important members of the health care team who can assist in the recognition of nutritional abnormalities and in their management.

Risk Factors

Patients at risk of malnutrition include

1. those who are grossly underweight or overweight, and when recent weight loss exceeds 10 percent of usual body weight, or 10 lb per month over several months

2. alcoholics
3. those without oral intake given ordinary IV solutions for 10 days; the elderly, for 5 days
4. those with nutrient losses from malabsorption, dialysis, fistulas, or wounds, or who have excessive needs because of hypermetabolism, infection, burns, trauma, or fever
5. those given drugs with antinutrient or catabolic properties such as corticosteroids and oral antibiotics

Stress

Sick, malnourished patients are especially stressed because of surgery, trauma, sepsis, or chemotherapy, and thus protein and energy needs are greater. The requirement for protein synthesis is increased for wound healing, increased production of white blood cells, and perhaps to meet the demands of tumor growth. In addition, there is increased demand for ATP to support protein synthesis, anaerobic metabolism, and tumor growth, as well as in the presence of fever. Adaptation to the stress state itself requires synthesis of a variety of enzymes. Nitrogen loss is accelerated with fever, or even with the stress of examination. Despite return of body temperature to normal, the rate of protein breakdown and resynthesis is accelerated for considerably longer periods, up to several weeks. Major surgery may result in 6 weeks of catabolism. Sepsis increases glucose requirements, especially those of the polymorphonuclear leukocyte, while fibroblastic activity in wound healing requires glucose for fuel as well. Nutritional intervention in these patients must meet energy demands and support optimal rates of protein synthesis.

Decreased Body Protein

The conditions most commonly associated with decreased body protein (wasting) are

- cardiopulmonary disease with hypoxia
- gastrointestinal disease
- neuromuscular impairment
- rheumatologic disorders
- organic brain syndromes
- febrile illnesses

CASE 13b: PROTEIN-ENERGY MALNUTRITION

A 23-year-old white woman was transferred from another hospital because of thrombophlebitis of the left leg. She had been hospitalized for the past 6 months for bilateral pneumonia and respiratory failure and had been bedridden for the last 4 months. During that time she was fed by the peripheral intravenous route and given enteral supplements. She was a heavy smoker and consumed a six-pack of beer daily along with a poor diet. She had lost weight from 54 kg to 33.5 kg, and was 168 cm tall (55 percent of ideal body weight). Her appetite was poor and her last menstrual period had been 6 months earlier.

She was depressed, emaciated-looking, and pale. Head hair was scant and reddish in color. Body hair was sparse, her tongue was smooth, and there were angular fissures at the corners of her mouth (see Fig. 14–4). Vibration sense was decreased in the lower extremities. She had wheezes and rhonchi in both lungs and evidence of deep venous thrombosis. She was unable to get out of bed or walk. Triceps skinfold was 6 mm and mid-arm muscle circumference was 15 cm. Her serum albumin was 1.8 g/dl, transferrin 90 mg/dl, hemoglobin 9.7 g/dl, and serum carotene 6 μg/dl. Alkaline phosphatase and glutamic-oxalacetic transaminase levels were elevated. A plasma zinc level obtained after treatment was 50 μg/dl.

She was treated with a high calorie, high protein diet in the form of meals supplemented with enteral preparations and therapeutic levels of multivitamins and minerals. The intake gradually was increased to 3700 kcal daily. Her deep vein thrombosis improved with anticoagulant therapy and she was discharged after 3 weeks.

Five months later she had gained 9 kg; her hair stopped falling out, and the hair growing in was sandy in color. Her appetite, strength, and mood improved. Serum albumin was 3.3 g/dl and hemoglobin 12.3 g/dl with a decrease in liver enzymes.

LESSON:

This patient had profound protein-energy malnutrition resulting from multiple causes: low socioeconomic status, alcoholism, cigarette smoking, poor diet, hospital malnutrition (sepsis plus lack of adequate food intake), unfamiliar surroundings and food compounding the anorexia of malnutrition, and malabsorption secondary to the malnutrition. Upon initial consultation it was suggested to evaluate this patient for anorexia nervosa! Her shallow effect was determined by psychiatric examination to result from her prolonged starvation. Of particular interest is the fact that she was rehabilitated with oral intake; a lot of attention and support resulted in her eating and drinking the enteral supplements rather than requiring tube feeding or TPN, which would have been provided if she had not improved so rapidly. It was only after her hair regrew that we realized that its red color was a sign of adult kwashiorkor.

Results of Nutritional Deficiency

The patient with secondary malnutrition may show the signs of marasmus or kwashiorkor similar to those found in patients with primary nutritional deficiencies of energy and protein. When accompanied by stress, protein depletion results in high mortality, deficiencies in wound healing and immunocompetence, and increases in infection and other complications of illness and trauma.

Organ systems may fail primarily because of malnutrition. Vulnerable systems include maintenance of body temperature, bone marrow function, and the gastrointestinal tract. Atrophy of intestinal mucosa occurs in protein malnutrition, with flattening of villi and disappearance of microvilli and malabsorption.

Inattention to nutritional considerations increases admission rates, duration of hospitalization, and mortality. Supporting statistics have been reported from university, community, and Veterans Administration hospitals.

Nutritional Requirements in Specific Disease States

Nutritional requirements in various disease states and provision of appropriate calories and protein are detailed in the chapters that follow.

CHAPTER 14

Nutrient Deficiency Diseases and Toxicities

A variety of diseases are caused by primary nutritional deficiency of one or another vitamin or mineral. In addition, specific symptoms and signs may be attributable to deficiency or excess of one specific nutrient. Finally, some clinical disorders appear related to single or multiple nutrient deficiencies.

This chapter includes the clinical manifestations of deficiency and toxicity, criteria and tests for diagnosis, treatment, and background information relating to pathophysiology, natural history, and prevention. Deficiency states of iron, cobalamin, and folic acid are presented in Chapter 15. Chapter 2 provides background information concerning requirements, sources, function, and metabolic fate of the nutrients.

VITAMIN DEFICIENCIES AND TOXICITIES

Predisposing Factors

Various factors may predispose individuals to vitamin deficiencies:

- inadequate dietary intake
- failure of endogenous synthesis (biotin, vitamin K, vitamin D)
- increased utilization (alcoholism)
- abnormalities in enterohepatic circulation and malabsorption (vitamin A, vitamin D, folate, vitamin B_{12})
- decreased storage capacity (vitamin A in liver disease)
- increased loss from the body
- defects in metabolism (vitamin D in liver disease)

Vitamins K and B_6 and biotin normally are produced by enteric bacteria, and deficiency based solely on inadequate dietary intake is uncommon. However, interference with their endogenous synthesis occurs, as with administration of antibiotics (see Case 16a, Anorexia Nervosa). A similar effect is seen with vitamin D, synthesized in the skin, where air pollution or lack of sunshine may inhibit production of this vitamin.

With vitamins that undergo an enterohepatic circulation (A, D, folic acid, cobalamin), an increased amount of the vitamin will be lost from the body when intestinal malabsorption is present because of lack of reabsorption, together with malabsorption of the vitamin ingested in food (see Chapter 21). Generally, vitamin and mineral requirements are increased in patients with malabsorption, regardless of the cause. Disorders that hinder the delivery of bile to the small bowel, such as obstructive jaundice or bile fistula, reduce absorption of fat-soluble vitamins. Deficiency can be prevented or relieved by administration of large doses of parenteral or oral vitamins, with added bile salts. Decreased storage of vitamin A is seen with chronic liver disease (see Chapter 22). Increased utilization may influence depletion of a variety of vitamins in the alcoholic, in whom malabsorption and poor dietary intake also interact and multiple deficiencies predominate (see Chapter 17).

Development of Deficiency State

The rate of loss of tissue function with vitamin deficiency depends on the nutrient (Fig. 14–1).

Stores—Water-soluble vitamins in limited stores are rapidly depleted within days of negative balance and depletion may be detected by declines in blood levels.

Cell metabolism—The effect of vitamin deficiency on cell metabolism is slower but may appear within 1 month.

Clinical defects—Become manifest over several months.

Anatomic defects—May not be apparent for 6 to 8 months.

Because of storage of fat-soluble vitamins and vitamin B_{12} in adipose tissue or liver, clinical deficiency of these vitamins is delayed and may take 2 years or more to develop.

Vitamin A

Night blindness was the first manifestation of vitamin deficiency described, in about 1500 B.C., in the Egyptian papyrus Ebers. Today vitamin A deficiency is common in South and Central America, Africa, India, and Southeast Asia, where it is the leading cause of blindness in children. Vitamin A deficiency may cause visual disturbances:

- night blindness (nyctalopia)
- dryness of the cornea (Bitot's spots)
- xerophthalmia
- keratomalacia (Fig. 14–2; see Case 14a)
- blindness

and also can lead to

- general symptoms of retarded growth
- hyperkeratinization of epithelial tissues (dryness of the skin)
- atrophy of odontoblasts with failure of tooth enamel

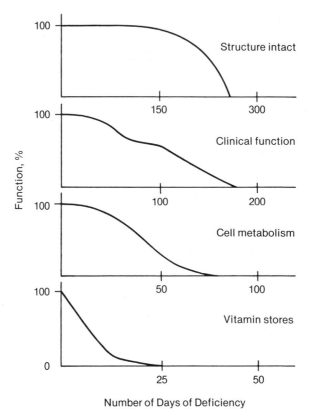

Figure 14-1. Time course of loss of function (100% to 0) in vitamin deficiency states in relation to rapid depletion of vitamin stores. Note the variation in time scales. Anatomic defects appear much later than symptoms of functional loss, which occur after cell metabolism is abnormal. Low levels of vitamin in blood precede depletion of tissue stores. (Adapted from Marks, J.: A Guide to the Vitamins. University Park Press, Baltimore, 1975, p. 10.)

Development of Vitamin A Deficiency

Vitamin A deficiency is primarily a disease of the young and is most prevalent in children 2 to 5 years of age. The deficiency also is more common in alcoholics. By contrast, oral contraceptives result in increased levels of vitamin A, which also may be increased in patients with end-stage renal disease.

In the development of vitamin A deficiency, liver stores of retinol decline gradually as they continue to supply retinol to the tissues; at this time blood levels of vitamin A remain normal. When liver stores are exhausted, blood

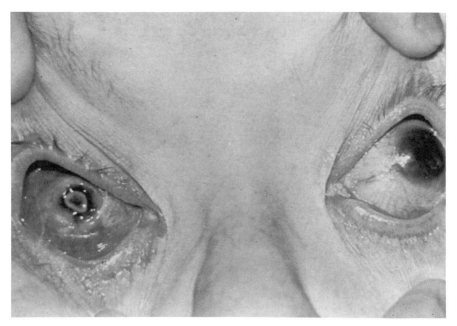

Figure 14-2. Keratomalacia and xerosis in the right and left eyes of a patient with vitamin A deficiency (Case 14a).

levels of vitamin A drop sharply. Because its half-life is longer than that of plasma retinol, retinol of the rhodopsin (the light-sensitive pigment of the retina) declines more slowly. At this stage night blindness, commonly the first symptom of vitamin A deficiency, sets in.

Xerosis results from squamous metaplasia and keratinization of the epithelial layer of the cornea that occur in the absence of retinol. The Bitot spot is a small, irregularly shaped, silver-gray plaque on the bulbar conjunctiva with a foamy surface. When it is accompanied by conjunctival xerosis, in young children, it is a sign of vitamin A deficiency. However, Bitot's spots are not a necessary stage in the progression of the disease. Keratomalacia due to vitamin A deficiency may occur without this sign.

Clinical Ophthalmologic Signs of Deficiency

Clinical ophthalmologic signs of vitamin A deficiency have been classified in five stages of increasing severity:

Stage	Effect On
0	Retina with poor dark adaptation
1	Conjunctiva with xerosis and Bitot's spots
2	Cornea with xerosis and superficial erosion

3   Cornea with irreversible ulcerations
4   Cornea with scarring and softening

The more severe eye defects are rarely encountered in the United States.

Other Signs of Deficiency

Plasma vitamin A levels are 10 μg per dl or lower when ophthalmologic and other clinical signs of vitamin A deficiency appear. Additional abnormalities are follicular hyperkeratosis, raised cerebrospinal fluid pressure, decrease in taste and smell, and abnormalities in vestibular function.

Cornification or keratinization occurs not only in the cornea, hair follicles, and epidermis but also in the trachea, urinary tract, vagina, sebaceous glands, salivary gland ducts, and pancreatic ducts. The lesions caused by the effects of vitamin A deficiency on epithelial growth and differentiation lead to invasion by microorganisms. Infection is the major cause of death resulting from vitamin A deficiency.

Rapid Dark Adaptation Test

This is a simple process in which subjects in dim light sort out white, red, and blue discs. The test is performed on the fully light-adapted eye. The time it takes the subject to sort the colored discs is a test of vitamin A function in adapting to scotopic, rod-mediated night vision. The rapid test is simpler than classic dark adaptation procedures that require 45 minutes and expensive, complicated instrumentation. The test is based on a shift of retinal wave length sensitivity as the eyes adapt (Purkinje's phenomenon), so that blue appears brighter than red when the rods begin to activate. Mean time for the rapid test is approximately 4^1/$_2$ minutes in individuals with sufficient vitamin A, increasing to more than 7 minutes in vitamin-deficient persons as measured by serum vitamin A levels less than 20 μg per dl.

Laboratory Tests

The plasma level of retinol can be measured to determine vitamin A status (Table 14–1). Carotene levels are measured as an index of intake or absorption.

Treatment of Deficiency

The deficiency is treated by enteral or parenteral administration of 30 mg (100,000 IU) of retinol. Vitamin A is available as capsules, 7.5 mg (25,000 IU); liquid, 1.5 mg per 0.1 ml (5000 IU); or by injection, 15 mg per ml (50,000 IU) in 5 ml vials. Corneal damage demands immediate treatment

Table 14-1. LIMITS OF NORMAL FOR LABORATORY TESTS
OF VITAMIN STATUS IN HEALTHY ADULTS*

Test	Level
Vitamin A, μg/dl	30–80
Carotene, μg/dl	100–200
Vitamin D, 25 OH, ng/ml	20–58
Vitamin D, 1,25 OH$_2$, pg/ml	26–65
Vitamin E, μg/dl	600–1200
Prothrombin time, sec	control +1.5
Vitamin C, mg/dl	0.3–2.0
Vitamin C, WBC, mg/dl	>15
Thiamin, urine, μg/g creatinine	>27
RBC transketolase AC[†]	<1.2
Riboflavin, urine, μg/g creatinine	>39
RBC glutathione reductase AC[†]	<1.4
Niacin metabolites,[‡] excretion ratio	1–4
Pyridoxine, ng/ml	>50
RBC aspartate-amino transferase AC[†]	<1.89
Folate, ng/ml	>3
Folate, RBC, ng/ml	>300
Vitamin B$_{12}$, pg/ml	≥200
Vitamin B$_{12}$, RBC, pg/ml	155–195
Biotin, pg/ml	200–500

*Values in plasma unless otherwise specified.
[†]AC = activity coefficient.
[‡]2-pyridone-5-carbox(yl)amide/N' methylnicotinamide.

with an initial high dose (30 mg, or 100,000 IU) followed by daily oral doses of 25,000 IU for several weeks. To be most effective, the patient's protein status must be normalized to provide for adequate synthesis of RBP.

CASE 14a: KERATOMALACIA

A 49-year-old woman was seen in the emergency room because of pain and presumed infection of her right eye (discharge and blurred vision) along with a productive cough, nausea, and vomiting. She had been a known alcoholic for many years, consuming a six-pack of beer daily. She had been hospitalized 2 years earlier with a diagnosis of scurvy and malnutrition. About 6 weeks before, she noted her eyes were "sore" but did not seek medical attention. Her dietary intake was reported by her family to be poor (cola and beer), but she denied this. She smoked one pack of cigarettes daily.

She weighed 57 kg; her height was 166 cm. Her right eye showed keratomalacia and endophthalmitis (Fig. 11–2), while the left eye showed xerosis. Suspicion of vitamin A deficiency prompted obtaining a blood sample (vitamin A level was 10 μg/dl with retinol binding protein 2 mg/dl and carotene 15 μg/dl) and intramuscular administration of 100,000 IU vitamin A followed by 25,000 IU orally daily for 3 weeks. The right eye was enucleated, and the left eye improved with treatment.

Her lung fields showed wheezes and rhonchi bilaterally, attributed to bronchitis. She exhibited ecchymoses over both forearms. The deep tendon reflexes were diminished. Anthropometric measurements were less than the 5th percentile (TSF 10 mm, MAMC 18 cm).

Hemoglobin was 11.3 g/dl with hematocrit 33 percent and MCV 101 fl. There was a mild leukocytosis and left shift. Blood chemistries and blood gases indicated a metabolic alkalosis. Serum albumin was 2.5 g/dl. Plasma prealbumin was 7 mg/dl and ascorbic acid level was 0.1 mg/dl (deficient = <0.2 mg/dl). The erythrocyte transketolase and glutathione reductase activity coefficients were elevated, indicating presumptive thiamin and riboflavin deficiency.

With treatment the vitamin A level increased in 2 weeks to 40 μg/dl and RBP to 5.1 mg/dl. Her calorie intake remained low.

Following her recovery from surgery, it was evident that she had manifestations of Korsakoff's psychosis. She was agitated and confused, disoriented as to time and place, delusional, and with memory loss. CT scan showed cerebellar and cerebral atrophy.

She responded to combined thiamin and Haldol therapy. Her oral energy intake improved to up to 2000 kcal daily. She was supplemented with vitamin A, thiamin, folic acid, iron, and zinc in addition to B complex and C. After 3 weeks, at discharge, her blood values had improved to carotene 79, vitamin A 66 μg/dl, RBP 9.9, and prealbumin 28 mg/dl.

Two months later the woman's vitamin A was 53 μg/dl, carotene 96 μg/dl, RBP 10.1, and prealbumin 36. Levels of transketolase activity, vitamins C and E, and selenium were within normal limits. Five months later she had gained 13 kg, her anthropometrics were TSF 14 mm, MAMC 24.4 cm, and she felt well.

LESSON:

This patient illustrates that alcoholism predisposes to multiple nutritional deficiencies that can manifest as classic vitamin deficiency syndromes—in this case vitamin A/keratomalacia, thiamin/Korsakoff's psychosis. Her nutritional collapse was precipitated by accompanying poor dietary intake and infection. Other nutritional deficiencies included protein, vitamins B_2, C, and E, iron, folate, zinc, and selenium. Refeeding and specific supplementation along with abstinence from alcohol resulted in rapid improvement except for the irreversible stage 4 vitamin A deficiency disease of the right eye.

Toxicity

Vitamin A is available in levels of up to 25,000 IU in over-the-counter tablets or capsules. Acute toxicity may result from ingestion of 500,000 to 2 million IU (150 to 600 mg) of the vitamin, and chronic toxicity (hypervitaminosis A) may follow daily intakes ranging from 25,000 to 300,000 IU (7.5 to 90 mg) for from 1 month to 2 years.

Acute vitamin A toxicity is associated with drowsiness, irritability, headache, and vomiting, whereas chronic toxicity is reflected by skin and lip desquamation, alopecia (that may be permanent), anorexia, nausea, bone pain and demineralization, hepatosplenomegaly, fatigue, and prominent eyes. Teratogenic effects have been observed in fetuses of women who consumed vitamin A at levels of 25,000 IU daily during pregnancy. In infants transient hydrocephalus with blurred vision and papilledema may occur. Among the minor symptoms of vitamin A toxicity are insomnia, weight loss, hypomenorrhea, sore tongue, anemia, and urinary frequency. Children may suffer growth retardation, and liver cirrhosis may develop. Plasma levels of vitamin A in the range of 5 to 30 times normal are diagnostic. Toxicity results when hepatic stores exceed 300 μg per g. Patients should stop intake of any vitamin A–containing supplements or liver or fish oils.

Severe acne has been treated with doses of vitamin A ranging from 50,000 to 100,000 IU per day. However, this treatment has been supplanted by use of retinoids—vitamin A analogues—which also are relatively toxic. Night vision is not improved by high doses of vitamin A except in deficient patients.

Vitamin D

Rickets and Osteomalacia

Rickets is caused by vitamin D deficiency. However, with adequate exposure to sunlight, the primary disorder is rare in the United States. Dietary rickets may be found where children are shielded from the sun, food is not enriched by vitamin D, and fish oils or vitamin preparations are not given. Rickets occurs in hereditary forms of vitamin D resistance and secondary to other diseases such as biliary atresia. The condition is diagnosed by radiographic changes, bone biopsy, and vitamin levels. Osteomalacia, or adult rickets, is metabolically identical to childhood rickets, and is seen primarily in malabsorption syndromes.

Physical Findings of Childhood Rickets. The physical findings include

- craniotabes
- chest deformity
- bowing of the long bones
- enlarged epiphyses of long bones
- greenstick fractures
- delayed dentition
- muscle weakness
- tetany
- impaired growth

In craniotabes the occiput is flattened, and there is bossing (thickening) of the skull over the frontal and parietal eminences. The sternum may be displaced anteriorly, forming a pigeon breast, or posteriorly with a trough. Harrison's groove is formed if the inferior ribs bend inward. A dorsolumbar kyphosis in early life may be replaced by a severe lordosis after the infant begins to walk. Back deformity and twisting of the tibia and femur cause the child to waddle. Bowed legs can be observed only in children who are already weight bearing (walking). Misshapen extremities include knobby deformities at the ends of the long bones, and displacement of the epiphysis so that posterior tilting of the lower tibial epiphysis by the weight of the foot results in the so-called saber-shin deformity. Displacement of the distal radial and ulnar epiphysis by the weight of the infant on his pronated hands results in a conspicuous bulging at the wrist.

Dentition is delayed and teeth may erupt out of order. Tooth enamel is thin, pitted, and occasionally absent in permanent teeth formed during the rachitic interval.

Biochemical Changes Caused by Vitamin D Deficiency. Characteristic biochemical changes of rickets include low plasma calcium and phosphate levels with high alkaline phosphatase. In mild cases, blood levels of calcium and phosphate are normal but enzyme levels are doubled. Defective calcium absorption often leads to secondary hyperparathyroidism in response to the low plasma calcium. Bone calcium is mobilized to restore serum calcium to normal, but parathyroid hormone causes hyperphosphaturia, leading to hypophosphatemia and finally failure of bone mineralization.

Symptoms Associated With Decreased Calcium or Phosphorus Stores. Vitamin D deficiency produces symptoms due to decreased body stores of calcium or phosphorus. Tetany results from hypocalcemia (low level of ionized calcium), while muscle weakness probably is due to a decrease in muscle phosphate. Defective bone mineralization with decreased calcification of newly formed bone and epiphyseal cartilage causes the skeletal manifestations of rickets. The organic matrix of both epiphyseal chondroblasts and osteoblasts fails to mineralize. The bone is not rigid, and the ends of long bones, the ribs, legs, and cranium are deformed. Wide osteoid seams (areas of uncalcified bone) are found as little calcium is deposited in the collagen matrix.

Radiographic Abnormalities in Rickets. Radiographs typically show concave cupping of the metaphysis. Stippling reflects incomplete deposition of calcium and phosphorus. Trabeculae of the bone appear coarse, the cortex is thin, and bone may be nearly translucent. The most useful radiologic manifestations of rickets appear at the lower ends of the radius and ulna. Changes may be similar to those of congenital syphilis or scurvy.

Osteomalacia. Osteomalacia results from decreased bone mineralization in vitamin D–deficient adults. Early bone disease may be seen with normal levels of blood calcium, while hypocalcemia and hypophosphatemia accompany severe bone disease. Only the shafts of the long bones and flat bones such as the pelvis are affected in osteomalacia, because longitudinal growth has stopped. Gross asymmetric deformity of the pelvis with narrowing of the outlet is typical, and pseudofractures of long bones also occur. Bone pain is especially felt in the spine, shoulders, and hips, and there is muscle weakness. Spontaneous fractures and pseudofractures occur. Inadequate exposure to sunlight, heavy skin pigmentation, and vegetarianism predispose to osteomalacia.

"Metabolic" Causes of Osteomalacia. Osteomalacia may be seen with the following conditions:

- end-stage renal disease (defective 1-hydroxylation)
- hepatic disease (defective 25-hydroxylation), common in alcoholics
- following intestinal resection with short bowel syndrome (decreased absorption of calcium)
- following gastrectomy (duodenum)
- with use of anticonvulsant medications

The severe bone disease of chronic renal failure is probably the most common defect in vitamin D metabolism and is much more common than dietary deficiency. Up to 30 percent of patients on long-term phenytoin/phenobarbital treatment for epilepsy may develop bone disease, accompanied by low circulating levels of 25-hydroxy vitamin D_3. The role of vitamin D deficiency in the etiology and management of osteoporosis is controversial.

Laboratory Tests. Vitamin D status can be assessed by measuring 25-hydroxy vitamin D_3 in blood (Table 14–1), with low levels (less than 8 ng per ml) indicating deficient status. The concentration in plasma is 5 to 10 times that in all other tissues except for adipose. 25-hydroxy vitamin D_3 is bound in plasma to a binding protein that binds all vitamin D metabolites.

Treatment of Vitamin D Deficiency. Both vitamin D and an adequate intake of calcium are required in the treatment of rickets. With early treatment, bone deformities can be avoided. Provision of 75 to 100 μg (4000 IU) of vitamin D daily is required until alkaline phosphatase is normalized, when the dose should be reduced to 10 μg daily for maintenance. The vitamin is available as calciferol in capsules containing 1.2 mg per ml (8000 IU). Calcitriol (1,25 dihydroxy cholecalciferol) is available in capsules containing 0.25 μg, and is recommended for use primarily in patients with renal failure. 25-

hydroxy vitamin D_3, available in 20 and 50 μg tablets, may be useful in treating osteomalacia by increasing the calcium content of bone. If there is malabsorption, the dose of vitamin D should be up to 1.25 mg (50,000 IU) daily and may be administered intramuscularly (see Chapter 21).

Hereditary Vitamin D–Resistant Rickets. Autosomal recessive vitamin D–dependent rickets occurs in two forms in children who demonstrate low plasma levels of the vitamin and develop rickets despite normal vitamin D intake. The metabolic defects lie either in the 1-hydroxylation of 25-hydroxy vitamin D_3, or in resistance to the vitamin. Rickets can be prevented by administration of 50,000 to 100,000 IU of vitamin D_3 daily. These children can also be treated with 1 mg per day of 1,25-hydroxy vitamin D_3 or somewhat higher levels of 1-hydroxy vitamin D_3.

Hypophosphatemic vitamin D–resistant rickets is an X-linked dominant defect in phosphate absorption in renal tubules. Treatment as yet is only partially successful. There also is a similar very rare autosomal dominant defect.

Toxicity

Patients with acute vitamin D toxicity present with anorexia, vomiting, polyuria, and headache, while chronic toxicity is associated with hypercalcemia and nephrocalcinosis. Because of a low therapeutic index, hypervitaminosis D may occur with doses four to five times the recommended 200 to 400 IU daily. Generally, over-the-counter preparations contain less than 2000 IU vitamin D per capsule.

Vitamin E (Tocopherol)

Deficiency

Vitamin E deficiency may cause hemolytic anemia in infants; in premature infants it is associated with thrombocythemia (elevated platelet count) and edema. Administration of vitamin E to infants is discussed in Chapter 8.

Low plasma tocopherol levels have also been observed in malabsorption syndromes (abetalipoproteinemia and short bowel syndrome), cystic fibrosis, chronic pancreatitis, ulcerative colitis, postgastrectomy, and with biliary obstruction. Vitamin E deficiency often is associated with symptoms of peripheral neuropathy in patients with hypobetalipoproteinemia and familial isolated vitamin E deficiency. Other neurologic abnormalities include ataxia and areflexia. Destruction of the nerves (axonal degeneration) may be a result of free radical damage.

Vitamin E deficiency is treated with 50 to 800 mg of the vitamin daily. Improved neurologic function, or arrest of deterioration, may require use of 400 mg to 10 g daily of vitamin E.

Laboratory Tests

The plasma or serum level of vitamin E can be measured (see Table 2–4). The deficiency is diagnosed by vitamin E levels in plasma less than 0.6 mg per dl. Current analytic methods determine the active form, α-tocopherol, and are indicative of vitamin E status. Ratios of serum vitamin E to total serum lipids should also be measured and interpreted with regard to hyperlipidemias and malabsorption.

Excess

In high doses vitamin E can interfere with vitamin K metabolism and lengthen prothrombin time, but the vitamin has relatively low toxicity.

Vitamin K

Deficiency of vitamin K causes bleeding. Clinical deficiency of the vitamin unrelated to anticoagulant drugs of the coumadin family usually is due to the combination of antibiotic therapy and poor dietary intake. (Case 16a illustrates vitamin K deficiency in a patient with anorexia nervosa treated with antibiotics for pneumonia.) Bile acid binding resins may also predispose to vitamin K deficiency. The one-stage prothrombin time is a measure of vitamin K adequacy (Table 14–1). Treatment is with 1 mg of vitamin K until the prothrombin time is normal. Weekly vitamin K may be prescribed with the bile acid binding resins.

Vitamin C and Scurvy

Scurvy is an ancient disease, first described by Egyptians in the papyrus Ebers about 1500 B.C., but uncommon today. A nutritional etiology was suspected as early as the 16th century, when it was noted that the condition could be prevented among seamen by eating lemons, oranges, berries, or sassafras.

Pathophysiology of Scurvy

The pathophysiology of scurvy may be described as a diminution or loss of the functions of ascorbic acid, including hydroxylation of proline, leading to defective collagen formation in capillary basement membranes, and of lysine, and precursors of catecholamines and other vasoactive and neurotropic substances.

Clinical Manifestations of Vitamin C Deficiency

Vitamin C deficiency is manifested by multiple symptoms, including

- fatigue
- weakness
- lethargy
- irritability
- bleeding gums
- muscle and joint pain
- weight loss

The first signs of deficiency may be bleeding gums (when teeth are present), gingivitis, and loose teeth. Gingival change is first seen at the base of the molars as interdental papillae become swollen and bluish-red and may develop secondary infection. In time the teeth fall out (see Chapter 20). These signs appear about 2 weeks after white cell levels of ascorbic acid become deficient (less than 2 mg per 10^8 cells), or 60 to 90 days after sustained deficient intake, with diets devoid of fresh fruits and vegetables.

Typical follicular hyperkeratosis, especially on the thighs and buttocks, with perifollicular hemorrhages, results from hair shafts poorly formed because of impaired protein synthesis. Brittle hair easily breaks off, with broken ends becoming impacted in the dry hair canal. Growing hair coils into a characteristic circle just beneath the superficial layer of skin. In more advanced cases the hair shaft is replaced by an irregular, horny material resembling a bit of broken fingernail. The presence of petechial hemorrhages in tissues surrounding the hair follicle is the most characteristic sign of the disorder in the adult (Fig. 14–3).

The psychologic effects of vitamin C deficiency include the triad of depression, hysteria, and hypochondriasis.

Other clinical manifestations of scurvy are loss of adrenocortical secretory functions in response to stress, neurologic impairment, cardiovascular malfunctioning, and, at times, edema. Poor resistance to infection probably is secondary to loss of secretions and disruption of mucous membranes.

Purpuric lesions coalesce to form ecchymoses that spread from the lower extremities to the rest of the body, especially to those areas exposed to trauma. Large interjoint and subperiosteal hemorrhages occur, and ultimately sudden death may follow from cerebral or cardiac hemorrhage.

In usual circumstances the onset of clinical scurvy in adults is delayed several months from the time dietary vitamin C is restricted. Plasma ascorbic acid reflects recent intake, falling to low levels in 3 or 4 weeks. Plasma ascorbic acid levels between 0.2 and 0.3 mg per dl are marginal; values less than 0.2 mg per dl with symptomatic scurvy indicate severe deficiency. The decline in white blood cell vitamin C occurs more slowly, reaching its nadir in 20 to 24 weeks.

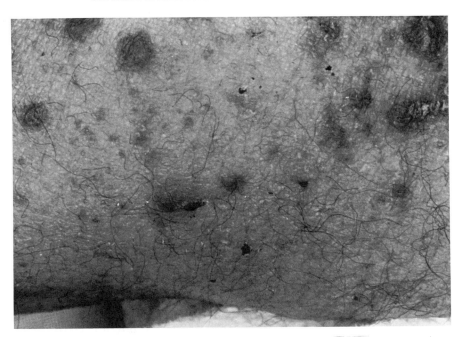

Figure 14–3. Perifollicular petechial hemorrhages of scurvy (Case 14b).

The deficiency of ascorbic acid may interact with iron and folic acid deficiency and with intercurrent infections, resulting in anemia. Because scurvy may result in sudden death due to large hemorrhages, treatment must not be delayed.

Laboratory Tests

Both plasma and white blood cell levels of ascorbic acid can be measured (see Table 14–1). Plasma ascorbic acid levels reflect intake but may be reduced in patients with chronic inflammatory diseases, in cigarette smokers, and in women taking oral contraceptives. Ascorbic acid in white cells is more closely related to body stores. Plasma ascorbate is generally used for evaluation of possible scurvy, with deficiency present at levels below 0.3 mg per dl.

Prevention and Treatment of Scurvy

Scurvy may be seen in alcoholics (Case 14b) and occasionally in the elderly ("bachelor's scurvy"). Preventive therapy is appropriate for patients with limited ascorbic acid intake, malabsorption, or increased need for vitamin C lasting more than 2 weeks. A daily intake of vitamin C as low as 10 mg will prevent symptoms of scurvy in normal individuals. Scurvy is treated with administration of 1 g ascorbic acid, available in tablets of 50 to 260 mg, as a liquid, or by injection, 500 mg per 1 ml ampule, given for 1 week, followed by maintenance intake and an improved diet.

CASE 14b: SCURVY

A 54-year-old white man with a history of heavy alcohol abuse presented to the VA Hospital on 6/11/87 with a 2-week history of jaundice and dark urine and swelling of his abdomen for 3 weeks. He gave an approximately 30-year history of heavy alcohol abuse, usually two to three pints of wine a day. Two months ago he began drinking 1 liter of gin a day. He ate one or two meals per week, usually a fast food hamburger and milk shake brought by his children, or a T.V. dinner. There was no recent hematemesis, melena, fever, chills, or nausea.

Past medical history included hypertension, treated with propranolol; previous icterus; an upper GI bleed, April, 1985, probably from esophageal varices; and gout, treated in the past with allopurinol.

The physical examination on admission revealed: temperature 100°F, pulse 86, respiratory rate 26, and blood pressure 110/62. The patient was severely icteric. Oropharynx: edentulous on the upper jaw, normal lower teeth; no gum lesions were noted. Chest exam revealed regular, unlabored respirations, bilateral breath sounds, no wheezes or rales. The heart rate and rhythm were regular with a II/VI systolic ejection murmur at the left lower sternal border that radiated to both carotids. The abdomen was protuberant with shifting dullness and a fluid wave. The liver edge was palpable 12 cm below the right costal margin and the spleen was ballottable through the ascites. Lower extremity exam showed perifollicular hemorrhages over both shins and an ecchymotic area over the left calf. There were multiple keratotic skin lesions and multiple spider angiomata. The neurologic exam was normal; the patient was alert and oriented, with no abnormalities of speech or thought processes.

Admission laboratory tests were (abnormal levels): hemoglobin, 12.1 g/dl; hematocrit, 35.8%; MCV, 114 fl, normal white blood cell count and differential and 89,000 platelets. Prothrombin time was normal and PTT was 30.9 with a control of 27.9 seconds. SMA-6 revealed (mEq/l): sodium, 125; potassium, 3.0; chloride 90; bicarbonate, 25; glucose, BUN, and creatinine were normal. Calcium (mg/dl) was 9.0; phosphate, 2.2; magnesium, 1.5. Serum enzyme studies revealed (units): lipase, 24; LDH, 229; SGOT, 178; SGPT, 32; alkaline phosphatates, 331; and gamma GT, 600. Bilirubin was 36 mg/dl. Total protein was 5.6 g/dl with an albumin of 2.3. Chest radiogram was normal.

The initial impression of the ward team was alcoholic hepatitis with jaundice and ascites. Initial therapy was correction of abnormal electrolytes with oral replacement. The patient was placed on 1500 cc fluid restriction and a 2 g sodium diet. Aldactone was given for diuresis. Because of the perifollicular hemorrhages, the Nutrition Service was consulted for evaluation of possible scurvy. Their initial impression was scurvy. After the blood had been obtained for laboratory tests, they recommended that the patient be started on ascorbic acid 500 mg plus two therapeutic multivitamins daily by mouth. They also recommended that the initially prescribed thiamin therapy be continued, and added folic acid 1 mg daily by mouth. The nutritional laboratory studies obtained included (mg/dl): a plasma prealbumin, 3.9; retinol binding protein, 0.6; transferrin, 129; vitamin C <0.10. In view of the very low RBP, 50,000 units of vitamin A by mouth were prescribed for 1 week. Later results showed retinol 5 μg/dl and zinc 50. There was gradual improvement in the perifollicular hemorrhages, with almost complete disappearance by 1 week. Jaundice and ascites were resolving, and the patient felt stronger. He was to be discharged directly to a detoxification unit.

LESSON:

The major manifestation of multiple vitamin deficiencies in a patient with alcoholic liver disease was clinical scurvy.

Excessive Doses of Vitamin C

Potential harmful consequences of excessive doses of vitamin C include development of renal calculi, especially in patients with gout, and development of calcium oxalate stones. The body may become conditioned to high levels of vitamin C, with scurvy developing when ascorbic acid intake is reduced to normal levels—a disorder observed in infants born to women who took high doses of the vitamin during pregnancy. Ascorbic acid in the stool may give a false positive result in the guaiac test for occult blood. There is no convincing objective evidence that vitamin C prevents or cures the common cold or other infections, or that it promotes wound healing (other than when given during deficiency).

Thiamin

The spectrum of thiamin deficiency ranges from early signs of peripheral polyneuropathy (dry or atrophic beriberi), to subacute or wet beriberi with cardiac signs, to Wernicke-Korsakoff encephalopathy and psychosis.

Although beriberi had been endemic in the Orient for over 4000 years, the disease was first recognized as a nutritional deficiency in Japan in the late 19th century, where polished rice was the major staple of the diet. In certain parts of Asia the incidence of beriberi may be further augmented by anti-thiamin factors in the diet (tea leaves, herring, shellfish, and raw carp).

Thiamin deficiency is common in alcoholics but has also been reported in patients on restricted diets for obesity (see Case 14c) or who receive total parenteral nutrition. Wernicke's encephalopathy recently was reported in a susceptible patient with diabetes mellitus and borderline thiamin reserves following correction of hyperglycemia with an oral hypoglycemic agent.

Dry Beriberi (Thiamin Intake 0.2 mg–0.3 mg per 1000 kcal)

The extremities of maximal use are most affected in the development of peripheral neuropathy. Manifestations include muscle tenderness, weakness and atrophy, and foot and wrist drop. Paresthesias, dysesthesias, hyperesthesia, anesthesia, and formication (a sensation of small insects crawling over the skin) occur. Deep tendon reflexes are initially increased, then progress from diminished to absent as the disorder becomes chronic. Important constitutional signs accompanying the peripheral neuropathy of thiamin deficiency (so-called dry beriberi) are

- fatigue
- decreased attention span
- impaired capacity to work

Gastrointestinal disturbances such as anorexia, nausea, vomiting, and constipation may also occur, along with oliguria.

Signs of chronic dry beriberi include

- flaccid paraplegia
- muscle wasting

Wet Beriberi (Thiamin Intake Less Than 0.2 mg per 1000 kcal)

Signs of wet beriberi include dependent edema and cardiovascular signs and symptoms in addition to the previously cited polyneuropathy. Beriberi heart disease develops over 30 to 120 days on a high carbohydrate diet with thiamin intake less than 0.2 to 0.3 mg per 1000 kcal (compared with the RDA of 0.5 to 1 mg per 1000 kcal). When dietary intake is very low, these cardiovascular signs are superimposed on the polyneuropathy. This form of the disease is still seen primarily in Southeast Asia, India, Brazil, and Africa.

Signs and symptoms include dull precordial and epigastric pain, pulsating neck veins, full bounding pulse, and systolic murmurs. The heart is dilated and there is high output failure; however, the patient usually exhibits normal sinus rhythm. The right side of the heart is particularly enlarged. Venous pressure is increased, but circulation time may be shortened or normal. Systolic hypotension, venous distention, and peripheral cyanosis occur. Therapy with thiamin may provide relief of cardiomyopathy, but neurologic symptoms may not respond rapidly.

Shoshin Beriberi. Fulminant cardiac failure may occur and has been termed "Shoshin beriberi," for the region in Japan where it was described. Patients with Shoshin beriberi have acute cardiovascular collapse, do not respond to digitalis or diuretics, and rapidly succumb with cardiac failure. Generally there has been gross dietary deficiency over a period of at least 3 months, with no other cause of heart disease present. Blood pyruvate levels exceed 0.75 mg per dl, and lactic acidosis is present. Red blood cell transketolase activity is decreased, and the activity coefficient is increased (see Table 14–1).

This type of severe congestive heart failure resulting from thiamin deficiency is very rare in the United States.

Wernicke-Korsakoff Syndrome

The most acute type of thiamin deficiency is Wernicke's encephalopathy, which occurs rarely in the Orient. The syndrome occurs primarily in alcoholics, half of whom have liver disease, and often is precipitated abruptly by administration of glucose to patients severely deficient in thiamin. If untreated, death is common; even with treatment, 17 percent die within 3 weeks. The Wernicke-Korsakoff syndrome, two related manifestations of thiamin deficiency, may occur only in patients with a genetic abnormality in the thiamin-dependent enzyme, transketolase. This may explain why only a minority of chronic alcoholics develop the syndrome. In the presence of starvation and famine, the syndrome does not develop, implying that a certain quantity of food is necessary for pathologic expression. The classic symptoms may not develop simultaneously. The patient with the syndrome often presents with global confusion. The patient is alert but not oriented to place and time, apathetic, with psychomotor retardation and lack of insight. There is considerable difficulty performing mental status testing with variable responses to questions over a short period of time. The memory deficit characteristic of Korsakoff's psychosis follows the initial confusional state. In addition, severe bilateral vestibular dysfunction (abnormal cold caloric test) may be present. The course usually evolves rapidly.

Wernicke's syndrome is characterized by incoordination and ataxia that involves principally the lower extremities and can range from mild (identified with tandem walking), to moderate (wide-based gait), or severe (patient is totally unable to ambulate). Individual limb movements are well preserved. The major ocular abnormalities of Wernicke's syndrome include weakness or paralysis of conjugate gaze or of individual extraocular muscles coupled with jerk nystagmus in horizontal and vertical directions. The earliest findings are nystagmus and lateral rectus weakness. The pupils are usually normal.

Korsakoff's psychosis impairs retentive memory and cognitive function, with confabulation a common characteristic. Korsakoff's psychosis encompasses impairment of learning and retrograde amnesia. This syndrome is not restricted to alcoholics nor a feature only of thiamin deficiency. A lessening of confabulation may result as the disorder progresses, but the impairment of learning may make independent living impossible. Recovery is poor in well-established psychosis. Mortality is secondary to non-neurologic causes and may be as high as 50 percent in debilitated patients.

In the Wernicke-Korsakoff syndrome, pathologic changes are found in the mammillary bodies around the third ventricle, aqueduct, and fourth ventricle. There is regional necrosis, petechial hemorrhages, and reactive gliosis associated with loss of myelin, neurons, and their axis cylinders.

Laboratory Tests

Thiamin in urine can be assayed chemically or microbiologically. Urinary thiamin levels reflect dietary intake; they do not assess body stores. At recommended intakes, urinary excretion of thiamin ranges from 40 to 90 μg per day. When intake is deficient, urinary excretion falls below 25 μg per day.

The chemical test for thiamin status involves erythrocyte transketolase which catalyzes the following reactions in the pentose phosphate pathway:

$$\text{xylulose-5-PO}_4 + \text{ribose-5-PO}_4 \rightarrow \text{sedoheptulose-7-PO}_4 + \text{glyceraldehyde-3-PO}_4$$

$$\text{xylulose-5-PO}_4 + \text{erythrose-4-PO}_4 \rightarrow \text{fructose-6-PO}_4 + \text{glyceraldehyde-3-PO}_4$$

The assay for transketolase is performed in the absence and presence of added thiamin and expressed as an activity coefficient. Values without added thiamin reflect the amount of coenzyme present in the red cells. The stimulation with added thiamin gives the measure of apoenzyme present that lacks coenzyme. Normal thiamin stimulation is less than 15 percent. In the deficient condition, thiamin stimulation exceeds 20 percent (see Table 14–1).

Prevention and Treatment of Deficiency

Thiamin is available in tablets of 25 or 100 mg, as an elixir, or in injectable form, 100 mg per ml. Wet beriberi should be treated with complete bed rest and administration of parenteral thiamin, 50 mg daily, for 3 days. This is followed by oral administration of 25 to 50 mg thiamin daily until recovery. The response is dramatic, with symptomatic relief within hours, the heart size becoming normal within a few days. A similar dosage schedule is used to initiate therapy for polyneuropathy, with less spectacular improvement. A good diet should be provided. The ocular manifestations of Wernicke's syndrome improve promptly, within hours, with administration of the large doses of thiamin, but the response of the Korsakoff's psychosis is slow and incomplete in the majority of patients. Preventive therapy should be given to patients with limited intake, malabsorption, or increased requirements lasting more than 2 weeks. The required dose approximates the RDA.

CASE 14c: WERNICKE'S ENCEPHALOPATHY

A 23-year-old elementary school teacher was transferred to the Neurology Service because of fainting spells and unsteady gait progressing over the previous 8 days. Symptoms included blurred vision and diplopia, and friends noted "her eyes were crossed."

During the preceding 10 months she had voluntarily restricted her energy intake and lost weight from 106 kg to her admission weight of 61 kg. Her height was 163 cm, and she was at 113 percent of her ideal body weight. Her diet had consisted of noncaloric soft drinks, with a hamburger and salad eaten about every fourth day. She had taken no vitamin supplements. For the 10 days preceding the onset of symptoms her total dietary intake had been noncaloric drinks.

She was torpid but awake and oriented, with coarse horizontal nystagmus observed in the primary position of gaze, accentuated with a quick component in the direction of gaze upon gazing laterally in either direction. The eye movements were dissociated at times. There was coarse vertical nystagmus on upward gaze. She had moderate trunkal dystaxia and inability to tandem walk. She tended to fall in Romberg's position. Deep tendon reflexes and sensory examination were normal.

Although the referral and initial diagnosis was of a possible posterior fossa neoplasm, Wernicke's encephalopathy was suspected by the attending neurologist, who prescribed 100 mg of thiamin hydrochloride for intravenous administration. Laboratory values showed 4+ ketonuria but otherwise were within normal limits. Ketonuria subsided with administration of $2^{1}/_{2}$ percent glucose IV. Within 48 hours the disconjugate eye movements disappeared and dystaxia was subsiding. The neurologic examination was normal 9 days after admission. The patient was maintained on a diet increased gradually to 1500 kcal (weight-maintaining) with therapeutic oral vitamin supplements replacing IV thiamin after several days.

LESSON:

This patient illustrated that Wernicke's encephalopathy is not confined to alcoholics and can result from unsupervised, self-prescribed weight reduction. Her condition worsened when she was treated at her local hospital for orthostatic hypotension, with 2 liters of 10 percent glucose in water.

Riboflavin

Riboflavin deficiency alone produces no specific disease syndrome, but the following symptoms, primarily oral or eye lesions, sometimes have been related to deficiency:

- photophobia
- tearing and itching of the eyes
- corneal vascularization
- soreness and burning of the lips, mouth, and tongue
- angular stomatitis (characterized by maceration and transverse fissures at the angles of the mouth)
- cheilosis involving the lip lines of closure (Fig. 14–4)
- geographic tongue and denudation of papillae
- desquamation of the skin and seborrheic dermatitis, especially in the nasolabial fold and scrotum
- hypochromic or normochromic anemia with erythroid hypoplasia

In the absence of riboflavin deficiency, similar lip and mouth lesions may result from drooling, poorly fitting dentures, or sensitivity to substances such as cosmetics and toothpaste. The tongue lesion (magenta tongue, Fig. 14–5) is also seen in deficiency of other B vitamins or iron, and occasionally with antibiotic therapy.

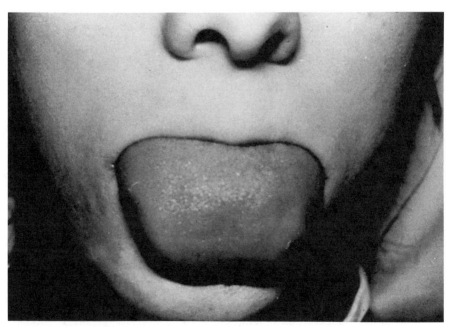

Figure 14–4. Angular fissures and glossitis (Case 13a).

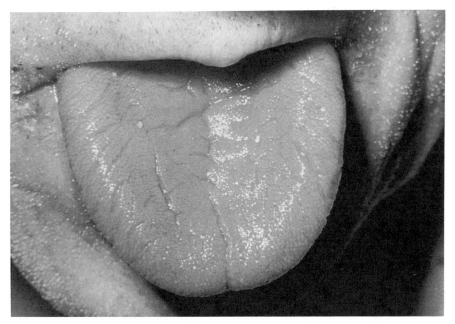

Figure 14-5. Glossitis in a patient with pernicious anemia (see Case 15a).

Laboratory Tests

The laboratory test for riboflavin status is measurement of erythrocyte glutathione reductase level and activity coefficient. Glutathione reductase catalyzes the following reaction:

$$NADPH + H^+ + GSSG \rightarrow NADP^+ + 2\,GSH$$

GSSG = oxidized glutathione   GSH = reduced glutathione

Like the functional assay for thiamin, this assay is performed in the presence and absence of the vitamin required, added flavin adenine dinucleotide (FAD). With riboflavin deficiency, stimulation of activity by added flavin exceeds 40 percent.

Treatment of Deficiency

Because the deficiency does not occur alone, patients should be managed with administration of an oral or intravenous therapeutic multivitamin preparation (B complex and C). No adverse effects of riboflavin treatment have been reported.

Niacin and Pellagra

Inadequate intake of niacin, usually associated with deficiency of other vitamins and minerals, and protein, leads to the disease known as pellagra. Early in this century, pellagra was epidemic in the southern United States in persons who ingested a diet high in cornmeal, exercised heavily, and were exposed to sun. Goldberger concluded in 1915–1917 that pellagra could be caused and cured by diet. In 1938, Sydenstricker treated pellagra patients with supplements of nicotinic acid. Deficiency occurs when dietary intake is between 9 and 15 mg, with the requirement increased as caloric intake rises. A governmental mandate for enrichment of flour has been the major factor in eradicating the disorder in the general population, by making foods such as bread good sources of niacin. However, alcoholics, elderly recluses, and others with bizarre eating habits remain at risk for pellagra. The disorder is occasionally seen in patients with malabsorption syndromes, thyrotoxicosis, diabetes mellitus, neoplasms, or carcinoid tumors (see Case 14d).

Niacin deficiency is commonly associated with deficiency of other nutrients. Thus patients with pellagra may also be deficient in protein, riboflavin, pyridoxine, thiamin, folic acid, vitamin A, magnesium, potassium, iron, and zinc. These associated deficiencies contribute to some of the clinical findings.

Signs and Symptoms of Pellagra

Pellagra is characterized by the four Ds:

- dermatitis
- diarrhea
- dementia
- death

The disorder affects all body systems, with the most significant signs involving the skin, nervous system, and gastrointestinal tract. Patients are apathetic, anorexic, and complain of pain in their extremities or over their body. The skin over exposed surfaces and pressure points may become thickened, hyperkeratotic, and hyperpigmented (Fig. 14–6). The characteristic rash of pellagra may resemble a severe burn and may become secondarily infected when niacin deficiency is severe. Classically the dermatitis appears as bilaterally symmetrical lesions over the back of the hands, the elbows, neck (Casal's necklace), and the anterior chest.

Oral and gastrointestinal involvement includes nonspecific lesions of cheilosis, angular fissures, glossitis, gastric achlorhydria, atrophy of the small intestinal mucosa, and nonspecific colitis. Anemia may be macrocytic and responsive to folic acid, or hypochromic and responsive to iron.

Neurologic manifestations of pellagra may predominate in less severe cases. They include peripheral neuropathy, diminished taste and smell, pro-

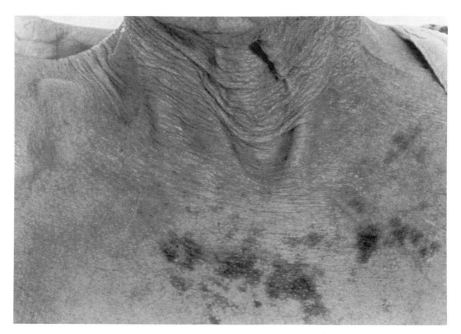

Figure 14–6. Dermatitis of upper chest (Casal's necklace) of a patient with pellagra (Case 14d).

prioceptive alterations, and encephalopathy. Depression is common. As the deficiency continues, cells of the motor cortex, peripheral nerves, and white matter of dorsal columns may degenerate. Psychiatric manifestations of pellagra accounted for a high proportion of admissions to mental institutions in endemic areas prior to the availability of nicotinic acid.

Diagnosis of Pellagra

The diagnosis of pellagra is usually clear in patients with the skin rash. However, the rash may be minimal or absent if the skin has not been exposed to sunlight or minor trauma. A careful dietary history is especially helpful in determining the diagnosis when patients present with only neurologic and gastrointestinal manifestations. A diet supplying less than 9.0 mg niacin daily or 4.4 mg per 1000 kcal is insufficient. Adults excrete 25 percent of the niacin as N1-methyl nicotinamide and 50 percent as the 2-pyridone metabolite. These metabolites can be measured in the urine, with low values indicating deficient intake (see Table 2–4). No reliable specific laboratory test is available for the diagnosis of the disorder, but low plasma levels of tryptophan may be suggestive of niacin deficiency.

Treatment of Pellagra

Treatment of pellagra should begin with 300 to 500 mg of niacinamide daily in divided doses, together with administration of other B vitamins. Intravenous niacin (50 mg) may be given initially. Later, 125 mg niacin daily will suffice. Initially, a soft diet may be helpful for the acutely ill patient because of mouth and gastrointestinal problems. However, the severely depleted patient may require enteral or parenteral nutrition (see Chapters 11 and 12). Large therapeutic amounts of nicotinic acid may be better provided in the form of nicotinamide, which does not produce a flushing reaction. Alternatively, pellagra may be treated with 600 mg on day one, 300 to 500 mg on day two, and 100 mg daily thereafter until symptoms resolve.

Hartnup's disease is a rare inborn error of metabolism that closely resembles pellagra. The underlying defect is in tryptophan transport in the intestine and renal tubule. Most patients respond well to treatment with nicotinamide.

CASE 14d: PELLAGRA

An 82-year-old male patient in a VA hospital was evaluated for possible pellagra. Pigmentation and flaking was present over the anterior chest, the dorsum of the hands and the pretibial areas (see Fig. 14–6). He had a history of lifelong alcohol abuse that had ceased 6 months earlier. He had developed anorexia and complained of dysphagia. He had undergone a Billroth II procedure for peptic ulcer disease 20 years earlier, with intermittent diarrhea and early satiety thereafter. He was depressed over his moderately severe coronary heart disease and was hospitalized for pacemaker battery change. His diet was generally poor and he had taken no vitamin supplements. In addition to the skin changes he was underweight; height 74 inches, weight 119 lb (62 percent of ideal). He was treated with niacin, 100 mg daily, and B complex vitamins for the duration of his hospitalization along with a nutritional regimen optimized by the dietitian to improve his oral intake. He was lost to follow-up.

LESSON:

Nutritional deficiencies are prone to occur in patients who are elderly, who are suffering from alcoholism, who have had resection of the gastrointestinal tract, and/or who are depressed. A combination of these circumstances is not uncommon; for example, the elderly are often depressed, gastrectomy is not uncommon in alcoholics, and so forth. Better clinical acumen should lead to recognition of problems before they become as severe as in this patient. Prevention is the most desirable approach.

Pyridoxine (Vitamin B_6)

Deficiency

Vitamin B_6 deficiency may occur in malnourished individuals, uremic patients, chronic alcoholics, and those with various forms of liver disease. Infants fed a commercial formula low in vitamin B_6 exhibited nervous irritability and seizures but responded well to pyridoxine therapy. Women taking oral steroid contraceptives may experience a decreased plasma concentration of pyridoxal phosphate, but it is not clear whether these agents produce a true vitamin B_6 deficiency. The administration of drugs with anti–vitamin B_6 properties such as isoniazid (INH), penicillamine, hydralazine, cycloserine, pyrazinamide, ethionamide, and L-dopa also can induce vitamin B_6 deficiency. In patients receiving the antituberculosis drug INH, pyridoxine should be prescribed.

Symptoms and signs associated with vitamin B_6 deficiency, which are unresponsive to riboflavin, include

- iron-resistant hypochromic anemia
- weakness
- irritability and nervousness
- insomnia
- peripheral neuropathy with impaired motor function later
- dermatitis resembling seborrhea, especially on the face
- occasional development of intertrigo under the breasts
- hyperpigmented, scaly pellagra-like lesions
- cheilosis, glossitis, and stomatitis indistinguishable from signs seen in pellagra and in riboflavin deficiency

Other vitamin B_6 deficiency syndromes have been reported in research studies. In one study subjects lost weight, and some showed apathy, somnolence, and increased irritability. There was a strong tendency to develop infections, especially of the genitourinary tract. High protein intake hastened the onset of pyridoxine deficiency.

Laboratory Tests

Pyridoxine status (see Table 14–1) can be tested by values of erythrocyte or serum glutamic-oxaloacetic or -pyruvic transaminase. In the transaminase reaction, added pyridoxal phosphate will always increase transaminase activity, but in healthy individuals the stimulated activity (activity coefficient) is less than 1.5. It was the observation of low SGOT that was normalized by adding pyridoxine in vitro in patients undergoing dialysis that led to the recommendation that patients with renal disease receive 25 mg daily of this vitamin.

Toxicity

Pyridoxine has recently been reported to cause sensory neuropathy in subjects who ingested maximum daily doses ranging from 2 to 6 g (1000 to 2700 times the RDA) over periods of 2 to 40 months. Symptoms included severely disabling ataxia with numb feet, followed by numbness and clumsiness of the hands, and finally perioral numbness. A "stocking-glove" distribution of sensory loss was nearly total, and nerve biopsy showed axonal degeneration. Patients had begun taking 50 to 100 mg of pyridoxine per day as self-imposed therapy for premenstrual edema, as treatment for behavioral disorders, or as dietary supplements. Symptoms improved markedly after a few months' abstinence but were not reversed completely.

The mechanism of pyridoxine toxicity may be because pyridines as a family are neurotoxic. In contrast to the unlimited gastrointestinal transport of pyridoxine, there is limited transport of the vitamin across the blood-brain barrier. The selective toxicity of pyridoxine for sensory fibers of peripheral nerves may be because the cell bodies of the fibers are located outside the blood-brain barrier. It is also possible that the massive dose of pyridoxine saturated the system converting pyridoxine to its active form, pyridoxal phosphate, resulting in a relative deficiency of the vitamin in its active form. Finally, there is a chance that at such a high dose of the vitamin, some contaminant may cause toxicity—a further indication of the hazards posed by indiscriminate use of megavitamins. Larger doses of pyridoxine may interfere with the therapeutic action of L-dopa in the treatment of Parkinson's disease.

Biotin

Biotin deficiency alone, although rare, has been noted in patients with prolonged total parenteral nutrition. Manifestations of the deficiency also have been observed in children with inborn multiple carboxylase deficiencies. Biotin deficiency is accompanied by scaling skin, maculopapular dermatitis, and alopecia but responds to pharmacologic doses of biotin. Biotin can be measured by a microbiologic assay in special laboratories (see Table 14–1).

The first demonstration of specific human biotin deficiency was described by Drs. Sydenstricker and Singal at the Medical College of Georgia in a study in which subjects were fed a raw egg white diet. A scaly dermatitis, atrophy of the lingual papillae, graying of mucous membranes, increasing skin dryness, depression, lassitude, muscle pains, paresthesia, anorexia, nausea, hypercholesterolemia, and abnormal electrocardiograms developed during a 10-week course of deficiency. These symptoms and signs were alleviated with provision of 150 to 300 μg of biotin by injection daily for a period of 3 to 5 days.

Excessive, huge doses of biotin used to treat biotin-responsive inborn errors of metabolism have been associated with hirsutism. Biotin in large doses thus has been touted as an unproven treatment for baldness!

Pantothenic Acid

No clear specific pantothenic acid deficiency syndrome has been reported in a human patient because it is so available in food. The best defined signs and symptoms of the deficiency have been noted in volunteer participants in a research study with a diet deficient in pantothenic acid and ingestion of an antagonist, omega methyl pantothenic acid. Subjects on this regimen developed vomiting, malaise, abdominal distress, and burning cramps. Later, tenderness in the heels, paresthesia in the hands and feet, fatigue, and insomnia occurred, and personality changes were also observed. These symptoms were reversed with large doses of pantothenic acid.

MINERAL DEFICIENCIES AND TOXICITIES

Calcium

Hypocalcemia and Low Calcium Status

Plasma calcium is regulated by parathormone, calcitonin and vitamin D, acting on bone, kidney, and intestine. Defects in this metabolic regulation are the most important causes of hypocalcemia.

Clinical Symptoms. Hypocalcemia results in increased neuromuscular irritability and tetany; clinical manifestations include tingling and carpopedal and laryngeal spasm with positive Chvostek's and Trousseau's signs. Symptomatic hypocalcemia is not uncommon in malabsorption syndromes (see Chapter 21). Cardiac arrhythmias may occur. (See Chapters 2 and 9 for discussion of calcium deficiency in bones and bone demineralization.)

Because of limited dietary sources, calcium deficiency is more common than deficiencies of magnesium or phosphorus. In addition, absorption of calcium also is limited, and its daily excretion in stool (300 mg) and urine (100 mg) is large compared with the body's exchangeable pool (1 g) and the daily flux from bone (200 to 300 mg). Hypocalcemia also is seen in renal failure (see Chapter 23).

Laboratory Tests. Urinary calcium excretion is an index of calcium intake and absorption. The usual excretion varies between 100 and 300 mg daily, approximately equal to net absorption. Serum or plasma ionized calcium is the free Ca^{++}, not bound to albumin, and about one half the total circulation. This fraction normally is maintained within a very narrow range by mobilization of calcium from bone and is low only with severe calcium, magnesium, or vitamin D deficiency or when alkalosis is present. Thus, vitamin D status should be evaluated in patients with calcium deficiency.

Treatment. Tetany is an emergency and should be treated with intravenous calcium gluconate (10 ml of a 10 percent solution), especially to prevent seizures. Calcium for chronic administration may be provided by mouth in the form of tablets of various salts, or as a liquid preparation. To avoid hypercalciuria and the potential for renal stones, the degree of supplementation (from 1 to 3 g daily of elemental calcium) should be monitored by checking urinary calcium twice a year. Vitamin D may be added to the regimen when there is malabsorption and increased fecal losses.

Hypercalcemia

Hypercalcemia usually is not of dietary origin unless associated with excessive vitamin D intake, but rather results from increased parathormone secretion or with malignancy. The acute condition may lead to weakness, stupor, and coma, while metastatic calcification, renal stones, or ileus are chronic features. Treatment is to induce diuresis with hydration and to administer calcitonin. Both high and low calcium levels in blood lead to cardiac arrhythmias; high calcium levels decrease the QT interval while low levels increase it.

Phosphorus

Hypophosphatemia

Phosphorus homeostasis is regulated by vitamin D and also is dependent on parathormone via their actions on bone and kidney. The clinical dysfunctions of phosphorus deficiency and hypophosphatemia usually are associated with depletion of ATP or of 2,3-diphosphoglyceric acid, leading to tissue hypoxia. Chronic deficiency of phosphorus also is a cause of rickets and osteomalacia. Phosphate deficiency alone may lead to acute ventilatory failure, decreased glucose utilization, and impaired hepatic function in cirrhosis.

Causes. Patients with symptoms of anorexia or vomiting may have greatly reduced phosphorus intake, with concurrent malabsorption caused by vitamin D deficiency. Severe hypophosphatemia most commonly occurs when there is a stimulus for movement of phosphate from plasma into cells:

- With anabolism, phosphorus is used for new tissue synthesis.
- Administration of glucose is a potent stimulus for phosphorus entry into cells for consumption during glycolysis.

- In diabetic ketoacidosis, treatment with unsulin and glucose and correction of acidosis results in rapid movement of phosphate into cells.
- In alcoholics, poor dietary intake, vomiting, malabsorption, heavy antacid use, excessive renal losses, electrolyte disturbances, and the diuretic effect of alcohol contribute to phosphate depletion.
- Respiratory alkalosis contributes to hypophosphatemia in patients with sepsis receiving parenteral or enteral nutrition.

Hypophosphatemia is seen in 15 percent of alcoholic patients and is heightened with nutritional repletion. Without a decrease in total body stores, hypophosphatemia is seen during nutritional repletion following starvation, especially with total parenteral nutrition.

Prolonged use of nonabsorbable aluminum antacid preparations interferes with phosphorus absorption and may lead to phosphorus depletion. Contrasted with calcium—since phosphate is abundant in the diet and its absorption is efficient—renal loss of phosphate is most often responsible for its clinical deficiency. Especially with renal tubular disease, phosphate loss can lead to depletion with symptoms of muscle weakness, malaise, and anorexia. Phosphate loss is also seen with use of diuretics and with concurrent electrolyte disturbances.

Clinical Symptoms. Nonspecific gastrointestinal complaints such as anorexia, nausea, and vomiting are often the first symptoms of hypophosphatemia. With severe hypophosphatemia (less than 1 mg per dl), muscle weakness, hemolysis, rhabdomyolysis, and cardiac failure may occur. Additional clinical symptoms of phosphorus deficiency include

- neurologic and psychiatric disorders (confusion, cranial nerve palsies, motor disturbances, seizures, coma)
- hypoparathyroidism
- joint stiffness
- hematologic disturbances

Laboratory Tests. Plasma levels of phosphate (Table 14–2) are more likely a reflection of renal or metabolic status than of body stores.

Treatment. Phosphate deficiency can be corrected with oral supplements in capsule or liquid form. Severe hypophosphatemia should be treated with intravenous phosphorus, with an initial dosage of 2.5 to 5.0 mg per kg body weight over 6 to 8 hours. Calcium, sodium, and potassium should also be monitored during this therapy.

Hyperphosphatemia

This disorder likewise commonly results from renal disease (see Chapter 23). Therapy consists of low phosphate intake and phosphate binders, an important component of management in chronic renal disease.

Table 14-2. LIMITS OF NORMAL FOR LABORATORY TESTS
OF MINERAL STATUS IN HEALTHY ADULTS*

Test	Level
Calcium, mg/dl	8.6–10.60
Ionized calcium, mg/dl, whole blood	4.73–5.21
Phosphate, mg/dl	2.5–4.8
Magnesium, mg/dl	1.3–3.0
Sodium, mEq/l	140–146
Potassium, mEq/l	4.0–5.5
Chloride, mEq/l	99–110
Iron, μg/dl	50–160 ♀
	65–170 ♂
Ferritin, ng/ml[†]	25, 61 ♀
(iron stores)	94, 90 ♂
Zinc, μg/dl	65-150
Copper, μg/dl	70–140
Selenium, μg/dl	6.2–14.6
Selenium, RBC, μg/ml	0.088–0.227
RBC glutathione peroxidase activity IU/g hemoglobin (selenium status)	12–41

*Values in plasma or serum unless specified otherwise.
†Figures represent <45 yr old, >45 yr old.

Magnesium

Deficiency

Causes. Magnesium deficiency is rare unless there is malabsorption, hyperexcretion, prolonged intravenous feeding, and diarrhea; it is almost invariably secondary to excessive loss from the kidney or gastrointestinal tract. Depletion of this element is seen in the following conditions:

- malabsorption
- chronic alcoholism
- parenteral feeding when there are increased gastrointestinal losses
- burns
- renal disease with tubular dysfunction
- diuretic use
- protein-energy malnutrition
- diabetic ketoacidosis
- hyperparathyroidism

Diuretics, especially furosemide and ethacrynic acid, and cardiac glycosides may promote renal loss of magnesium.

Clinical Symptoms. Severe hypomagnesemia may be asymptomatic, with marked, persistent signs developing only in the presence of hypocalcemia. Positive Chvostek's sign, positive Trousseau's sign, or both, can be observed. Clinical manifestations include

- muscle twitching and tremor
- muscle weakness
- convulsions
- delirium
- depression
- cardiac arrhythmias
- tetany

Hypocalcemia and hypokalemia are frequent in magnesium deficiency.

Laboratory Tests. Urinary excretion reflects intake and absorption of magnesium. Serum magnesium (Table 14–2) does not directly reflect body stores.

Treatment. Replacement is achieved with appropriate salts (e.g., $MgSO_4$ IV, Mg gluconate or oxide taken orally) with attention to renal function.

Hypermagnesemia

Hypermagnesemia may occur in patients with renal insufficiency, especially with use of magnesium-containing antacids (see Chapter 23). Paradoxically, hypermagnesemia may induce hypercalcemia.

Sodium

Deficiency

Causes. Causes of hyponatremia (plasma sodium concentration less than 135 mEq per liter) include

- chronic wasting illness
- major multiple trauma
- excessive water intake (usually iatrogenic) with abnormal external loss of sodium without adequate replacement
- dietary restriction
- diuretics

Sodium depletion occurs in uncontrolled diabetes mellitus, Addison's disease (adrenal insufficiency), acute renal failure in the diuretic phase, and chronic renal failure.

Symptoms. The appearance of symptoms (oligemia, fall in blood pressure) usually indicates that there has been a reduction of at least 10 percent in volume of extracellular fluid (ECF). (Normally, ECF volume is about 20 percent of body weight.) When the loss is severe (20 percent of ECF), the effects may be accompanied by other metabolic consequences. Thus, loss of gastric secretion may be followed by hypochloremia and alkalosis; severe diarrhea may lead to metabolic acidosis or, in less severe cases, alkalosis.

An experimental 11-day regimen of a salt-free diet combined with sweating and ad libitum water intake decreased the serum sodium of healthy volunteers (the investigator and three medical students) from 147 to 131 mEq per liter and the serum chloride from 100 to 83 mEq per liter. The subjects experienced the following symptoms:

- nausea, anorexia, and abdominal discomfort
- loss of sense of taste
- widespread muscle cramps
- breathlessness and fatigue followed by general exhaustion
- apathy and nightmares

The central nervous system effects of hyponatremia appear not only with sodium depletion but also with water intoxication. These effects may include lightheadedness and headache, followed by weakness, lethargy, restlessness, confusion, delirium, and psychosis. Other signs referrable to low serum sodium level are aphasia, hyporeflexia, generalized rigidity, ataxia, staggering, focal hemiparesis, and unilateral Babinski's sign. Brain damage may be permanent if severe symptomatic hyponatremia is not treated.

Laboratory Tests. The serum sodium level reflects the relationship between total body sodium and ECF volume. Urinary sodium reflects intake and body stores in the normal state. Excess sodium is excreted promptly.

Treatment. In the study cited earlier, the sense of taste returned with the first meal containing salt; the exhaustion was dissipated after the first day of repletion, and normal energy was present within 48 hours. Oral intake is preferable. Care must be taken not to raise serum sodium too rapidly in order to avoid fatal neurologic damage (central pontine myelinolysis) by IV administration.

Hypernatremia

Hypernatremia (plasma sodium greater than 150 mEq per liter) can occur with dehydration (desiccation) without adequate water replacement, excessive solute loading without adequate supplemental water intake, or the production of a large volume of dilute urine. It occurs only when thirst is impaired or when the patient does not have access to water or is comatose. It is particularly likely when water losses are enhanced. Thus, it may occur with burns, with high protein tube feedings and a large excretion of urea, or in semicomatose, febrile patients.

Symptoms are primarily neurologic, including central nervous system depression, with letharge progressing to coma. Seizures and muscle weakness also may be seen. Permanent brain damage may develop, especially in children with fever. Lowering plasma sodium should be slow, over 2 to 3 days.

Potassium

Hypokalemia

Causes. Common causes of hypokalemia (plasma potassium levels less than 3.5 mEq per liter) include

- metabolic alkalosis following loss of acid gastric juice
- renal potassium loss following administration of diuretics
- renal wastage of potassium with prolonged acidosis or alkalosis
- urinary loss of potassium in excess of nitrogen and reduced potassium intake following multiple trauma
- chronic renal tubular acidosis with wasting of potassium
- hyperadrenalcorticism or administration of adrenal steroids
- rehydration after dehydration, particularly after insulin treatment of diabetic ketoacidosis
- prolonged parenteral fluid therapy with inadequate potassium replacement, particularly with gastrointestinal losses (vomiting, diarrhea)

A pre-existing deficit of total body potassium in wasting diseases, loss of body cell mass, and expansion of extracellular fluid enhance these conditions.

Clear liquid diets are low in potassium (about 750 mg) and may lead to deficiency after prolonged use. If renal excretion is increased, potassium losses may reach 150 to 300 mEq per day. A loss of body potassium of between 200 and 300 mEq corresponds to a decrease in serum potassium of 1 mEq per liter if not altered by metabolic factors.

Symptoms. With loss of body potassium stores exceeding 10 percent, a decrease in membrane potential impairing muscle contraction results in muscle weakness. Such symptoms usually are not experienced until serum potassium falls to 2.5 mEq per liter or less. The weakness is most prominent in the legs, especially the quadriceps muscles. Muscle cramps and paresthesias may also be troublesome. Other signs and symptoms of severe potassium depletion may include

- respiratory failure from involvement of respiratory muscles; death is possible
- ECG abnormalities including depressed ST segments, flattened or inverted T waves, and presence of U waves
- myocardial necrosis
- postural hypotension
- signs of latent tetany (Chvostek's and Trousseau's signs)
- lethargy, apathy, drowsiness

- an acute brain syndrome with memory impairment, disorientation, and confusion
- glucose intolerance
- anorexia, nausea, vomiting, with ileus

Chronic potassium depletion can result in muscle atrophy. A predisposition to rhabdomyolysis is particularly evident after prolonged exercise. Also, renal concentrating ability is impaired and results in polyuria. Such chronic depletion is sometimes due to laxative addiction (see Case 14e).

Laboratory Tests. Serum potassium levels (Table 14–2) reflect total body stores and glucose utilization as facilitated by insulin, rather than dietary intake.

Treatment. Hypokalemia is treated by oral replacement, if possible, in order to replete serum potassium slowly in equilibrium with the intracellular compartment. Potassium supplements, primarily potassium chloride, are available as powders, liquid, and tablets. Ample water should be provided. With severe depletion, potassium chloride can be given intravenously, with administration not exceeding 40 mEq per hour. Virtually all changes in the electrocardiogram are reversed rapidly when the potassium deficit is corrected.

CASE 14e: HYPOKALEMIA

A 21-year-old female clerk was referred because of a recent hospitalization in an intensive care unit in another hospital for adult respiratory distress syndrome associated with severe hypokalemia (K = 2 mEq/l) resulting in respiratory failure. She was approximately at her ideal body weight but had a history of laxative abuse (20 to 30 cascara tablets daily), which an older sister also practiced. She was counseled regarding the serious medical implications of this habit. Several months later she reported an episode of profound muscle weakness confirmed by neurologic examination. Her serum potassium was 1 mEq/l. She denied using laxatives but admitted ingesting diuretic tablets. She was lost to follow-up.

LESSON:

The patient's bizarre behavior illustrates how eating disorders combined with laxative and/or diuretic abuse can be life-threatening and how difficult it is to modify such behavior.

Hyperkalemia

Causes. Common causes of hyperkalemia (potassium greater than 6.0 mEq per liter) include

- renal failure
- acute dehydration

- massive trauma
- severe acidosis and shock
- major sepsis, hemorrhage, and other massive catabolic states
- excessive rapid infusion of potassium

Excessive potassium intake can occur from the use of salt substitutes or potassium penicillin.

Symptoms. Hyperkalemia may produce an electrocardiogram showing high-peaked T waves, prolongation of the PR interval, and widening of the QRS complex. Complete heart block may occur, and in severe instances the cardiac effects progress to ventricular fibrillation or come to a standstill. Very high potassium levels also may produce rapidly ascending muscular weakness leading to flaccid quadriplegia, as a result of the depolarization block at the neuromuscular junction and failure of propagation of the muscle impulse.

Treatment. The immediate treatment includes intravenous administration of sodium bicarbonate, glucose with insulin, or calcium gluconate. Chronic treatment includes elimination of potassium from parenteral infusions and from food (see Chapter 2 for sources), and the use of resins.

Chloride

Common causes of hypochloremia (plasma chloride less than 98 mEq per liter) include

- dilution (accompanied by hyponatremia)
- chloride loss from the gastrointestinal tract, primarily from the stomach but common from all levels
- diuretics
- adrenal steroids
- compensation for respiratory acidosis
- hypokalemic acidosis
- chronic renal disease and acute renal failure

The chloride ion concentration in the plasma is closely tied to the concentration of sodium, such as in dilutional hyponatremias (when both are decreased) and in desiccation dehydration (when levels of both are elevated). The normal plasma sodium-to-chloride ratio is slightly less than 3:2. Deviations from that ratio are usually due to excessive chloride loss from the gastrointestinal tract or kidneys, or to chloride retention in renal disease or ureterointestinal anastomoses.

Chloride deficiency results in H^+ wasting and metabolic alkalosis. Major hemodynamic and neurologic abnormalities (convulsions, coma) result when there is a marked increase in pH. Hyperchloremia may also be iatrogenic with excessive administration of ammonium chloride or hydrochloric acid.

Laboratory Tests

Normal chloride values (Table 14–2) reflect fluid, electrolyte, and acid-base balance.

Zinc

Deficiency

Causes. Zinc deficiency can result from

- inadequate dietary intake, especially in some children and pregnant women and with prolonged intravenous feeding
- malabsorption, especially in gastrointestinal disease when there is massive loss of intestinal secretions
- increased losses in urine and feces as in alcoholism and Crohn's disease
- chronic liver or renal disease of alcoholism
- chronic hemolytic anemia
- anabolic phases such as repletion of patients with protein-energy malnutrition
- zinc-chelating agents such as penicillamine
- burns or trauma

Symptoms. A syndrome of zinc deficiency was described in male adolescents from Egypt and Iran who ingested a high phytate cereal diet with little meat. Levels of zinc in plasma, red blood cells, hair, and urine were decreased. The patients were dwarfed, with hematosplenomegaly and hypogonadism with primary pituitary dysfunction. Other studies indicate that zinc deficiency may lead to loss of taste (hypogeusia) or smell (hyposmia).

Acrodermatitis enteropathica is a rare inborn error of metabolism in which weaned infants develop alopecia, pustular and bullous skin lesions on the face and extremities (Fig. 14–7), diarrhea, photophobia, psychologic changes, and infection, and fail to thrive. If untreated, the disease is fatal. Plasma zinc levels are low. This condition has been found to be a defect in zinc absorption, transmitted as an autosomal recessive trait.

Patients receiving long-term total parenteral nutrition may develop bullous skin lesions that respond to added zinc.

Laboratory Tests. Plasma and red blood cell concentrations can be measured (Table 14–2), but values correlate poorly with zinc nutriture.

Treatment. A response to therapy is probably the most reliable way to diagnose zinc deficiency in humans. Zinc deficiency can be treated by oral administration of 1 mg zinc per kg body weight as the sulfate or acetate salt. Such treatment has been effective in reversing symptoms such as skin lesions, including increasing the growth of zinc-deficient children.

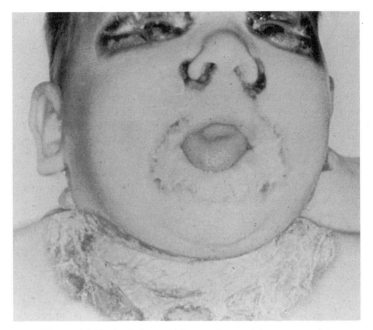

Figure 14-7. An infant with acrodermatitis enteropathica.

Toxicity

Excessive ingestion of zinc may occur from consuming food or beverages stored in galvanized containers. Diarrhea is the most common symptom, along with nausea, vomiting, abdominal cramps, and fever. Inhaled zinc oxide fumes also produce similar acute toxicity.

Copper

Deficiency

Causes. Copper deficiency is unusual other than in inborn errors of metabolism, or in prolonged dietary intake of cow's milk as a sole diet, or of a low copper infant formula for repletion after protein-energy malnutrition. Other conditions that may be associated with this deficiency are

- prolonged diarrhea
- malabsorption
- long-term parenteral nutrition without copper
- long-term use of chelating agents (e.g., D-penicillamine)

Symptoms. Copper deficiency may be indicated by

- neutropenia and anemia unresponsive to iron
- bone changes similar to those in scurvy
- anorexia
- failure to thrive
- depigmentation of hair and skin
- skin lesions
- dilated superficial veins

Serum copper and ceruloplasmin concentrations are decreased.

Premature infants are especially at risk of copper deficiency and may show

- refractory sideroblastic anemia
- neutropenia
- osteopenia
- hypotonia
- psychomotor retardation
- visual impairment
- depigmentation of skin and hair

See Chapter 8 for further discussion of the nutritional needs of such infants.

Menkes' Kinky Hair Syndrome. Copper metabolism is severely deranged in Menkes' kinky hair syndrome, an X-linked defect in copper transport. The condition results in progressive fatal degeneration of the central nervous system, absence of aortic media elastin, and accumulation of collagen. The features of this rare syndrome result from enhanced copper binding by the intestine, leading to a deficiency of the various copper-containing enzymes. The disease does not respond to copper supplementation.

Laboratory Tests. Plasma copper (Table 14–2) does not correlate with intake and only roughly reflects body stores. Urinary copper does not reflect body stores.

Toxicity

Copper toxicity is uncommon except for deliberate ingestion of an excessive amount of elemental copper. An exception is Wilson's disease, an autosomal genetic disorder characterized by excessive accumulation of copper in the liver, brain, kidney, and cornea, and decreased levels of ceruloplasmin in serum. Deposits of copper around the cornea (Kayser-Fleischer green rings) are diagnostic. Liver damage (cirrhosis) usually precedes parkinsonian-like neurologic symptoms and psychiatric symptoms in the condition, which is treated with a low copper diet and administration of D-penicillamine. The effects of the condition on the liver are further dealt with in Chapter 22.

Selenium

Marginal selenium nutriture has been associated with a number of chronic diseases including cardiovascular disease, myotonic dystrophy, celiac disease, cystic fibrosis, cancer, liver disease, multiple sclerosis, and protein-energy malnutrition. However, there is no evidence yet that low selenium (Se) status is a factor in causing these disorders. In selenium-deficient patients, plasma and red blood cell selenium levels are decreased and selenium-dependent glutathione peroxidase levels are also low; a significant linear relationship has been observed between plasma selenium and RBC glutathione peroxidase.

Selenium in blood can be measured, with plasma levels reflecting recent intake. Selenium status can be evaluated by measuring red blood cell or platelet Se-dependent glutathione peroxidase activity (Table 14-2). Urinary selenium excretion reflects dietary intake.

Symptomatic selenium deficiency is largely limited to geographic areas with low soil selenium concentrations, such as mainland China. Keshan's disease, a selenium-responsive cardiomyopathy of children, is found in areas where the daily selenium intake does not exceed 10 μg per day for children and 16 μg for adults. The cardiomyopathy is global, with a dilated heart and areas of focal necrosis, swelling of mitochondria, and microspherical particles. Mild pathologic changes are also noted in skeletal muscle. The disorder has been prevented by administration of sodium selenite, which can be added to salt.

In New Zealand, another low selenium area, white discoloration of the nails has been observed.

Iatrogenic Se deficiency has recently been reported in patients receiving parenteral nutrition and in children fed chemically defined diets for treatment of inborn errors of metabolism. For this reason, selenium supplementation is now recommended in patients receiving prolonged parenteral nutrition.

Selenium toxicity, or selenosis, has been observed in miners and after excess intake of supplements. Symptoms include loss of hair and nails.

Iodine

Deficiency

In iodine deficiency, the thyroid gland enlarges to form a simple goiter in response to release of feedback inhibition of thyroid-stimulating hormone secretion. Adults who are deficient in iodine may develop mild hypothyroidism, but infants born to iodine-deficient mothers may develop a serious thyroid hormone deficiency (cretinism) in utero. The mother's iodine level should be improved prior to conception in order to prevent the condition.

Toxicity

When excess iodine is ingested, iodine uptake by the thyroid is decreased and iodine is excreted in the urine. Hyperthyroidism may be exacerbated. With gross excess, thyrotoxicosis may occur. Iodine is used in treatment of hyperthyroidism to inhibit hormone release and in preparation for thyroidectomy.

Chromium

Chromium deficiency may produce impaired glucose tolerance in infants and adults; ataxia and defective peripheral nerve conduction have also been found. These symptoms developed in patients following 3 to 5 years of total parenteral nutrition, but they were successfully reversed by chromium administration (250 μg $CrCl_3$ daily intravenously). At present the analytic techniques to measure chromium accurately are not available generally but only in specialized laboratories. Administration of trivalent chromium has been reported to improve control of their disease in some patients with diabetes mellitus, presumably by increasing sensitivity to insulin.

Manganese

Manganese deficiency, which is rare, results in weight loss, skin lesions, nausea, decrease in hair growth, change in hair color, ataxia, and striking hypocholesterolemia. Low serum manganese levels have been associated with some inherited forms of epilepsy. Low sodium, low protein diets are also low in manganese. At present the analytic technique to measure manganese accurately is available only in a few specialized laboratories. While ingestion of toxic levels of manganese in food is unknown, miners have developed toxic symptoms of psychosis and parkinsonism.

Molybdenum

Possible deficiency of molybdenum has been demonstrated in one patient undergoing long-term parenteral nutrition. There were high levels of sulfur-containing amino acids in blood and urine, which decreased with administration of molybdenum. The patient's low serum uric acid also rose, and symptoms of encephalopathy were reversed.

Excess molybdenum exposure has been associated with development of gout in the Soviet Union.

ESSENTIAL FATTY ACIDS

Function

Essential fatty acids (EFA) are necessary to platelet function, prostaglandin synthesis, wound healing, immunocompetency, and integrity of skin, hair, and myelin. (Chapter 1 discusses EFA more fully.) The linoleic acid in the diet is converted to longer chain, more polyunsaturated fatty acids, which are essential components of membranes.

Occurrence of EFA Deficiency

Deficiency of essential fatty acid (EFA) is seen primarily in patients receiving parenteral nutrition without lipid. (See Chapter 12 for more information on parenteral nutrition.) Biochemical signs of EFA deficiency may occur as early as 2 to 10 days after omission of linoleic acid, more rapidly in premature infants. Clinical signs of EFA deficiency are also observed in adults after several weeks of administration of lipid-free parenteral nutrition. Clinical symptoms and signs include

- dry, scaly dermatitis
- sparse hair growth
- increased metabolic rate
- impaired wound healing
- increased susceptibility to respiratory and other infection
- reduced growth rate and weight gain
- diarrhea
- increased capillary permeability
- increased red blood cell fragility
- increased platelet aggregation
- thrombocytopenia

Biochemical Diagnosis

EFA deficiency is diagnosed by an increase in the ratio of 5,8,11-eicosatrienoic (triene, 20:3) to arachidonic acid (tetraene, 20:4) in plasma phospholipids to more than 0.4. Mean content of linoleate (18:2) and arachidonate falls, while 18:1 and 18:3 acids increase.

Prevention and Treatment of Deficiency

For adult patients receiving total parenteral nutrition, infusion of a 500 ml unit of 10 percent emulsion three times weekly may replete depleted patients; 1 to 2 units weekly may prevent the deficiency. Dietary linoleate requirement is 2 to 4 percent of dietary calories and cannot be met with medium chain triglycerides. EFA deficiency may be prevented in adults by ingestion of 30 ml daily of a polyunsaturated oil (see Fig. 19–10). Cutaneous application of EFA-rich oils will not prevent EFA deficiency and may not correct it.

CHAPTER 15

Nutritional Anemias

Anemia is a disorder characterized by decreased circulating hemoglobin with poor oxygen transport capacity of blood. Nutritional anemias result primarily from diminished production of red blood cells attributable to deficiency of iron, folate or vitamin B_{12}, alone or in combination. (The function, requirements, sources, and metabolism of these micronutrients are presented in Chapter 2.) Inadequate dietary intake, maldigestion, malabsorption, inadequate storage, and excessive demands are among the causes of depletion of these nutrients initially, leading in time to symptomatic deficiency states.

(See Chapters 7 and 8 for special needs of children and pregnant and lactating women.) Other nutrients—pyridoxine, copper, vitamin E, zinc, protein—also are involved in hematopoiesis and may contribute to the development of anemia. Symptoms of anemia are weakness and pallor.

IRON

Function and Stores

The bone marrow needs iron to synthesize hemoglobin for new red blood cells. Hemoglobin contains most of the body's "functional iron" associated with energy metabolism and about two thirds of the total body iron. Iron reserve stores must be depleted before changes in functional iron status are reflected in changes in various hematologic indices (Table 15-1).

Table 15-1. TYPICAL FINDINGS IN ANEMIA

	Normal Women	Deficiency			Anemia of Chronic Disease
		Iron	Folate	B_{12}	
Hemoglobin, g/dl	12–16	7	7	7	7
Hematocrit, %	36–47	28	22	22	
Red blood cells ×10⁶/cmm	3.9–5.6	3.5	2.0	2.0	
Mean corpuscular hemoglobin concentration, %	30–36	25	32	32	<30
Mean corpuscular hemoglobin, pg	27–32	20	35	35	
Mean corpuscular volume, fl	75–95	<80	110	110	<80
Plasma folate, ng/ml	>7		<3	11	
Plasma B_{12}, pg/ml	>200		>200	<100	
Plasma iron, µg/dl	115	<40	↑	↑	<50
Transferrin iron binding capacity, µg/dl	330	410			<350
% Saturation	35	<15	↑	↑	15
Ferritin, µg/l	35,70	10	↑	↑	>30
Red blood cell folate, ng/ml	>150		<100	<100	
B_{12} binding capacity % Saturation	40		40	<10	

The body's iron content is relatively stable, with loss occurring only when cells are lost. Red blood cells are broken down at the end of their 120-day life, and released hemoglobin iron is reutilized by the bone marrow. Thus, a minimal amount of additional iron is needed from the daily diet of the healthy adult.

Effect of Inadequate Transport Iron

Hemoglobin is composed of iron (0.33 percent by weight), protoporphyrin, and globin. When transport iron is inadequate, red blood cells produced in the bone marrow are reduced in number and are microcytic (decreased mean corpuscular volume) and hypochromic (low mean corpuscular hemoglobin) (Table 15-1). Similar-appearing blood cells are seen in the anemia of chronic disease, the thalassemias, hemoglobin C or E disease, lead poisoning, and in sideroblastic anemias.

Causes of Iron Deficiency

Iron deficiency is the major nutritional cause of anemia worldwide. Iron deficiency anemia is seen in 15 percent of menstruating women in the United States, and depletion of iron stores without anemia may be present in half. Dietary intake may be inadequate to meet increased iron requirements caused by menstrual blood loss. Iron deficiency in adult men and nonmenstruating women should be considered secondary to blood loss (gastrointestinal), unless proved otherwise. In many parts of the world, hookworm disease is the major predisposer to gastrointestinal blood loss. Factors exacerbating iron deficiency include dietary inadequacy (see Chapter 2), malabsorption (see Chapter 21), and pica (see Chapter 7).

Laboratory Tests

Largely bound to transferrin, serum iron undergoes a diurnal variation with morning values (see Table 14-2) 30 percent higher than evening values. Ferritin is the major storage form of iron. Serum ferritin levels reflect total body iron stores and correlate with the stainable iron in bone marrow specimens.

Development of Iron Deficiency Anemia

With depletion of iron stores (ferritin, hemosiderin), bone marrow storage iron and plasma ferritin fall, and the iron-binding capacity and degree of unsaturation rise. This is followed by iron deficiency erythropoiesis, with a fall in serum iron and further fall in transferrin saturation. The percent of iron-containing cells in the marrow also falls. The characteristic red blood cell morphology may be seen when anemia finally develops. When iron deficiency is combined with deficiency of vitamin B_{12} or folate, or both, red blood cell indices may be normal, or the cell population may be mixed.

In addition to symptoms of anemia, iron deficiency may result in glossitis, characterized by a pale, smooth tongue, and in brittle, dry, flattened-to-concave nails (koilonychia).

Iron Therapy

The reticulocyte count will increase in 3 to 10 days with administration of iron. Oral iron therapy will bring normal laboratory test results within several months, although 6 months of therapy may be required to replenish body iron stores. Ferrous sulfate—300 mg after meals and at bedtime—is an inexpensive iron preparation.

Adverse effects of iron therapy include nausea, vomiting, diarrhea, and crampy abdominal pain. Such symptoms may respond favorably to reduction of dose and prescribing with meals. Parenteral iron—which is expensive—may cause pain at the site of intravenous or intramuscular injection, with local inflammation and numerous other adverse effects.

If the cause of iron deficiency can be eliminated, iron therapy may be discontinued when iron balance is normal. Patients should be re-evaluated for folate or vitamin B_{12} deficiency after 1 month of iron therapy.

ANEMIA OF CHRONIC DISEASES

The anemia of chronic diseases is a moderate decrease in hemoglobin that may accompany infection, inflammatory disorders, collagen diseases, or neoplasm. Such anemias are differentiated from iron deficiency anemia by their low serum iron, low iron-binding capacity, increased unsaturation and tissue iron stores, and relative bone marrow failure with near-normal cellular pattern (Table 15-1). The extent of hypochromia or microcytosis is rarely as severe as in iron deficiency anemia. With coexisting chronic blood loss or iron malabsorption, iron stores decrease and only the transferrin level will distinguish between the two disorders. A therapeutic trial of oral iron may be indicated for differential diagnosis.

Folate

Symptoms of Megaloblastic Anemia

Megaloblastic anemia with macro-ovalocytes and hypersegmented neutrophils (more than 5 percent with five or more lobes) is caused by folate and/or vitamin B_{12} deficiency in 95 percent of patients. (Iron deficiency may also be present.) In addition to the usual symptoms of weakness and fatigue, patients may exhibit

- sore tongue
- glossitis
- diarrhea
- mental changes
- anorexia
- weight loss
- cytologic abnormalities in various epithelia
- megaloblastic bone marrow

Associated symptoms include

- leukopenia and thrombocytopenia
- fever
- pallor
- icterus
- splenomegaly
- vitiligo

Characteristic Cell Changes in Megaloblastosis

Megaloblastosis refers to marrow disorders caused by defective DNA synthesis, with megaloblastic erythropoiesis, granulopoiesis, and thrombopoiesis. Cells are abnormally large, with a higher than normal ratio of cytoplasm to nucleus. Red blood cells vary widely in size and shape and may manifest stipling and other inclusions. The anemia is normochromic and macrocytic. With severe anemia, nucleated megaloblastic cells may appear in the blood. Bone marrow is cellular and often hyperplastic, with striking megaloblastic changes primarily in the erythroid series but also in myeloid and platelet precursors. The myeloid-erythroid ratio drops to 1. The megaloblastic changes in the bone marrow may be obscured by a few days' ingestion of nutritious hospital food. Serum lactate dehydrogenase (LDH) isozyme-1 activity exceeds that of LDH-2, a reversal of the usual pattern.

Megaloblastic anemia is associated with ineffective erythropoiesis and moderate hemolysis. Plasma iron is elevated and iron accumulates in marrow stores, liver, and other tissues (Table 15–1).

Table 15–2. CAUSES OF FOLATE DEFICIENCY

Abnormality	Cause
1. Inadequate food ingestion	Poor diet, chronic alcoholism
2. Inadequate absorption	Blind loop
3. Inadequate absorption due to defective folate polyglutamate hydrolysis	Congenital or acquired conjugase deficiency, conjugase inhibitors in foods or drugs, low pH
4. Defective intestinal mucosal transport	Congenital, diphenylhydantoin, ethanol, high pH
5. Malabsorption syndrome	Gluten enteropathy, tropical sprue
6. Inadequate utilization	Folate antagonists, ?anticonvulsants, enzyme deficiency, B_{12} deficiency, alcohol, dietary amino acid excess, uremia, sex steroids
7. Increased requirements	Pregnancy, lactation, malignancy, prematurity, hemolysis, chronic blood loss, hypermetabolism, Lesch-Nyhan syndrome, drugs
8. Increased excretion	?B_{12} deficiency, ?liver disease, dialysis, oral contraception
9. Increased destruction	?Scurvy, ?oxidants

Adapted from Goodhart, R.S., and Shils, M.S. (eds.): Modern Nutrition in Health and Disease, ed 6. Lea and Febiger, Philadelphia, 1980, pp. 236–237.

Causes of Folate Deficiency

Folate deficiency is commonly caused by inadequate diet, especially when accompanied by significant alcohol consumption (see Chapters 2 and 17). Deficiency may also result from inherited or acquired abnormalities of absorption and utilization, and from increased requirements, destruction, and excretion (Table 15–2).

Laboratory Tests

The level of folate can be measured in plasma and red blood cells (see Table 14–2). Red blood cell folate concentrations reflect tissue stores while serum folate reflects the recent dietary intake. Folacin circulates as 5′-methyl tetrahydrofolic acid, about two thirds of which is protein bound. About 90 percent of this is loosely attached to albumin and α-2-macroglobulin, with 10 percent specifically bound to other proteins. Laboratory tests are summarized in Table 15–1.

Development of Folate Malabsorption and Deficiency

Folate malabsorption results from small bowel disease. Such drugs as hydantoins and alcohol may cause folate malabsorption or inhibit its metabolism, while malnutrition may also impair its absorption. Tests of folate absorption are not generally available, but malabsorption may be inferred by demonstration of a malabsorption syndrome in the folate-deficient patient (see Chapter 21). In the absence of alcohol, folate deficiency alone may impair jejunal absorption. Increased demand for or utilization of folate may be associated with anemia of pregnancy or low birth weight infants (see Chapters 7 and 8).

Effects of Folate Deficiency

Folate deficiency in the bone marrow reduces DNA synthesis and replication and the rate of cell division; the more rapid the rate of cell division, the greater the requirement for folate, as in the hemoglobinopathies and hemolytic anemias. Thus, folate is usually prescribed for patients with sickle cell anemia.

Development of Anemia

Anemia with dietary folate deficiency develops rapidly after about 20 weeks of deficiency, preceded by low serum folate (at 3 weeks), hypersegmentation in blood neutrophils (at 7 weeks), low red blood cell folate (at 17 weeks), and megaloblastic marrow (at 19 weeks). Reticulocyte count commonly is 1.5 to 8 percent.

The hematologic manifestations of folate and vitamin B_{12} deficiencies are indistinguishable. Specific neurologic abnormalities are not seen in pure folate deficiency.

Treatment of Folate Deficiency

Deficiency is treated with oral or parenteral administration of 1 mg folic acid per day. Toxicity has not been reported. Vitamin B_{12} status should be evaluated as adequate before folate is administered.

VITAMIN B_{12} (COBALAMIN)

The megaloblastic anemia of vitamin B_{12} deficiency is identical to that resulting from folate deficiency. However, because of body stores, vitamin B_{12}

deficiency takes years to develop. In addition, the neurologic damage associated with vitamin B_{12} deficiency ("combined system disease") is unique.

Role of Vitamin B_{12}

Vitamin B_{12} coenzymes are implicated in a variety of metabolic systems, mostly well defined in bacteria. In human (animal) cells, adenosyl cobalamin-dependent methylmalonyl CoA-mutase (intramolecular acceptor-donor of hydrogen) and methylcobalamin-dependent methyltetrahydrofolate-homocysteine methyltransferase (methionine synthesis, conversion of N^5-methyltetrahydrofolate to tetrahydrofolate) are systems that have been well described.

Development of Megaloblastic Anemia

The megaloblastic anemia of vitamin B_{12} deficiency is a consequence of impaired DNA synthesis without impaired RNA synthesis. The metabolic derangement may result from accumulation of N^5-methyltetrahydrofolate ("methylfolate trap"), sequestering folate, and preventing production of the essential metabolite cofactor of thymidylate synthetase.

Disorders Causing Vitamin B_{12} Deficiency

Specific deficiency syndromes include "Addisonian" pernicious anemia due to genetically acquired defective secretion of intrinsic factor (IF), presumably because of an autoimmune mechanism (Table 15–3). Antibodies to gastric parietal cell cytoplasm, to IF, or to the IF-B_{12} complex are common. Many of these patients also have thyroid auto-antibodies, or have thyrotoxicosis, hypothyroidism, or Hashimoto's thyroiditis.

Gastric atrophy is present and does not change with vitamin B_{12} therapy. Megaloblastosis occurs in epithelial cells throughout the body. Patients typically are over 40 years of age, female, and of northern European extraction.

Selective malabsorption of vitamin B_{12} and congenital intrinsic factor deficiency are among other vitamin B_{12} deficiency disorders. More commonly partial gastrectomy may result in iron deficiency anemia, with megaloblastic anemia developing 5 to 6 years after total gastrectomy without vitamin B_{12} supplementation. The vitamin should be administered by injection prophylactically to all patients following total gastrectomy.

Additional disorders predisposing to vitamin B_{12} deficiency include ileal resection or disease, tropical sprue, gluten enteropathy, blind loop syndrome, fish tapeworm infestation, and vegetarianism (vegans who do not consume meat, fish, eggs, or dairy products).

Table 15-3. CAUSES OF COBALAMIN DEFICIENCY

Abnormality	Disorder
1. Inadequate ingestion	Vegans, chronic alcoholism, fads
2. Impaired food digestion	Gastrectomy, achlorhydria
3. Decreased secretion of intrinsic factor (IF)	Pernicious anemia, hereditary failure, gastrectomy, gastric atrophy
4. Impaired transfer to IF	Pancreatic insufficiency, Zollinger-Ellison syndrome
5. Abnormal IF	Decreased ileal binding
6. Competition for uptake	Bacterial overgrowth (blind loop), fish, tapeworm infestation
7. Impaired attachment to ileal receptor	Ileal disease or resection, gluten enteropathy, tropical sprue, drugs
8. Impaired passage through ileal cell	Familial cobalamin malabsorption
9. Impaired uptake into blood	Transcobalamin II deficiency, abnormal B_{12} binding protein
10. Inadequate utilization	B_{12} antagonists, protein malnutrition, neoplasm, hepatic/renal disease, enzymatic defects
11. Increased requirement	Hypermetabolism, pregnancy, malignancy
12. Increased excretion	Hepatic/renal disease
13. Increased destruction	?Excessive intake of vitamin C

Adapted from Seetharam, B., and Alpers, D.H.: Absorption and transport of cobalamin (vitamin B_{12}). Ann Rev of Nutr 2:360, 1982.

Neurologic Effects of Vitamin B_{12} Deficiency

Demyelination may result from impaired synthesis, excessive destruction, or some as yet unknown abnormality. Efforts to relate these effects to the known functions of vitamin B_{12}–dependent enzymes have so far been unsuccessful. The fully developed neurologic syndrome of vitamin B_{12} deficiency includes

- increased deep tendon reflexes
- increased muscle tone
- Babinski's toe sign
- paresthesias
- impaired vibration and position sense
- ataxia
- degenerative changes in dorsal and lateral columns of the spinal cord

These signs do not necessarily correlate with the degree of anemia, and the syndrome is relatively infrequent.

CASE 15a: PERNICIOUS ANEMIA

A 63-year-old man was hospitalized on the Neurology Service because of ataxia for 4 weeks. He had a 2-year history of numbness in his hands and feet. Neurologic examination showed a slapping gait with difficulty in tandem walking and rapid movements of the lower extremities, weakness of the legs, and positive Babinski's toe sign. Vibration sense was absent from toes to knees and position sense was lost in the toes. His tongue was swollen, smooth and reddened (see Fig. 11–5), and he reported some soreness for 1 month.

He had been prescribed supplements of multivitamins and folic acid (5 mg daily) by his local physician because of macrocytic anemia. His dietary intake was good.

On admission he weighed 62.5 kg and his height was 165 cm. His hemoglobin (13.8 g%) and hematocrit (41 percent) were normal; his red blood cell count was 3.2 million/mm^3; indices were macrocytic (110) and hyperchromic (37). His serum vitamin B_{12} level was low (100 pg/ml). An abnormal Schilling test (0.3 percent excretion) confirmed the diagnosis of pernicious anemia, with increase to normal excretion with intrinsic factor. Serum folate was 20.5 ng/ml (upper limit of normal). Achlorhydria after histamine was present. There were a few hypersegmented polymorphonuclear leukocytes on blood smear. He was treated with vitamin B_{12}, 1 mg IM daily at first, followed by monthly injections after discharge. Two years later his neurologic status was unchanged; his MCV was 88.

LESSON:

This patient provides a classic example of the failure to recognize vitamin B_{12} deficiency as a cause of megaloblastic anemia and the increased hazard of combined systems disease with inappropriate partial treatment with folic acid alone.

Diagnosis of Vitamin B_{12} Deficiency

Methylmalonic aciduria is a specific feature and a reliable index of vitamin B_{12} deficiency, although the best evidence for diagnosis is a decreased serum vitamin B_{12} level (see Table 15–1). This may be seen after 2 or 3 years of deficiency, preceded by hypersegmentation of neutrophils and accompanied by a megaloblastic bone marrow, low red blood cell folate, and normal or elevated levels of serum folate.

Levels of vitamin B_{12} can be measured in plasma or red blood cells (see Table 14–2). The Schilling test measures absorption of ingested radiolabeled vitamin B_{12} in the absence and presence of intrinsic factor. Following the test dose, isotope excretion in urine is measured. A level less than 7 percent is clearly low, and over 10 percent is clearly normal. Antibodies to IF also can be detected and quantitated.

Treatment of Vitamin B$_{12}$ Deficiency

Intramuscular injection of 100 μg vitamin B$_{12}$ may be given daily for 2 weeks, followed by injections twice weekly, then monthly (1000 μg). Larger (250 μg), more frequent doses (twice weekly) for 6 months are suggested for patients with neurologic disease.

Response to parenteral vitamin B$_{12}$ is rapid, with conversion of bone marrow to normoblastic within 72 hours, followed by reticulocytosis maximal in 4 to 10 days. The deficient patient will not respond to a physiologic dose of folate (100 to 400 μg per day) but will develop reticulocytosis with large doses of folic acid (5 to 15 mg per day), which may accelerate the development of neurologic disease.

CHAPTER 16

Obesity, Anorexia Nervosa, and Bulimia

OBESITY

It is estimated that 14 percent of men and 24 percent of women in the United States are obese, making this the most common nutritional disorder in this country. Defining obesity as body weight exceeding 120 percent of ideal or using a critical level of a body mass index is imprecise, and there is a need for a suitable data base relating body weight by gender, age, and frame size to morbidity and mortality in order to establish a desirable range of body weight. Obesity may also be defined as an excess of body fat, but the means to ascertain this parameter accurately may not be available for common use.

Caloric Requirements

Caloric requirements vary according to age, gender, body size, energy expenditure, climate, and race. The recommended energy intake for age and gender may vary as much as 1800 calories, or almost 100 percent among young individuals (Table 16–1). Adult allowances are set within a range of plus or minus 400 calories.

Theories of the Etiology of Obesity

Many factors may contribute to obesity. Although a few rare diseases serve as models for study of the etiology of the disorder, they do not explain the mechanisms of the usual problem (see Table 8–14). There is a substantial genetic component that may involve single dominant or recessive genes, or be polygenic. Obesity is more prevalent in black women of low socioeconomic status, is found in 80 percent of children of two obese parents, and is influenced by cultural and ethnic factors. Environmental causes include overfeeding, inactivity, the cooking and dietary habits of the family, their socioeconomic status, and the palatability of the diet. Psychologic causes relate to body image and include depression, providing food as a "reward," use of food as entertainment, and relation of food intake to stimulate endorphins. Thus, the disorder probably reflects a composite of heterogeneous factors. Underlying mechanisms may be associated with disordered metabolism of adipose tissue, defective energy balance involving energy intake, or processing as expenditure or storage. In the end, energy balance must be positive before obesity can develop. Endocrine causes of obesity are rare, but excessive body fat may result from hyperinsulinism, excess cortisol, or thyroid hormone deficiency.

Obesity theories relate to the classification of excess fat deposition into two categories: hypertrophic with increase in the size of fat cells, and hyperplastic with increase in the number of adipocytes. In normal growth and development, the *number* of fat cells increases until adolescence; however, fat cells can increase in *size* throughout life. Variations in the stimulus to hyperplasia or hypertrophy, age of onset, and response of adipose tissue to these factors may be critical in the etiology of obesity, and may play important roles in the response to treatment and control of overweight. Genetic and endocrine factors are more commonly seen in childhood obesity (see Chapter 8). With early age of onset (infancy, childhood, or adolescence), reversal of obesity to normal weight is difficult.

Table 16-1. RECOMMENDED ENERGY INTAKE

Gender	Age (Yr)	Weight kg	Weight lb	Height cm	Height in	Energy Needs (kcal) Mean	Energy Needs (kcal) Range
Male	11–14	45	99	157	62	2700	2000–3700
	15–18	66	145	176	69	2800	2100–3900
	19–22	70	154	177	70	2900	2500–3300
	23–50	70	154	178	70	2700	2300–3100
	51–75	70	154	178	70	2400	2000–2800
	76+	70	154	178	70	2050	1650–2450
Female	11–14	46	101	157	62	2200	1500–3000
	15–18	55	120	163	64	2100	1200–3000
	19–22	55	120	163	64	2100	1700–2500
	23–50	55	120	163	64	2000	1600–2400
	51-75	55	120	163	64	1800	1400–2200
	76+	55	120	163	64	1600	1200–2000

Thermogenesis

Metabolic changes in energy expenditure may occur by way of dietary thermogenesis, or may be explained by the concept of luxuskonsumption, that is, wasteful, inefficient energy metabolism in some people, keeping them thin. The thermic effect of food may be substantial, owing to increases in metabolic rates. Energy may be dissipated as heat, without storage. Calories generally, and especially carbohydrate-rich diets, may increase activity of the sympathetic nervous system with an enhanced norepinephrine response (Fig. 16–1). Changes may also occur in thyroid function in response to dietary intake. Defects in thermogenic response to meals have been reported in obese persons together with blunted response to norepinephrine. Thus, their increased efficiency, or "thrift," may slightly reduce energy requirements. This innate defect may interact with excessive appetite and food intake, leading to their obesity.

Brown Adipose Tissue. The thermogenic defect has been linked to a lack of brown adipose tissue, which is found in the interscapular region and along the aorta. This tissue is active in human infants, young animals, and animals awakening from hibernation. In animals, brown adipose tissue thermogenesis is induced by carbohydrate feeding by way of sympathetic activation. This has given rise to the hypothesis that lean individuals have more responsive brown adipose tissue than do preobese persons, so that in the former, fat is oxidized more readily than stored.

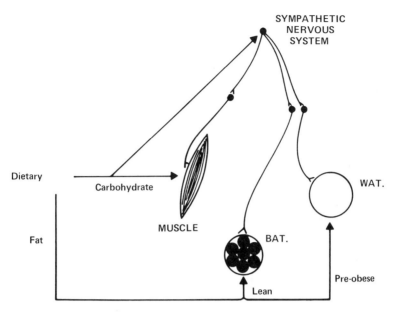

Figure 16-1. Hypothetical integration of carbohydrate-induced and fat-induced thermogenesis in individuals with differing constitutional predispositions to obesity. BAT = brown and WAT = white adipose tissue. (From James, W.P.T.: Energy requirements and obesity. Lancet 2:388, 1983, with permission.)

Other Metabolic Alterations

Deficient sodium pumping across cell membranes is another manifestation of altered metabolic efficiency in obese persons. The sodium content of cells is increased by a defect in the sodium-dependent ATPase. Increased adipose tissue lipoprotein lipase, which increases the uptake of fatty acids into adipose tissue, is another metabolic alteration in obesity (see Chapter 19). Increased glucose uptake into adipose tissue has also been demonstrated.

Differences in Energy Requirements

Recently, differences in energy requirements have been emphasized in attempts to explain the development of obesity. Despite great variations in energy expenditure among different individuals, the expenditure of a particular individual is relatively consistent. By contrast, energy (or food) intake can vary widely and may fluctuate from week to week. Also, methods of measuring energy expenditure are more precise than those used in measuring food intake. Cues that trigger unconscious regulation of food intake to compensate for variations in energy content are poorly understood. Changes in levels of catecholamines or thyroid hormones, or both, may regulate food intake. Whether small, consistent changes in exercise patterns influence weight change is unknown, as is the possible role of spontaneous activity (e.g., fidgeting) as a mechanism for controlling energy balance. Exercise *does*, however, raise the overall metabolic rate in addition to the actual exercise expenditure per se.

Decrease in Basal Metabolic Rate With Increasing Age

Contributing to the development of obesity later in life is the decline in basal metabolic rate with age (2 percent per decade), so that the daily caloric requirement declines by about 200 kcal from age 50 to 75 (about 100 kcal per decade). For those over age 75, the decrease in energy expenditure is even greater (minus 500 kcal in men and minus 400 kcal in women). (Chapter 9 discusses nutrition and the elderly in greater detail.)

Defects in Control Mechanisms for Eating

Eating behavior in the obese may be abnormal because of a defect in one or more controlling mechanisms, including hypothalamic controls of food intake and energy expenditure. Central regulation of calories is determined over the long term by the ventromedial nucleus of the hypothalamus, and short term by the lateral hypothalamus via adrenergic receptors. The paraventricular nucleus has also been implicated. These nuclei may respond to levels of fuels such as glucose, amino acids, fatty acids, and/or glycerol; to hormones (insulin, glucagon, cholecystokinin); and to environmental cues such as time of day and light intensity, as well as the availability and tastiness of food.

Complications of Obesity

The many complications of obesity include the following:

- **diabetes mellitus** (Fig. 16–2): The prevalence of diabetes mellitus type II triples as relative weight increases from normal to 150 percent of ideal. (The important relation of this type of non–insulin-dependent diabetes to obesity is described in Chapter 18.)
- **hypertension** (Fig. 16–3): Systolic and diastolic blood pressure increase about 15 and 10 mm respectively as relative weight increases to 150 percent of ideal. (The effects of obesity and weight reduction on hypertension, hyperlipidemia, and cardiovascular disease are reviewed in Chapter 19.)

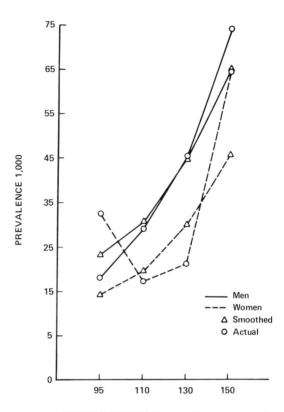

Figure 16–2. Prevalence of diabetes mellitus by relative weight. Framingham Study: men and women (age-adjusted rates: 45 to 64). (From Kannel, W.B., Gordon, T., and Castelli, W.P.: Obesity, lipids, and glucose intolerance. The Framingham Study. Am J Clin Nutr 32:1241, 1979, with permission.)

- **atherosclerosis:** The Framingham study of cardiovascular epidemiology concluded that obesity is an independent risk factor for the development of atherosclerosis or coronary heart disease.
- **osteoarthritis**
- **gout**
- **mentrual irregularities**
- **gallbladder disease and gallstones**
- **increased prevalence of endometrial cancer** (see Chapter 24)
- **increased prevalence of kidney stones**
- **sleep apnea and Pickwickian syndrome:** Grossly obese persons may develop the Pickwickian syndrome of alveolar hypoventilation, characterized by hypoxia, secondary polycythemia, pulmonary hypertension, cor pulmonale, and somnolence. Emergency treatment may require hospitalization with the patient placed on a respirator. Potential for the sleep apnea syndrome should be evaluated with appropriate

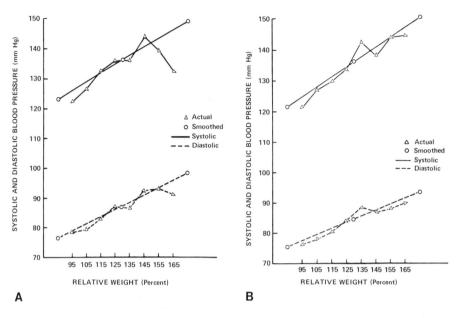

Figure 16-3. A, Regression of systolic and diastolic blood pressures on relative weight in men ages 45 to 54. B, Regression of systolic and diastolic blood pressures on relative weight in women ages 45 to 54. (From Kannel, W.B., and Gordon, T.: The Framingham Study. In Bray, G.A. (ed): Obesity in America. Washington, DC USDHEW NIH Pub. 79-359, 1979, with permission.)

pulmonary tests. Tonsillar obstruction should be looked for and surgical correction performed, including, if needed, tracheostomy (see Case 16a and Fig. 16–4).

- **heart failure:** With severe obesity, the heart enlarges, with increases in cardiac output, stroke volume, and blood volume; however, this may be reversed with weight loss.

CASE 16a: MORBID OBESITY

A 27-year-old man was referred for weight loss. He had been overweight all of his life. He weighed 310 lb at high school graduation and gradually gained over 300 lb since then, weighing 565 lb 2 years ago and 628 lb at present. He was 75 inches tall. He had been unable to work for 2 years because of limited exercise tolerance (shortness of breath). He noted fitful sleeping, waking up with a sense of choking, lifelong snoring, and increasing daytime sleepiness over the past year. He took two to three 1-hour naps daily. He fell asleep anytime he was sitting. His wife noted periods of apnea during sleep. All day long, he had difficulty breathing through his nose. He was short of breath even

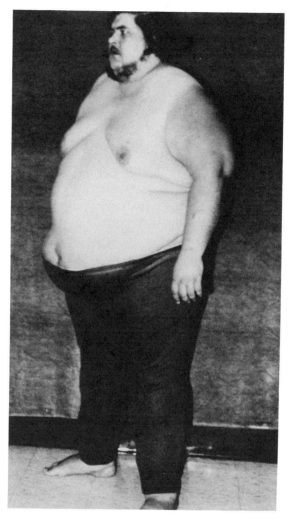

Figure 16–4. 27-year-old man with morbid obesity and sleep apnea syndrome (Case 16a). Height 75 inches, weight 628 lb.

with talking and had pleuritic chest pain with exertion. He had had significant swelling of the lower extremities, morning headache, and occasional sexual problems.

His father had died at age 41 of a myocardial infarction. His mother was alive, age 50 years, and obese. Six siblings were all living, in good health and not obese. He had no children. He had smoked two packs of cigarettes daily for 12 years and rarely used alcohol. Positive findings on physical examination included a redundant oropharynx, end-expiratory wheezes throughout both lung fields, and minimal leg edema. Blood glucose, blood lipids, and thyroid function tests were normal.

He underwent two sleep studies to evaluate the possibility of a sleep disorder. The impression was of obstructive sleep apnea syndrome with very severe nocturnal oxygen desaturation. His nocturnal hypoxemia was the worst ever seen at the sleep laboratory. The recommendation was to perform uvulopalatoplasty and provide oxygen therapy. A second sleep study with continuous positive airway pressure (CPAP) showed total control of the sleep apnea syndrome by 7 cm pressure but continued oxygen desaturation. Further recommendations were to lose weight and stop smoking. He was discharged with home oxygen and CPAP and placed on a protein-sparing modified fast regimen with vitamin and mineral supplements. He lost 23 lb in 25 days. The urine ketones were moderately positive.

Mortality increases with increasing relative weight, so that life expectancy is decreased 11 percent in men and 7 percent in women, with body weight 110 percent of ideal. With body weight 120 percent of ideal, life expectancy decreases 20 percent in men and 10 percent in women. One index of body mass, weight:height^2, has been categorized as follows: 20 to 25, normal; 25 to 30, cosmetic; greater than 30 ↑mortality and morbidity; 35, mortality 2 times normal; greater than 40, ↑↑morbidity and mortality. (Fig. 16–5).

Evaluation of the Obese Patient

Alterations in endocrine and metabolic status that occur in association with obesity should be evaluated (i.e., hypothyroidism, Cushing's disease, cystic ovaries). Measurements of height, weight, waist and hip circumferences, and skinfold thicknesses should be taken, and thyroid status evaluated. Women should be observed for possible virilization. Assessment of cardiovascular function should include measurement of blood pressure and pulmonary function as well as performance of a stress test. To avoid incorrect measurements in the very obese, blood pressure should be taken using a long, wide cuff. Glucose tolerance should be determined, and lipids, lipoproteins, and uric acid measured. Ultrasonography may be used to check for gallstones.

The amount of body fat and the growth of adipose tissue can be evaluated. Excess body fat commonly is interpreted on the basis of excess weight, and overweight typically does derive from an increase in the adipose tissue compartment. Measurement of skinfold thickness yields an approximation of body fat, most accurately done by combining four sites: triceps, subscapular, biceps, and iliac (see Chapter 3). Body density measurements by underwater weighing determine the proportion of fat. Other methods of estimating body

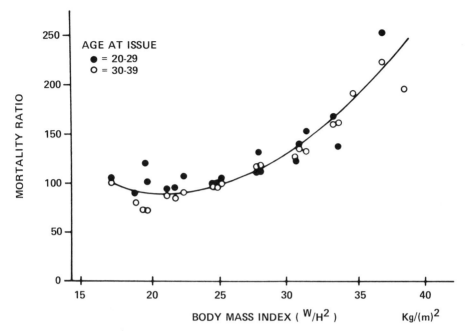

Figure 16–5. Relation of the body mass index to mortality. Adapted from data in the Build and Blood Pressure Study of 1959. As body mass index rises above the normal (25), the excess mortality (> 100) increases. (From Bray, G.A. (ed): Obesity: Comparative Methods of Weight Control. Technomic Publishing Co, Westport, CT, 1980, p. 4, with permission.)

fat include isotopic measurement of whole body potassium content or water dilution, or total body electrical conductivity or impedance. These measurements correlate with body water; calculations yield lean body mass and fat. These measurements can be followed and evaluated as patients follow weight loss regimens.

Recently the pattern of body fat distribution has been reported to be an important determinant of morbidity and mortality. Upper body obesity (excess fat in neck, shoulder, arm, and upper trunk) is associated with hypertension, diabetes mellitus, and hyperlipidemia and may be a marker for risk of coronary heart disease, stroke, and death. Lower body obesity (hips, thighs, and buttocks) is not predictive of these conditions. Cardiovascular risk increased sharply when the ratio of waist to hip circumferences exceeded 1.0 in men and 0.8 in women.

Treatment

Motivation

Unless the patient is highly motivated, the likelihood of successful weight reduction is poor. The dieter must learn to ingest a balanced variety of foods in the form of three or more meals per day and maintain this regimen over a long period. Motivation may be strengthened by a self-help or group program, preferably professionally directed, that may involve the family. Behavior modification techniques include developing an awareness of eating cues so as to reshape eating behavior. This technique deals with the antecedents, behavior, and consequences of eating patterns, with emphasis on the location and atmosphere of meals and eating slowly. A contract involving rewards and penalties may be agreed upon by the patient and supervisor.

Weight Reduction Diets

Various weight reducing diets have been employed to provide the limited, reduced numbers of calories. These may be nutritionally balanced or unbalanced (see Chapter 6). In general, the patient learns to count calories and to become familiar with food groups and exchanges (see Chapters 4 and 10). Diets at very low energy levels—800 calories or less—should provide at least 55 g of high quality protein (see Chapter 1). In other diets the proportions of macronutrients are varied:

- the ketogenic diet, low in carbohydrate and calories, induces a marked diuresis (this may be an all-protein diet)
- a high fiber diet
- a monotonous diet with emphasis on a "special" food
- fasting (rarely indicated, if ever)

These diets are often self-imposed and may, therefore, be hazardous. In a well-balanced diet, protein should provide 15 to 20 percent of total caloric intake and fat less than 30 percent.

Low Calorie Diets. Since treatment of significant obesity usually is difficult, goals should be set with a target loss determined at the outset of a treatment program. In most cases this is achieved by a slow, steady loss of 1 to 2 lb per week. Since on average a deficit of approximately 3500 kcal is required to yield 1 lb of weight (fat) loss, a daily deficit of 500 to 1000 kcal (usually resulting in prescription of a 1000 to 1200 kcal diet) is necessary. Factors to be considered when prescribing the low calorie diet include meeting specific nutrient needs with supplements, adapting to the patient's tastes and habits, trying to achieve satiety, and satisfying the rest of the patient's family. Long-term suitability of the diet must be evaluated with the aim of developing a lifelong eating pattern that involves both food choices and eating habits.

Very Low Calorie Diets. At lower calorie levels—800 kcal or less—individuals may develop weakness, fatigue, nausea, vomiting, dehydration, postural hypotension, or gout. Such diets should be restricted to the morbidly obese, often only when hospitalized or under close medical supervision (see protein-sparing fast, further on). Since it is difficult to meet daily requirements of many vitamins and minerals on a diet of less than 1300 kcal, a vitamin-mineral supplement should be prescribed, usually a one-a-day over-the-counter preparation (see Chapters 2 and 14).

Starvation and Modified Fasts

The protein-sparing modified fast should be reserved for the severely obese patient in whom rapid weight loss is vital. The development of cardiac arrhythmias is a serious potential side effect of this regimen, which generally involves administration of 300 to 400 kcal as high quality protein (1 to 1.5 g per kg ideal body weight), with total intake of less than 500 calories. Protein may be ingested as powder or supplement, or as foods such as tuna fish and turkey. It has not been proved that pure-protein regimens are more effective than carbohydrate-containing diets in reducing appetite or in sparing body nitrogen. These diets are supplemented with minerals and trace elements (calcium, magnesium, potassium, iron) and vitamins.

Hospitalized patients on a semistarvation regimen will develop hypotension and protein loss and will become depleted in fluids, electrolytes, and vitamins, including folate, vitamin B_{12}, and vitamin B_6. Additional side effects include severe ketosis, hyperuricemia, hypoglycemia, and alopecia. (See Chapter 13 for a more complete description of the effects of fasting.) Since the safety of such diets is questionable, they should be reserved for patients of at least 130 percent of ideal body weight who are under medical supervision and ongoing surveillance and who are expected to maintain weight loss with a balanced diet. Use for more than 3 months is not recommended.

Exercise/Activity

Increase in activity, with an exercise program, is very important. Energy expenditure increases as follows:

Activity	kcal/min
Sleep	0.8
Very light	1.5–2.0
Light (walking, golf)	2.0–3.5
Moderate (bicycling, tennis, swimming, dancing)	3.5–7.0
Heavy (basketball, jogging, skiing)	7.5+

Medications

The use and efficacy of anorectic drugs remains controversial, with problems of safety, addiction, and tolerance. Generally, drugs are of only limited, short-term usefulness (less than 3 months).

Surgery and Invasive Procedures

Surgery should be reserved for patients under 50 years of age with life-threatening obesity who are at least 100 pounds overweight, or twice ideal weight, and who have repeatedly and seriously attempted to lose weight. Surgical procedures include gastric reduction by bypass or stapling, jejunoileal bypass (no longer recommended), and jaw wiring. Jejunoileal bypass appears to result in diminished food intake and a malabsorption syndrome with steatorrhea (see Chapter 21). Potential complications of the jejunoileal bypass include

- diarrhea
- malnutrition (hypoproteinemia, decrease in vitamins B_{12}, A, and E)
- potassium loss
- decrease in serum calcium and magnesium, possibly producing tetany
- fatty liver or cirrhosis, or both
- intestinal bacterial overgrowth with pseudo-obstruction
- urinary calculi (oxalate stones)
- migratory polyarthritis

Some of these complications are sufficiently serious to warrant reanastomosing the small intestine, with reversal of symptoms.

Gastric bypass and vertical banded gastroplasty construct a small (15 to 50 ml) pouch connected through a small (28 to 32 French) stoma to an outflow tract. Patients eat small amounts slowly and take no liquids with meals. Average weight loss is about 100 pounds. Potential complications include

- vomiting
- epigastric pain
- thiamin, vitamin B_{12}, and folate deficiency
- hair loss
- bone demineralization

Follow-up Weight Maintenance Programs

Follow-up weight maintenance programs are best done in a group setting (e.g., Weight Watchers). Regardless of the modality, only 25 percent of patients sustain a 20 lb loss for 2 years. Therefore, a weight maintenance plan must be a major component of any weight reducing regimen.

ANOREXIA NERVOSA

Epidemiology and Pathogenesis

Anorexia nervosa is a chronic eating disorder characterized by severe, self-induced restriction of calories. It is seen primarily in adolescent and young white women, usually within 7 years of menarche, and less commonly, prior to menarche. Men also may be affected. Persons at high risk include dancers, models, and long-distance runners. The disorder is largely confined to middle- and upper-middle class individuals with unusually high self-expectations. The condition is believed to be caused by psychologic factors, and is almost invariably accompanied by endocrine disturbances that are not all reversed by adequate weight gain. The central nervous system (hypothalamic-pituitary axis) is believed by some investigators to be involved in the pathogenesis. Associated hypothalamic defects occur in the gonadal axis, and in fluid and temperature regulation. There is a decrease in sympathetic nervous system activity and associated changes in emotions and locomotion.

Clinical Presentation and Diagnosis

Criteria for the diagnosis of anorexia nervosa include

1. loss of at least 25 percent of original body weight without a known physical illness to account for the loss
2. a distorted, implacable attitude toward eating that overrides hunger
3. an intense fear of obesity
4. a distorted body image

Anorectics also may show these signs and symptoms:

- amenorrhea, which may precede weight loss
- impotence (in males), decreased libido
- lanugo
- bradycardia
- periods of intense hyperactivity and exhaustive exercise regimens
- laxative or diuretic abuse
- cold intolerance
- dry skin
- hypothermia and abnormal thermoregulation
- hypotension
- yellow palms accompanied by carotenemia
- edema with altered fluid regulation
- episodes of bulimia or self-induced vomiting or both (in a subgroup of anorectics)

Some patients with anorexia nervosa never binge and are "restricters," as differentiated from bulimic anorectics.

Anorectic patients may have a low basal metabolic rate, presumably an adaptive response to starvation. In other studies, caloric expenditure is excessive. Results of other laboratory tests tend to be inconsistent. Normal or increased levels of plasma cortisol with normal diurnal rhythm are characteristic. (Patients with panhypopituitarism or Addison's disease have low plasma cortisol levels.)

Disorders such as inflammatory bowel disease, malignancy, and autoimmune conditions or chronic infection should first be considered as possible causes of weight loss. A thorough history frequently pinpoints the diagnosis, usually eliminating the need for a costly, extensive work-up.

Treatment

There is no single treatment regimen for anorexia nervosa. Hospitalization is necessary when protein-energy malnutrition (PEM) is life threatening (see Chapter 13). Although treatment is primarily psychiatric, enteral or parenteral feeding is required for life-threatening PEM. Most therapies combine nutritional repletion with individual and family psychotherapy, including behavior modification techniques. Those with loss exceeding 30 to 40 percent of prior weight are at increased risk and must be refed with extreme care to avoid refeeding edema and cardiac arrhythmias.

Prognosis

Mortality rate is 4 to 6 percent, and long-term follow-up reveals the persistence of psychiatric and weight problems in the majority of patients.

CASE 16b: ANOREXIA NERVOSA

An 18-year-old woman was referred to the Psychiatry Service for progressive weight loss and vomiting for 1 year. Ten months earlier she had complained to her family physician about stomach aches, worse after eating, postprandial vomiting, anorexia, and increasing weakness, because of which she had changed her diet to clear liquids. Four months earlier she weighed 44 kg (height 167 cm), having lost 8 kg over the preceding 6 months. One month before admission she developed pleuritic chest pain and hospitalization was recommended. Her last menstrual period occurred 4 months before admission. She complained of palpitations. She was hostile and denied being undernourished.

Her blood pressure was 85/50. She weighed 29 kg (50 percent of ideal body weight), with triceps skinfold thickness of 4 mm and mid-arm muscle circumference 14.5 cm. She was emaciated and had a flat affect. Breath sounds were decreased bilaterally. Her serum albumin was 2.7 g/dl, prealbumin 13 mg/dl, retenol-bonding protein 2.7 mg/dl, and potassium 3 mEq/l. Prothrombin time was prolonged to 24 seconds with a control of 12 seconds. Vitamin A level was marginal (28 μg/dl). Her chest radiogram showed an infiltrate on the right lung and sputum examination showed gram-negative rods. White blood cell count was 8100/mm^3.

Her aspiration pneumonia was treated with two courses of penicillin. Intake was less than 700 kcal/day and nasogastric tube feeding was begun. Serum phosphorus fell to 0.5 mg/dl. Ecchymoses developed, which were attributed to vitamin K deficiency, which was treated with Synkayvite and improved rapidly. Her weight increased slowly and the tube feeding was replaced with an enteral supplement by mouth containing about 2500 kcal daily with 70 g protein. Two months after admission she weighed 36 kg. Serum albumin was 4.2 g/dl. She still avoided high calorie foods.

LESSON:

This patient with anorexia nervosa illustrates the pitfalls of refeeding even via the enteral route and the development of vitamin K deficiency because of inadequate dietary intake with superimposed antibiotic therapy.

BULIMIA

Clinical Presentation and Diagnosis

Bulimia, or binge-eating, is a recently recognized syndrome of unknown pathogenesis. It is characterized by recurrent eating episodes in which massive amounts of high calorie foods are consumed in a discrete, finite period of time (Table 16–2). Such binges terminate in sleep, abdominal pain, or self-induced vomiting and purgation. They may begin as a group or family activity, but most often are done in secret as a solitary activity. Bulimics frequently attempt to lose weight on severely restricted diets and/or by using diuretics or laxatives. Bulimics have a body weight distribution that straddles the norm, without the extreme weight loss seen in anorectics. Individuals' weight frequently fluctuates more than 10 pounds as a result of bingeing and fasting. Eating patterns are egodystonic; patients are depressed and have self-deprecating thoughts after bingeing, with strong fears about their loss of control. The disorder is suspected when the complications are observed or other people report the abnormal eating behavior.

Table 16–2. DIARY OF AN
EATING BINGE,
3:30 P.M. UNTIL BEDTIME*

kcal	Food
700	T-bone steak, 10 oz
140	baked potato
100	with butter
100	salad with oil and vinegar
210	3 slices bread
100	and butter
32	2 coffees, sugar (1 tsp/cup)
340	2 beers
340	2 big cola drinks
350	1 slice cheesecake
450	1 slice carrot cake, cream cheese frosting
—	mushrooms
2862	
210	3 scoops of ice cream
160	caramel sauce
80	whipped cream
16	1 coffee, sugar
310	ice cream sandwich
776	
900	2 ice cream sundaes
340	1 ice cream
70	cone
981	3 dishes (1/2 cup) of bread pudding, ice cream, cola drink
2291	
140	wheat crackers
200	and cheese
280	4 oatmeal cookies
200	10 honey sesame candies
280	2 English muffins,
200	butter
1300	

Temperature next A.M. 99.6° F

TOTAL 7229 CALORIES

*Data provided by Dr. Diane K. Smith.

Complications

Complications of bulimia include pancreatitis, enlarged parotid glands, gastrointestinal injury, anemia, amenorrhea, electrolyte disturbances, ipecac cardiotoxicity, and other complications of vomiting, such as erosion of tooth enamel.

Treatment

Treatment of bulimia is difficult, consisting primarily of individual psychotherapy, antidepressants, and nutritional counseling. Return to normal eating habits is likely, although there may be relapses for years after successful treatment.

Prognosis

Management may be more or less successful than treatment of anorexia nervosa. Best therapeutic results are achieved using the addiction model.

CHAPTER 17

Alcoholism

Alcoholic beverages, especially wine and beer, are commonly ingested in moderate quantities to quench thirst, and may be enjoyed for their taste, relaxing qualities, and as accompaniments to good food, especially during social events. The pharmacologic effects of excessive alcohol, however (sedation, mood change, anesthesia, coma), and its addictive properties produce physical and mental illness and contribute significantly to morbidity and mortality, especially in young adults. In our society, alcoholism is the single most important factor in producing nutrient deficiencies and the relatively rare nutritional deficiency diseases (see Chapters 14 and 15). Alcohol consumption may relate to the prevalence of obesity (see Chapter 16); hypertension, hyperlipidemia, and cardiomyopathy (see Chapter 19); diseases of the gastrointestinal tract, liver, and pancreas (see Chapters 21 and 22); and cancer (see Chapter 24).

Alcohol dependence is defined by the World Health Organization as consumption exceeding limits accepted by the culture or injuring health or social relationships. Alcoholism affects 30 to 50 percent of the patients seen in a general hospital, but much of the time the diagnosis can be missed. The condition generally develops over a period of 10 to 15 years, or more. Although it has been suspected, genetic vulnerability to alcohol addiction has not been established with certainty but is likely in males.

Approximately half of the United States adult population consumes one or more alcoholic drinks per month, with mean and modal daily intakes of 25 g and 34 g (32 to 40 ml), respectively. Heavy alcohol intake (exceeding 50 g or 64 ml per 70 kg daily) affects 15 percent of males and 9 percent of females. The incidence of cirrhosis rises steeply when daily alcohol intake exceeds 80 g in men. Alcohol is associated with 250,000 deaths per year and is involved in one third to one half of all fatal motor vehicle accidents.

This chapter briefly reviews

- the metabolism of alcohol (ethyl alcohol or ethanol)
- alcohol intoxication and withdrawal syndromes
- the effects of alcohol in inducing nutritional deficiencies and specific metabolic disorders
- alcohol's effects on the digestive, cardiovascular, and nervous systems

ALCOHOL METABOLISM

Nutritional Value of Alcohol

When metabolized efficiently, alcohol yields 7 kcal per g. It provides from 5 to 10 percent of the calories in the usual diet in the United States. Its caloric value can be calculated as 0.8 × proof × ounces; one fifth of whiskey thus yields about 1500 calories. Alcoholic beverages contain from 30 to 300 g alcohol per liter of water, with insignificant amounts of vitamins and minerals, thereby providing "empty" calories. Small amounts of congeners are formed during fermentation; these include methanol, propanol, isobutyl alcohol, isoamyl alcohol, ethyl acetate, ethyl formate, acetaldehyde, ethers, fusel oils, and volatile acids. The role of these toxic substances in the etiology of hangover is unknown.

Absorption

Alcohol is primarily absorbed in the intestine and small intestine (90 percent). Fat and milk delay absorption, which may take place in a period of 5 to 90 minutes, depending on whether beer, wine, or stronger beverages are consumed straight or diluted and with or without food. The absorbed alcohol is metabolized in the liver at a usual rate of 7 to 8 g per hour in the 70 kg person, representing 75 to 150 mg alcohol per kg body weight per hour. This corresponds to metabolizing 15 to 22 mg per dl blood alcohol concentration per hour, or the equivalent of ingesting two thirds to 1 oz of 90 proof whiskey.

Oxidation

Alcohol is oxidized to carbon dioxide and water (98 percent), with minimal amounts excreted in urine or via respiration. It is first metabolized via alcohol dehydrogenase (cytoplasm) to acetaldehyde and then to acetate, which in turn yields carbon dioxide and water via the mitochondria. Alcohol oxidation produces 16 moles of ATP (-2 ATP for acetyl CoA) and is therefore 90 percent efficient. A microsomal ethanol oxidizing system (MEOS) does not involve phosphorylation, generates free energy, and is less efficient than the alcohol dehydrogenase-mitochondrial pathway. This alternate oxidative mechanism is more common in regular alcohol users. Through its production of acetate, alcohol is ketogenic.

Blood Levels of Alcohol

Alcohol is detectable in the blood at levels of 10 mg per dl or above (Table 17–1). Social drinkers' blood levels typically are fivefold higher. Following ingestion of 6 oz of whiskey (or the equivalent 48 oz beer or 20 oz wine) on an empty stomach, an average-size individual's blood alcohol level reaches 100 mg per dl. Variations in legally defined limits of ethanol may range as high as 180 mg per dl. (Frank intoxication is present at that level.) Severe intoxication, stupor or coma, and even death are associated with progressive increases in blood alcohol up to 500 mg per dl. Thus, the ratio of blood levels from social to fatal is of the order of 10. Fatal levels may be reached with an ingestion of 20 oz of whiskey.

Table 17-1. BLOOD ALCOHOL
LEVELS AND CLINICAL STATE

State of Subject	Blood Alcohol Level (mg/dl)
Detectable level	10
"Social" drinking	50–75
6 oz whiskey—empty stomach	100
Severe intoxication	200
Stupor, coma	400
Fatal	500

ALCOHOL INTOXICATION AND WITHDRAWAL

Alcohol Intoxication

Acute alcohol intoxication (drunkenness, excitement, coma) affects fluids, electrolytes, body temperature, and ventilation, and may be associated with hypoglycemia. Since alcohol causes cutaneous vasodilatation, hypothermia may occur, especially in cold weather.

Alcohol may cause diuresis (decrease in antidiuretic hormone), thirst, and dehydration. Hangover possibly results from increased blood levels of pyruvic acid. Sodium and water retention is common in alcoholics with chronic liver disease. Decreased magnesium in skeletal muscle, hypocalcemia, hypophosphatemia, and hypokalemia may occur in acute or chronic alcoholism, with resultant rhabdomyolysis and acute renal failure (see Chapter 14).

Withdrawal Syndromes

"Shakes," "fits," and delirium tremens are characteristic withdrawal syndromes. Tremulousness may be seen within 1 to several days following a patient's abrupt withdrawal from alcohol and may last 3 days, with peak occurrence in 1 to 2 days. Treatment at this stage may prevent the occurrence of seizures and delirium tremens. Patients may be superalert, easily startled, flushed, sleepless, irritable or excitable, with tachycardia and tremor—symptoms related to catecholamine release. Hallucinosis occurs in one fourth of patients. Treatment is with thiamin (50 mg IM) and chlordiazepoxide, 50 to 100 mg stat, or 25 mg qid, or diazepam 10 mg two to four times daily.

Fits—grand mal seizures, postictal confusion, and somnolence—may be seen within a few days following alcohol withdrawal. Seizures are treated with phenytoin or carbamazepine. Because one third of these seizure patients progress to delirium tremens, anticipatory hospitalization with vigorous treatment is recommended.

Delirium Tremens

Characterized by profound disorientation, severe agitation, vivid hallucinations, delusions, sweating, tachycardia, fever, and hypertension, but rarely seen in patients under age 30, delirium tremens occurs 3 to 4 days after alcohol withdrawal and lasts about 72 hours. The syndrome may occur as late as 1 week after alcohol is stopped. About 9 percent have seizures and 15 percent of patients die. Patients should be hospitalized and observed for signs of infection, especially pulmonary and genitourinary. The condition may be accompanied by hypoglycemia or by head injury, and frequently is associated with alcohol-related disease of the liver or pancreas, or use of other drugs (see Chapter 22). There also is a defect in cell-mediated immunity induced by alcohol.

In the management of delirium tremens, it is essential to monitor hydration, electrolytes (potassium), magnesium, and phosphate and acid-base balance, and to maintain the airway. Treatment includes administration of 50 to 100 mg thiamin and use of benzodiazepines (chlordiazepoxide), loading with 100 to 400 mg, and tapering by 25 percent per day. Smokers may require higher doses of tranquilizing drugs. The goal of therapy is to keep the patient awake and calm. Shorter acting drugs (oxazepam or lorazepam), or beta blockers may be useful in managing withdrawal symptoms in patients with liver disease. Those with malnutrition are at higher risk for morbidity and mortality from delirium tremens than are well-nourished alcoholics.

DISEASES AND METABOLIC ALTERATIONS ASSOCIATED WITH CHRONIC ALCOHOL ABUSE

Nutritional Disorders

Nutrient abnormalities and malnutrition with multiple causes are common in the alcoholic (Fig. 17–1).

- Inadequate food intake is due in part to spending money on "booze" rather than food.

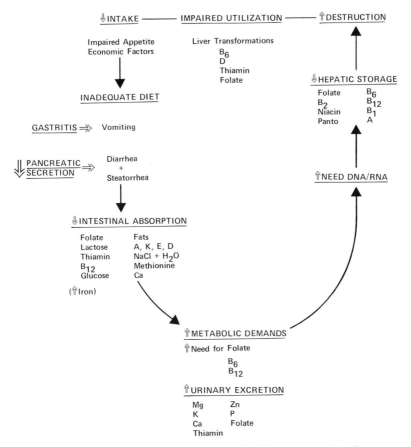

Figure 17-1. Mechanisms of nutritional deficiency in alcoholics.

- Alcoholics tend to choose meals poorly, predominating in carbohydrates, with inadequate protein and vitamin content.
- Maldigestion may be caused by pancreatic insufficiency (see Chapter 22).
- Malabsorption (see Chapter 21) has been reported in 50 percent of hospitalized alcoholics, but is reversible.
- Hyperexcretion and malutilization of nutrients may also be present.
- Nutrient requirements may be increased, especially for vitamin-dependent metabolic reactions.

It is not known whether alcoholics' nutrient requirements differ from those of healthy individuals. Possible impairment of protein synthesis and release from the liver may be an influencing factor.

CASE 17A: PROTEIN-ENERGY MALNUTRITION AND SEPSIS

A 66-year-old white woman with a history of chronic ethanol abuse presented to the MCG-ICA obtunded, responsive only to deep pain. The history was given by her intoxicated husband, who reported her to have been lying on the couch for the past month ingesting only beer and crackers. She had not eaten for 3 days prior to admission. She was brought to the ICA because she was unable to drink and would not respond to her husband. The past medical history, social and family histories, and review of symptoms were unobtainable.

The admission physical examination was: blood pressure 84/ palpable, respiratory rate 32, pulse 92, temperature 36.4°C. The patient was diaphoretic with multiple ecchymoses over the forearms, arms, and thighs. There were excoriated areas on both axillae, buttocks, and back, and necrotic areas over both posterior thighs. The patient also had head lice and multiple maggots and roaches over her body. Her head was nontraumatic; her mouth revealed poor hygiene with dry mucous membranes. Positive gag was present. The lung examination showed diffuse rhonchi, greater on right than left. No bowel sounds were audible over the abdomen. The extremities demonstrated poor tone. The neurologic examination showed the patient to be disoriented to person, place, and time. Nuchal rigidity was absent with full range of motion of the neck. The remainder of the examination was within normal limits. An ECG showed normal sinus rhythm with no acute changes. The chest radiograph showed a right lower lobe infiltrate. The SMA-18 was abnormal with a serum sodium of 114 mEq/l, potassium 5.6 mEq/l, BUN 33 mg/dl, creatinine 0.8 mg/dl, albumin 2.2 g/dl, phosphorus 5.0 mg/dl, alkaline phosphatase 179 mU. The white blood cell count was 26,700/mm^3, hemoglobin 11.4 g/dl, hemocrit 36.7 percent, MCV 97.9 fl. There were 68 segmented polys, 26 bands, 1 lymphocyte, 4 monocytes. Serum alcohol was negative. Prothrombin time 10.9 seconds, control 11.3; PTT 25.9, control 29.1. Fibrin split products < 10, fibrinogen 460 mg/dl. Arterial blood gas was pO$_2$ 214 mm, pH 7.26, pCO$_2$ 28.5 mm, HCO$_3$ 12.4 mEq/l. Urinalysis showed moderate bacteria with gram-negative rods. A sputum Gram stain showed many gram-positive cocci and moderate gram-negative rods. TSF 12 mm, MAC 25 cm, ht 162 cm.

The initial assessment was volume depletion, hyponatremia, profound protein calorie malnutrition, sepsis with urinary tract infection, RLL aspiration pneumonia and metabolic acidosis, generalized necrosis of thighs and buttocks. Cautious repletion of calories, 1200, due to patient's starvation status was advised.

Vigorous rehydration and electrolyte repletion was initiated. Debridement was also completed with the patient placed on a Clinitron bed. Fifty percent ventimask with suctioning q hour was accomplished.

Broad spectrum antibiotics were initiated. Multiple consults were obtained which included a nutrition consult. Hyperalimentation TPN was initiated with 2 liters D_{10}, 4.25 percent amino acids, and 500 cc 10 percent Intralipid. Multivitamins were given in addition to high doses of vitamin A, niacin, and ascorbic acid. A nutrition screen was obtained prior to nutritional supplementation. Abnormal were: plasma retinol 7 $\mu g/dl$, plasma α-tocopherol 95 $\mu g/dl$, plasma copper 64 $\mu g/dl$, plasma selenium 4.4 $\mu g/dl$, prealbumin 2.4 $\mu g/dl$, retinol binding protein 0.75 mg/dl, transferrin 91.0 mg/dl.

Despite aggressive and heroic attempts with intravenous fluids and antibiotics, the patient had a progressive decline. At the request of the family, aggressive and extensive resuscitation efforts were not attempted, and the patient expired at 6:50 A.M. the morning after admission.

Vitamins

Folate Deficiency. Folate deficiency may be found in up to 80 percent of alcoholics, who will present with megaloblastic anemia (see Chapter 15). Inadequate intake, malabsorption, and impaired liver storage are factors contributing to this condition. The deficiency contributes to impaired sodium and water transport in the small intestine, resulting in diarrhea.

Thiamin Deficiency. The neurologic signs of thiamin deficiency—that is, polyneuropathy (dry beriberi) and Wernicke-Korsakoff syndrome—and the cardiovascular signs—high output heart failure (wet beriberi)—are discussed under Neurologic Syndromes, p. 416.

Vitamin B_6, Niacin, and Vitamin C Deficiencies. Vitamin B_6 deficiency occurs in about half of alcoholics. Metabolism of this vitamin may be disturbed by the oxidation of alcohol and in niacin deficiency, which is found in one third of alcoholics (see Chapter 14 for a description of pellagra). Low levels of vitamin C are common in alcoholics, with occasional cases of scurvy (see Chapter 14).

Vitamin A, D, and K Deficiencies. Overt deficiency of fat-soluble vitamins is less common, but vitamin A storage is significantly impaired in the presence of alcoholic liver disease (see Chapter 22). Vitamin A levels are decreased owing to impaired absorption, steatorrhea, decreased storage, and decreased activation (see Chapter 2). Alcoholics may thus manifest impaired dark adaptation or frank xerosis, xerophthalmia, and keratomalacia (see Chapter 14). Hepatic disease, as well as decreased vitamin D intake, absorption, clearance, hydroxylation, degradation and storage lower vitamin D levels, resulting in decreased absorption of calcium and increased urinary losses. Osteopenia in males with no antecedent history of bone disease usually is due to alcoholism, and one half of chronic alcoholics show bone loss. Vitamin K deficiency with resultant prolongation of prothrombin time and bleeding can stem from dietary deficiency, malabsorption, and/or decreased bacterial synthesis of vitamin K.

Minerals

Alcoholism also has adverse effects on trace mineral status, with increased urinary loss of zinc and increased iron absorption with increased iron stores.

Fluid and Electrolyte Disturbances

Electrolyte depletion may occur with acute intoxication. Disorders of water and electrolyte metabolism may occur in alcoholics with chronic liver disease (sodium and water retention, low body potassium stores). Severe hypomagnesemia is a rare occurrence in chronic alcoholics.

Malabsorption

Malabsorption in the alcoholic is characterized by weight loss, anorexia, nausea, epigastric discomfort, abdominal pain, diarrhea, and flatulence. The condition may result from the direct, toxic effect of alcohol on the small intestine, or may be secondary to alcohol-induced malnutrition, especially protein (Chapter 13) and folate deficiencies or bacterial overgrowth (Chapter 21). Any or all of these factors may operate in the etiology of the malabsorption syndrome. Lactase deficiency is common. Steatorrhea is found in 50 percent of patients but usually is mild and is attributable to fat maldigestion resulting from inadequate pancreatic lipase. Absorption of D-xylose and water-soluble vitamins is impaired. Fecal nitrogen is increased owing to impaired amino acid transport resulting from decreased Na/K ATPase activity.

Treatment of the malabsorption includes providing a high protein diet and vitamin supplements. Pancreatic function will also improve after several weeks of this therapy.

Metabolic Disorders

Ketoacidosis, hypoglycemia, hyperglycemia, and hyperuricemia are among the other metabolic problems resulting from alcohol abuse. Ketoacidosis results from increased production of lactate and acetate. Hypoglycemia is related to a decrease in liver glycogen resulting from inhibition of gluconeogenesis, together with autonomic dysfunction and other abnormalities. Diabetes mellitus may develop, with abnormal glucose tolerance, increased insulin, and abnormal response to glucagon. In addition, hyperuricemia and gout may result from decreased renal excretion of urate, owing to increased lactate levels.

Liver Disease

The liver is the principal site of alcohol metabolism and a common site of injury. Alcohol-related liver disease includes the entities of fatty liver, alcoholic hepatitis (including hepatic encephalopathy), and cirrhosis. Alcohol is a direct hepatotoxin. In addition, associated malnutrition may increase the liver's susceptibility to injury from alcohol as well as accelerate the rate of progression of liver disease. It is important to keep in mind that no nutritional regimen (supplemental vitamins, protein, and so forth) can be relied on to prevent liver damage in the presence of persisting use of substantial amounts of alcohol. (The features and management of liver disease are discussed thoroughly in Chapter 22.)

Pancreatitis

Alcoholism is also related to the development of acute and recurrent pancreatitis, resulting in abnormal pancreatic exocrine and endocrine secretion, malnutrition, and malabsorption (see Chapter 22).

CASE 17b: ALCOHOL MALABSORPTION SYNDROME

A 46-year-old man was hospitalized with diabetic ketoacidosis. His past history included six prior episodes of chronic recurrent pancreatitis over 12 years and the development of insulin-dependent diabetes mellitus 6 years earlier. He was prescribed 30 units NPH insulin daily. He had been drinking 1 pint of whiskey daily for several years, and had lost 14 kg in the previous 3 months. Two weeks before admission he developed pain on swallowing. He had chronic epigastric pain. His sole dietary intake for 2 weeks consisted of red beans, rice, and grits. He had chronic diarrhea and malodorous stools, and had noted decreasing night vision, dry skin, and soreness of his tongue, lips, and mouth. He was unable to stand up from a squatting position and both legs were numb.

He was cachectic and emaciated—weight 44 kg, height 173 cm (63 percent of ideal body weight). Triceps skinfold thickness and mid-arm muscle circumference were 33 and 75 percent of standard, respectively. His skin was dry and flaking, and his head hair was dry, dull, and easily pluckable. Conjunctivae showed bitemporal xerosis. Angular fissures, cheilosis, and a smooth, magenta tongue were present. The scrotal skin was erythematous, the epigastrium was tender, and signs of peripheral neuropathy were noted.

Serum glucose was over 700 mg/dl and serum acetone was positive. His serum albumin was 2.9 g/dl with prealbumin 5 mg/dl. Plasma vitamin A level was 11 µg/dl, carotene 13 µg/dl, vitamin C 0.42 mg/dl, and vitamin E 305 µg/dl. Plasma zinc was 55 µg/dl. He exhibited the fatty acid pattern of essential fatty acid deficiency. After his ketoacidosis was corrected, he was given a high calorie, high protein, low fat diet. Addition of pancreatic enzymes permitted his fat to be increased to normal. He was given parenteral thiamin, vitamin A, B complex, and vitamin C, as well as 3 units of 10 percent fat emulsion intravenously over 3 days.

LESSON:

This patient illustrates the effect of alcohol abuse in causing pancreatic exocrine and endocrine insufficiency and resultant multiple nutritional deficiencies. Not only did the patient exhibit protein-energy malnutrition but also he had signs of specific vitamin deficiencies (fat- and water-soluble). His skin lesions presumably resulted from a combination of protein, essential fatty acid, and zinc deficiencies.

Neurologic Syndromes

Polyneuropathy

Thiamin deficiency is seen to 30 to 80 percent of alcoholics and is characterized primarily by polyneuropathy, especially peripheral neuropathy (see Chapter 14). Also contributing to the development of neuropathy are deficiencies of vitamin B_6, pantothenic acid, niacin, riboflavin, and vitamin B_{12} (absorption of vitamin B_{12} may be impaired). Polyneuropathy is associated with discomfort and fatigue of the anterior tibial muscle, paresthesias in the feet, and weakness in the ankles and toes. There is "stocking-glove" sensory disturbance (hypesthesia, anesthesia, and/or hypalgesia), with decreased fine movements, impaired vibration sense, and diminished ankle jerks.

Wernicke-Korsakoff Syndrome

This syndrome is another sign of thiamin deficiency (see Chapter 14). Wernicke's encephalopathy is characterized by disordered eye movements, irregular, poorly reactive pupils, ataxia, gait and stance disturbances, drowsiness, and global confusion. There is horizontal and often vertical nystagmus, ophthalmoplegia or paralysis of the external recti, and paralysis of conjugate gaze. The syndrome is abrupt in onset and may be lethal. Prompt treatment with parenteral thiamin is essential; abnormal eye signs can improve within 6 hours.

Korsakoff's psychosis is characterized by anterograde and retrograde amnesia, disordered time sense, confabulation, and cognitive deficits. Fewer than one third of these patients recover. There are symmetrical lesions of petechial hemorrhages in the periaqueductal gray and perivestibular areas, the mammillary bodies of the midbrain, and the cerebellum. The disorder is associated with abnormal brain transketolase that has a decreased affinity for the cofactor thiamin pyrophosphate (see Chapter 14 and case histories).

It is important to be aware that thiamin deficiency is likely in the alcoholic, and that administration of glucose can precipitate its symptoms. Thiamin administration should therefore be routine when handling the alcoholic patient.

Other Neurologic Syndromes

Other neurologic syndromes in alcoholics include dementia with brain atrophy and memory loss, cerebellar ataxia, central pontine myelinolysis, and skeletal myopathy. Brain damage from alcohol may antedate severe liver injury. Amblyopia is another feature of alcohol's adverse nutritional effects.

Cardiovascular Disease

Cardiovascular diseases induced by alcoholism include alcoholic cardiomyopathy, cardiovascular (wet) beriberi (see Chapter 14), and hypertension (alcohol ingestion raises the blood pressure in hypertensives—see Chapter 19).

Alcoholic Cardiomyopathy

Alcohol toxicity may product a dilated (congestive) cardiomyopathy, usually after 10 or more years of abuse. This cardiomyopathy results in low output heart failure (in contrast to beriberi), arrhythmias, tachycardia, and thromboembolism. It is characterized by cardiomegaly, gallop rhythm, narrow pulse pressure, peripheral vasoconstriction, elevated end-diastolic pressure, and decreased stroke volume. Patients usually complain of chest pain and palpitation. It is important to distinguish between this type of cardiomyopathy and coronary heart disease. Abstinence from alcohol is required for effective treatment; however, in patients with severe heart failure, the prognosis is poor.

Plasma Lipoproteins and Cholesterol

Modest to moderate amounts of alcohol will raise levels of HDL cholesterol, but excessive alcohol consumption may result in hypertriglyceridemia, with production of type 4 hyperlipoproteinemia or conversion of type 4 to type 5. Ingestion of alcohol by patients with type 5 hyperlipoproteinemia can precipitate episodes of acute pancreatitis (see Chapters 19 and 22). Alcohol induces increased synthesis of hepatic lipoproteins and fatty acids and fatty acid oxidation. Finally, cholesterol synthesis also is enhanced by alcohol.

Anemia and Other Hematologic Disorders

Anemia in the alcoholic may be caused by folate deficiency, increased iron utilization, dietary deficiency of protein, copper, and iron, gastrointestinal bleeding, and a direct toxic effect of alcohol on the bone marrow. Anemia or bone marrow abnormalities are found in about 75 percent of patients hospitalized with alcoholism. The direct toxic effect of alcohol on the bone marrow may also result in thrombocytopenia and granulocytopenia.

Cancer

Alcohol intake has been associated with the prevalence of some cancers, notably esophageal cancer, whose incidence increases twofold to fourfold with ingestion of 41 to 80 g of alcohol per day and 18-fold with over 80 g per day. In addition, colon cancer has been related to beer consumption.

Disease Associated With Alcohol Contaminants

Other aspects of alcohol consumption may also contribute to disease. For example, nonbonded alcoholic beverages may be contaminated with arsenic or cobalt, contributing to cardiomyopathy, or with lead, which causes saturnine gout.

Fetal Alcohol Syndrome

The fetal syndrome of microcephaly, mental deficiency, growth retardation, anomalies primarily of the face (epicanthal folds, short palpebral fissures, and maxillofacial hypoplasia), and cardiac septal defects results from excessive alcohol consumption during pregnancy (see Fig. 7–5). Prevalence is estimated to be 0.42 to 1.25 cases per 1000 pregnancies. Increased neonatal death and low birth weight infants have also been associated with alcoholism in pregnancy (see Chapter 7).

SECTION V

Nutritional Aspects of Acute and Chronic Diseases

It is no exaggeration to say that the composition of the blood is determined not by what the mouth takes in but by what the kidneys keep.

Homer W. Smith, 1895–1962, *From Fish to Philosopher*, Ch. 1

Moving on from Section IV's chapters on overnutrition and undernutrition, Section V examines the role of nutrition in various acute and chronic clinical situations—in particular, diabetes mellitus and oral/dental, gastrointestinal, liver, pancreas, and kidney disease. The section concludes with a chapter on the interaction of nutrition and cancer, followed by a chapter on the nutritional needs of patients stressed by trauma, surgery, burns, and sepsis.

Chapter 18—**Diabetes Mellitus**—begins by focusing on the disease itself, its complications, appropriate nutritional management, and the nature of the defect in type I and type II diabetes. The chapter then turns to the diabetic diet, delineating key principles of the diet and discussing metabolic responses to different foods. The chapter concludes with other recommendations and considerations, including new monitoring and insulin delivery techniques.

In Chapter 19—**Cardiovascular Diseases**—we first look at epidemiologic studies, then provide information on blood lipids and lipoproteins. After discussing the hyperlipidemias and hyperproteinemias, we turn to a coronary heart disease and its relationship to diet and lipids. The chapter concludes with a section on hypertension, followed by a brief discussion of the relationship of other dietary constituents to heart disease.

Chapter 20—**Oral and Dental Diseases**—begins by delineating the nutrients required for the development and maintenance of normal oral tissues. Next, the special nutritional needs during oral diseases and oral wound healing are presented. Finally, the chapter explores the oral cavity as a reflection of disease and the effects of excess fluoride on the oral cavity.

Chapter 21—**Gastrointestinal Diseases and Malabsorption**—discusses diseases of the esophagus, stomach, small intestine, and colon. The chapter includes a thorough examination of the malabsorption syndrome, including lactose and other intolerances, clinical tests, and other syndromes involving malabsorption.

In Chapter 22—**Hepatic and Pancreatic Disease**—we first describe metabolism in normal liver function, then discuss dietary management of patients with liver disease. Defects in the secretion of bile and pancreatic juice are covered next. The chapter concludes by presenting guidelines for the management of acute and chronic pancreatitis.

Chapter 23—**Acute and Chronic Renal Failure**—starts by detailing normal kidney function, then describes the etiology, clinical manifestations, pathophysiology, and management of acute and chronic renal failure. Finally, nutritional therapy for the dialysis patient is thoroughly explained, and the chapter ends with a brief discussion of other renal diseases.

In Chapter 24—**Cancer**—we examine the evidence linking specific dietary constituents and cancer. We then look at the nutritional status of the cancer patient, including the adverse effects of cancer, cancer cachexia, the effects of therapy, and, finally, nutritional interventions.

Chapter 25—**Trauma and Critical Care**—concludes Section V. Here we briefly discuss the body's general response to stress, then deal specifically with trauma and surgery, the burned patient, and sepsis.

CHAPTER 18

Diabetes Mellitus

THE DISEASE

Diabetes mellitus is the third leading cause of death in the United States. The disease currently is found in 15 percent of those over age 60, and is increasingly affecting a greater proportion of the general population. It has been simply defined as hyperglycemia, or an increase in blood sugar (greater than 140 mg per dl) in the fasting subject. There are two main types of diabetes: insulin-dependent (type I) and non–insulin-dependent (type II), with the latter much more common. Table 18–1 outlines the characteristics of both types. Diabetes in pregnancy and diabetes in children are discussed in Chapters 7 and 8, respectively, while diabetes secondary to pancreatitis is reviewed in Chapter 22.

THE DISEASE

Diabetes is a catabolic process that occurs in the absence of effectively functioning insulin, a primary hormone that controls anabolism and growth.

421

Table 18-1. CHARACTERISTICS OF TYPES
OF DIABETES MELLITUS

	Insulin-Dependent	Non–Insulin-Dependent
Age of onset, yr	Childhood–40 yr	>40
	Any	
Ketonemia	+	−
Hyperglycemia	Severe	Mild/Moderate/Severe
% IBW	Normal	Majority obese
Serum lipids	Abnormal	Abnormal
Insulin requirement	++	− ±
Insulin secretion	↓ 0	~ Normal
Onset	Sudden	Gradual
% of diabetes	5–10	70–95
Genetic component	HLA types	Very strong, frequent
Environmental factors	β cytotoxic virus	Adiposity { Overeating / Weight gain
	Autoimmune	Aging
	Chemical toxins	Pharmacologic
Pancreas lesion	β cell destruction "insulitis"	↓ β cell response to glucose
Special considerations of nutrition	Timed, consistent food intake	Encourage caloric restriction
Exercise	Regular activity	Regular exercise
		Improves receptor function
Other defects		Cell receptor or postreceptor response to insulin
		↓ hepatic uptake of glucose
Life expectancy	50% Normal	70% Normal
Rates of atherosclerosis	Excessive	Excessive
Cause of death	Renal failure	Coronary disease

The Defect in Diabetes

The underlying defect may be

- a lack of insulin because of pathology involving destruction of the beta cells of the pancreas, which secrete insulin
- a defect in the cell receptor or postreceptor response to insulin
- a decrease in the hepatic uptake of glucose

Insulin is the hormone that controls fuel storage and metabolism, events occurring primarily in liver, skeletal muscle, and adipose tissue. With insulin deficiency, glucose uptake and oxidation in muscle are decreased, muscle glycogen is lost, and glycogenesis is defective. Amino acids are released by muscle, primarily in the form of alanine, supplying the liver with substrate for gluconeogenesis. In adipose tissue, fatty acid uptake together with glucose uptake is decreased, and lipolysis is increased. These events result in lack of glycerophosphate for triglyceride synthesis in adipose tissue. Many of these events are similar to those seen in starvation (see Chapters 1 and 13). Fatty acids released from adipose tissue are metabolized in the liver and glycogenolysis is enhanced. There is thus an excess of glucose in the circulation resulting from a combination of overproduction and underutilization.

Type II Diabetes

Two defects characterize type II diabetes: (1) a relative lack of insulin and insulin resistance (accentuated by obesity) because of a decrease in insulin receptors, and (2) multiple defects in postreceptor intracellular insulin responses. Obese patients have increased levels of circulating insulin from enhanced secretion together with impaired glucose tolerance or frank diabetes. Elevated blood glucose combined with high insulin levels reflects insulin resistance. Insulin exerts its effects after binding to cell surface receptors. These receptors are decreased in obese patients, partially accounting for the insulin resistance. However, it is unclear whether the peripheral insulin resistance or the islet cell defect is the primary event (see Chapter 16). Seventy to 90 percent of these patients are obese.

The symptoms of diabetes include polydipsia, polyuria, and polyphagia. Presence of the disease may be heralded by the development of skin infections with furuncles and carbuncles. In women, the glycosuria predisposes the patient to vaginitis with Candida infection.

In the adult onset, non–insulin-dependent form of diabetes, complications may be symptomatic before any appreciation of hyperglycemia. These symptoms in the adult man may include the development of impotence. Diabetes is also associated with loss of vision resulting from cataracts and retinopathy.

This disorder may be treated with insulin injections or with oral hypoglycemic drugs. Approximately 25 percent of known diabetics in the United States are receiving insulin, which may be administered as short- or long-acting forms, or as some combination of the two. Injections may be given before breakfast, before each meal, before breakfast and supper, or at bedtime. The nature of the insulin and the time of its administration influence the timing and content of meals.

To monitor the effects of treatment, patients can test their urine for sugar and acetone; blood glucose can be measured by patients with a glucometer or sent to the laboratory, and levels of factors related to metabolic control can be measured, such as the level of hemoglobin A_1C (normal 4 to 7 percent, and up to 20 percent with hyperglycemia).

Severe Clinical Symptoms

With the advent of insulin the usual clinical problem and cause of death—diabetic ketoacidosis—has become less prevalent. Untreated type I diabetics may present with this problem, with its classic somnolence progressing to coma. Brittle diabetics (less than 5 percent of insulin-dependent patients) and those with insulin resistance continue to be clinical problems. Management of patients with diabetic ketoacidosis is achieved primarily with administration of insulin in adequate amounts, together with fluid and appropriate electrolytes (see Chapters 2 and 11).

Another clinical syndrome of the diabetic is hyperosmolar nonketotic coma, with extremely high blood glucose levels, which must be treated even more aggressively with fluid.

Complications of Diabetes

Hyperlipidemia, renal failure, and gastrointestinal problems are all possible complications of diabetes. Diabetic neuropathy may be of vascular or degenerative origin, with accumulation of sorbitol in the nerves possibly responsible for the pathology. Use of B complex or other vitamins in high dosage has no place in the treatment of these complications, other than the usual need for therapeutic supplementation when the diet has been and continues to be inadequate. Optimum control of the blood sugar by diet and insulin seems the best means of preventing, or possibly reversing, the diabetic triopathy of nephropathy, retinopathy, and neuropathy.

NUTRITIONAL MANAGEMENT

Nutritional management of diabetes is an example of the use of diet in treating a disease: a therapeutic diet. The physician specifies the diet prescription and the dietitian determines its nutrient components and translates them into foods and meals. The dietitian may use an exchange system of foods (the Exchange List for Meal Planning) developed by the American Diabetes Association for implementing the diabetic diet. This principle has since been extended to other types of modified diets. A team consisting of the physician and dietitian or nutritionist and often a nurse is involved in explaining the diet to the patient and in educating and supporting the patient and family. This chapter discusses general principles and theoretical aspects of the diet. Some details of the diet and exchange system are found in Chapter 10.

1986 Revision of Nutrition Recommendations

In 1986, a committee of the American Dietetic Association and the American Diabetes Association revised the exchange lists. Changes emphasize a high carbohydrate, high fiber diet (doubling fiber intake) and alter nutritive values for starch/bread and fruit lists. A new simplified meal plan for initiating patient education divides food choices selected by diabetics into six food groups. The nutrition recommendations were updated in 1986 as follows:

- Calories—prescribed to achieve and maintain desirable body weight.
- Carbohydrate intake:
  1. Liberalized to 55 to 60 percent of total calories, individualized according to blood glucose and lipid responses and eating patterns.
  2. Substitute fiber-containing foods for highly refined foods.
  3. Modest amounts of refined sugars may be acceptable, depending on metabolic control and body weight.
- Protein intake—should follow the RDA, but requirements may be greater for elderly subjects, or reduced in patients with incipient renal disease.
- Total fat and cholesterol intake—should be restricted to less than 30 percent of total calories and less than 300 mg per day, respectively. Replacement of saturated fat with unsaturated fat, or eicosapentaenoic acid and monounsaturated fats may be desirable.
- The use of various alternative sweeteners is acceptable.
- Salt intake is recommended at 1000 mg sodium per 1000 kcal, not to exceed 3000 mg sodium per day. Hypertensive individuals should reduce salt intake, but severe sodium restriction may be harmful in individuals with poor diabetic control, postural hypotension, and fluid imbalance.
- Alcohol should be used with caution. Specific problems with its use include hypoglycemia or hyperglycemia, obesity, hyperlipidemia, and/or neuropathy.
- Vitamins and minerals should meet the RDA, except that vitamin and mineral supplements may be warranted with very low calorie diets. Calcium supplements may be necessary under special circumstances.

Goals for Diabetes Management

Goals include restoring normal blood glucose and optimal lipid levels in order (1) to prevent hyperglycemia or hypoglycemia, or both, (2) to prevent or delay the long-term complications associated with diabetes, and (3) to contribute to a normal pregnancy for diabetic women. The plan should maintain normal growth rate in children and adolescents, permit the attainment and maintenance of reasonable body weight in adolescents and adults, and provide adequate nutrition for pregnant and lactating women and for the fetus. Consistent timing of meals and snacks should prevent inordinate swings in blood glucose levels for insulin users. The meal plan should be appropriate for the patient's lifestyle and allow integration of insulin therapy with the eating and exercise pattern. Weight management in the non–insulin-dependent diabetic involves changes in food intake and eating behavior as well as increased activity level. The success of these approaches is dependent on continued support and follow-up by qualified health professionals. Overall health of the diabetic should improve through optimal nutrition.

Methods to achieve these goals include the following components:

- a simple, individualized meal plan introducing the basics
- continued nutrition counseling by a nutritionist at least once or twice a year
- a team approach to education and counseling integrating family members
- an individualized, realistic and flexible program appropriate to the patient's lifestyle, age, educational level, and prior nutrition knowledge
- a daily aerobic exercise program is recommended

Principles of Good Nutrition in Diabetes

Carbohydrates, Fiber, and Glycemic Index

Diets high in soluble fiber (including supplements) offer some improvement in carbohydrate metabolism, and lower total cholesterol and low density lipoprotein cholesterol. A practical goal is to double the intake of most individuals by gradually increasing fiber intake to 40 g per day, or 25 g per 1000 kcal, with a maximum intake of 50 g. Fiber supplementation appears beneficial only when given with a diet of at least 50 percent of calories as carbohydrate. Foods to be selected include legumes (peas, beans), lentils, roots, tubers, green leafy vegetables, whole grain cereals (wheat, barley, oats, corn, and rye) and raw fruits and vegetables (see Table 1–9).

The long-term safety of high-fiber diets is not known. Postmenopausal women, the elderly, or growing children may require supplements of calcium and trace minerals. People with abnormal upper gastrointestinal function may develop bezoars and should avoid a diet high in leafy vegetables. To avoid hypoglycemia the insulin dose must be reduced if there is a radical change in fiber intake. Starting with small servings and increasing portions gradually can minimize abdominal cramping, diarrhea, and flatulence.

Table 18-2. SOME FOODS WITH
LOW GLYCEMIC INDEX,*
% RELATIVE TO GLUCOSE

Type	Food	Index
Grain	Spaghetti, white	50
	Spaghetti, whole meal	42
Cereal	Oatmeal	49
Vegetable	Potatoes, sweet	48
Legume	Beans, butter	36
	Beans, navy	31
	Beans, kidney	29
	Lentils	29
Fruit	Apples	46
	Pear	47
	Peach	40
	Plum	34
Other	Fructose	25

*Two-hour blood glucose response area to a portion containing
50 g carbohydrate.

Classifying foods by their effects on blood glucose (glycemic index) and use of this information in day-to-day management may result in favorable effects. Glycemic index tables (Table 18–2) identify the starchy foods with lower glycemic potential that may be offered on trial to diabetics.

Hyperlipidemia

Plasma lipids and lipoproteins, risk factors for atherosclerosis, are targets for dietary alteration (see Chapter 19). Hyperlipidemia in diabetes usually involves an increase in serum triglyceride and very low density lipoprotein cholesterol and triglyceride, with a decrease in high density lipoprotein cholesterol levels. Treatment of hyperglycemia results in improvement in plasma lipoprotein concentrations, especially when associated obesity is also treated. Thus, patients with diabetes should be prescribed a fat-modified diet in which total fat is restricted to less than 30 percent of total calories: saturated fat less than 10 percent, polyunsaturated fat 6 to 8 percent, and the rest as monounsaturated fat. The cholesterol content should not exceed 300 mg per day. This diet is comparable to that recommended by the American Heart Association for the general public. In this diet, the intake of unrefined carbohydrate is liberalized; this also may improve the management of hyperlipidemia. Details of the stricter diets recommended for patients with disorders of lipoprotein metabolism are found in Chapter 19.

Alternative Sweeteners

The use of caloric sweeteners such as fructose and sorbitol may lead to weight gain because their caloric contribution may be substantial.

Diet for the Insulin-Dependent Patient

The meal plan is important for maintaining metabolic balance and avoiding hyperglycemia and preventing hypoglycemia. Consistency of food intake is very important. The individualized meal plan should consider

- timing and consistency of food dictated by individual needs that depend on blood glucose monitoring, lifestyle, physical activity, insulin effect, and administration
- meal plan composition
- energy content—Total daily energy intake should be distributed consistently throughout the day with at least three regular meals, a bedtime snack, and one or more between-meal snacks. The flexibility in meals must be determined by the type and number of injections of insulin and be based on the results of blood glucose monitoring.
- dietary adjustment for exercise—Energy intake and insulin dosage should be adjusted to day-to-day variations in physical activity. Vigorous exercise should be undertaken only when the blood glucose level is between 100 and 200 mg per dl and there is no ketosis. To avoid hypoglycemia, supplemental carbohydrate-containing snacks may be taken before and during exercise and up to 24 hours after. Any adjustment of insulin dosage should be done after consultation with the physician and health care team.

Diet for the Non-Insulin-Dependent Patient

Weight reduction of obese diabetic patients results in a reduction in hyperglycemia, hyperlipidemia, hypertension, and proteinuria. More general benefits are described in Chapter 16. The need for oral hypoglycemic agents or insulin may be reduced or eliminated with reduction of caloric intake. The long-term prognosis may be improved with delay of onset or prevention of complications.

The diet should be balanced and nutritionally complete, with moderate caloric restriction (500 to 1000 kcal below usual). The use of very low calorie diets in which there is need for rapid, significant weight reduction is discussed in Chapter 16, along with the necessary maintenance program. Even modest caloric restriction may have positive effects on blood glucose and requirements for insulin and oral hypoglycemic agents.

Those individuals with upper body fat localization may have higher glucose levels, increased insulin resistance, more abnormal lipoproteins, and increased cardiovascular risk.

Summary

Nutrient needs of diabetics usually can be met without the use of special dietetic or diabetic foods. The need for essential nutrients is the same for diabetics as for nondiabetics of the same age, size, and gender. The high risk of vascular disease in patients with diabetes and associated hyperlipidemia dictates a need to restrict the intake of total fat, saturated fat, and cholesterol. The recommendations of the American Diabetes Association are similar to those advocated by diabetic associations throughout the world and by the American Heart and Cancer Associations and the American Academy of Pediatrics.

OTHER RECOMMENDATIONS AND CONSIDERATIONS

Chromium

Especially in the form of brewer's yeast, chromium can improve glucose metabolism. Chromium deficiency may be a factor in some persons with decreased glucose tolerance receiving total parenteral nutrition without added chromium. To date there is no clinical indication for the use of chromium in the treatment of diabetes.

New Monitoring and Insulin Delivery Techniques

Complications of microangiopathy include the diabetic triopathy mentioned earlier. Accumulating evidence shows that control of the blood sugar level reduces the severity or delays onset of these serious problems. Newer modalities for monitoring blood sugar and insulin delivery are improving treatment of diabetes. Some examples are

- availability of human insulin, which should be less antigenic than the usual beef or pork sources
- home glucose monitoring with a reflectance meter, allowing the patient to monitor blood sugar levels at frequent intervals
- the insulin pump with open or closed loop feedback systems for automatic delivery
- transplantation of the pancreas or pancreatic islet cell implants

With identification of some viruses, drugs, or other environmental factors that damage the pancreas, as well as autoimmune factors, it may be possible in the future to prevent or ameliorate the damage and pathologic events leading to diabetes.

CHAPTER 19

Cardiovascular Diseases

Nutrient excesses or deficiencies have been implicated as causing or contributing to cardiovascular diseases, particularly

- atherosclerosis
- hypertension
- cardiomyopathy

The nutritional factors affecting the cardiovascular system include calories, macronutrients and micronutrients, and alcohol (Table 19-1). The interaction between diet and cardiovascular disease includes conditions unquestionably due to nutrient deficiency (such as beriberi heart disease resulting from thiamin deficiency), conditions in which the deficiency occurs in conjunction with other environmental factors (such as the cardiomyopathy of Keshan's disease relating to selenium deficiency), or conditions in which the dietary factor is present in excess (such as alcoholic cardiomyopathy).

More common, however, are disorders in which the nutrient relates to diseases of unknown etiology via unknown mechanisms, such as the connection between dietary fat and atherosclerosis, or between sodium intake and hypertension. These diseases are the major causes of morbidity and mortality in affluent Western societies. Evidence of a nutrition connection is derived from epidemiologic data, from studies of migrants, from studies of inborn errors of metabolism in humans and animals, and from animal experiments. Despite the absence of conclusive evidence that excessive amounts of nutrients cause the disorders directly, health professionals advise limiting dietary intake of nutritional factors consumed in excess of physiologic requirements.

EPIDEMIOLOGIC STUDIES

Epidemiologic studies track the intake of dietary factors of interest to correlate with various aspects of a disease. The usual aim is to quantitate a specific nutrient or determine the pattern of food consumption of individual or group. These data then can be used to evaluate the effects of an intervention program. Nutrient intakes can be estimated from data related to food production, consumption, or intake. Data may be collected by a 24-hour recall of foods eaten, a food record or diary over a period of 1 week, or determination of the frequency of consumption of certain foods. The data bases available for determining the nutrient content of foods, however, may be limited or regional, e.g., for trace minerals. The disease parameter for correlation should be precise (e.g., myocardial infarction diagnosed by specific criteria; sudden death; elevated blood pressure defined and measured under controlled conditions).

Such data first described strong relationships between the dietary intake of cholesterol and saturated fat and mortality from coronary heart disease, and an association between intake of sodium or salt and hypertension. These

Table 19-1. NUTRIENTS IMPLICATED IN CAUSING
CARDIOVASCULAR DISORDERS

Atherosclerosis Coronary Heart Disease Peripheral Vascular Disease	Hypertension Intracranial Hemorrhage	Cardiomyopathy Heart Failure
Calories	Calories	Calories
Fat		
Saturated fat	(Polyunsaturated fat ↓ Blood pressure)	
Cholesterol		
Alcohol	Alcohol	Alcohol
Animal protein		↓ Protein
↓ Fiber	Sodium	Sodium
	Sodium:Potassium	↓ Potassium
	↓ Selenium	↓ Selenium
	↓ Calcium	↓ Thiamin

correlations do not, however, indicate cause and effect; other factors differing among communities but correlated with nutrient intake may be the primary determinants of the disease. Such analyses also preclude comparison of the relationships of nutritional intake, biochemical measurements, and disease for specific individuals within a population. The variation within the individual as well as between individuals also magnifies the difficulties of testing the relationship of amount of nutrient and risk of disease. Such studies are carried out better in animal models.

BLOOD LIPIDS AND LIPOPROTEINS

Excessive levels of blood lipids have been related to the development of cardiovascular disease. The lipids in plasma include cholesterol, free and esterified with fatty acid; triglycerides (triacylglycerols); phospholipids (lecithin or phosphatidylcholine, phosphatidylethanolamine, sphingomyelin, phosphatidylserine, and phosphatidylinositol); and unesterified or free fatty acids. Small amounts of monoglycerides and diglycerides, bile acids, and sterols other than cholesterol also are present in the blood.

The lipids are transported in plasma in the form of lipoprotein particles, which are classified according to their physical and chemical properties (Table 19-2). The plasma lipoproteins are

- chylomicrons
- very low density lipoproteins (VLDL)
- intermediate density lipoproteins (IDL, or beta-VLDL)
- low density lipoproteins (LDL)
- high density lipoproteins (HDL)

Table 19-2. PLASMA LIPOPROTEINS IN HUMANS

| Class | Particle Diameter (nm) | Flotation Density | Electrophoretic Mobility | Apoproteins | Chemical Composition | | | | |
| | | | | | Surface | | | Core | |
					Proteins	Phospho-lipids	Cholesterol %	Cholesterol Esters	Triglyc-erides
Chylomicrons	80–500	0.93	α2	B, E, A-I, A-IV, C	2	7	2	3	86
VLDL	30–80	0.95–1.006	pre-β	B, E, C	8	18	7	12	55
IDL	25–35	1.006–1.019	slow pre-β	B, E	19	19	9	29	23
LDL	22	1.019–1.063	β	B	22	22	8	42	6
HDL$_2$	10	1.063–1.125	α1	A-I, A-II, C, E	40	33	5	17	5
HDL$_3$	7.5	1.125–1.210	α1	A-I, A-II, C	55	25	4	13	3

(From Feldman, E.B. (ed.): Nutrition and Heart Disease, Vol. 6: Contemporary Issues in Clinical Nutrition. Churchill-Livingstone, New York, 1983, p. 48, with permission.)

Cholesterol

Cholesterol is a sterol that is both synthesized in the body (see Fig. 1–6) and obtained in the diet. Levels of cholesterol in plasma vary with age, increasing in men from puberty to about the fourth decade and in women until the fifth decade (Table 19–3). Plasma cholesterol levels in women generally are lower than those of men until the middle or later years. Among adults in the United States, plasma cholesterol levels range (5th to 95th percentile) from 120 to 300 mg per dl, with averages between 160 and 230 mg per dl depending on age and gender. Mean serum cholesterol levels in adults have declined recently by 2 to 20 mg per dl depending on age and gender. About two thirds of the plasma cholesterol is transported as LDL; levels of LDL parallel those of total cholesterol. HDL cholesterol levels average about 45 mg per dl in men and are 9 to 17 mg per dl higher in women. Diseases such as diabetes mellitus, hypothyroidism, the nephrotic syndrome, renal failure, pancreatitis, and obstructive liver disease—as well as some drugs and hormones, especially thyroid and gonadal hormones—influence plasma cholesterol levels, usually raising levels that will respond to appropriate treatment or altering medication.

Table 19-3. AVERAGE LEVELS OF CIRCULATING LIPIDS*

	White Men					White Women			
				mg/dl					
Age (yr)	Total C	LDL C	HDL C	TG		Total C	LDL C	HDL C	TG
15–19	152	93	46	68		157	93	51	64
20–24	159	101	45	78		165	102	51	80
25–29	176	116	44	88		178	108	55	76
30–34	190	124	45	102		178	109	55	73
35–39	195	131	43	109		186	116	53	83
40–44	204	135	43	123		193	122	56	68
45–49	210	141	45	119		204	127	58	94
50–54	211	143	44	128		214	134	62	103
55–59	214	145	46	117		229	145	60	111
60–64	215	143	49	111		226	149	61	105
65–69	213	146	49	108		233	151	62	118
70+	214	142	48	115		226	147	60	110

*50th percentile. C = cholesterol; LDL = low density lipoprotein; HDL = high density lipoprotein; TG= triglycerides.
(Adapted from Lipid Research Clinics Prevalence Study.)

Triglycerides

Circulating triglyceride levels average about 100 mg per dl in young adults and are somewhat lower in women. Triglycerides increase by 50 to 75 percent with age (see Table 19–3). Median triglyceride levels range from 80 to 130 mg per dl; levels in the population (5th to 95th percentile) range from 40 to 320 mg per dl, depending on age and gender. Levels are influenced by genetic and dietary factors (calories, fat, carbohydrate, alcohol) and disease (diabetes, pancreatitis, nephrotic syndrome).

Apoproteins

The apolipoproteins, or apoproteins, are the primary determinants of the metabolic fate of individual lipoprotein particles and also maintain the solubility of lipoprotein lipids in the aqueous environment of the plasma. They include A-I and A-II, B (big or B-100 and little/small B-48), C-I, C-II, and C-III, D, and three isoforms of E (2, 3, and 4), as well as F and G. The distribution in lipoproteins and the normal levels in plasma of some apoproteins are shown in Tables 19–2 and 19–4. Apoprotein measurements, together with lipid levels, may aid in diagnosing disorders of lipoprotein transport—the dyslipoproteinemias—and may be useful predictors of the risk of developing coronary heart disease or other cardiovascular disease. Survivors of

Table 19–4. NORMAL LEVELS
OF APOPROTEINS IN PLASMA
(mg/dl)

Apoprotein	X ± SD
A-I	120 ± 20 (men)
	135 ± 25 (women)
A-II	33 ± 5 (men)
	36 ± 6 (women)
B	100 ± 20
C-I	7 ± 2
C-II	4 ± 2
C-III	13 ± 5
D	6 ± 1
E	5 ± 2

(From Albers, J.J.: The determination of apoproteins and their diagnostic value in clinical chemistry. In Kaiser, E., Gabal, F., Muller, M.M., et al. (eds.): XIth International Congress of Clinical Chemistry. Walter de Gruyter and Co., Berlin, 1982, p. 226, with permission.)

myocardial infarction, for example, have low levels of apo-A-I and increased levels of apo-B. Apoprotein levels or changes in size or amino acid composition may thus turn out to be better predictors of coronary heart disease than lipid levels, and may correlate with the severity of the disease.

Lipoproteins

Each lipoprotein contains specific amounts of the various lipid components as well as apoproteins. The ratio of lipid to protein determines the hydrated density of the lipoprotein particle and is the basis for some separation procedures. It also determines the name given to the lipoprotein. Thus,

$$d < 1.006 \text{ g per ml} = \text{VLDL}$$
$$d\ 1.006-1.019 = \text{IDL}$$
$$d\ 1.019-1.063 = \text{LDL}$$
$$d\ 1.063-1.21 = \text{HDL}$$

The HDLs are further subdivided as follows:

$$d\ 1.063-1.125 = \text{HDL-2}$$
$$d\ 1.125-1.21 = \text{HDL-3}$$

Preparative ultracentrifugation permits separation of the lipoprotein particles; their composition and the concentration of their lipid and protein constituents may then be determined.

Chylomicrons

Chylomicrons are lipoprotein particles formed in the intestine when triacylglycerol esters of long chain fatty acids are ingested. They are present in plasma only after a fatty meal and are not observed in the fasting state (12 to 14 hours after the last meal). Chylomicrons in plasma kept refrigerated in a test tube may be seen as a creamy top layer. Chylomicrons usually are present in the blood only when triglyceride levels exceed 700 mg per dl and approach 1000 mg per dl. (Plasma appears turbid when triglyceride levels exceed 200 mg per dl.)

The chylomicron is the primary transporter of exogenous triglyceride and consists predominantly of triglyceride, with small amounts of phospholipids, cholesterol, and apoproteins (see Table 19-2). Chylomicrons are absorbed from the small intestine into the lymphatics and then into the blood. They are removed from the circulation by the action of lipoprotein lipase, an enzyme located in the capillary endothelium of extrahepatic tissues, thereby producing the chylomicron remnant. The remnant particle is taken up by the

EXOGENOUS PATHWAY

ENDOGENOUS PATHWAY

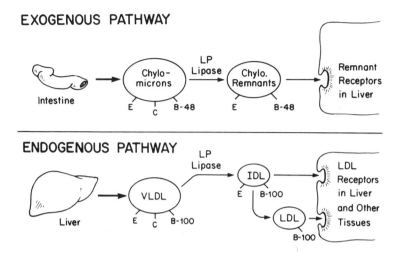

Figure 19–1. Receptor mediated pathways of lipoprotein transport indicating the specific roles of the apoproteins. LP = lipoprotein. (From Brown, M.S., and Goldstein, J.L.: Lipoprotein receptors in the liver. J Clin Invest 72:744, 1983, with permission.)

liver, which has receptors that specifically recognize the apoprotein constituents (Fig. 19–1).

VLDL

VLDL is produced by the liver and contains a B apoprotein (apo-B) of approximately twice the molecular weight (B-100) of the apo-B of the chylomicron (B-48). VLDL is the main transporter of endogenous triglyceride that is produced from carbohydrate precursors in the diet. The VLDL particle is smaller and contains less triglyceride, more cholesterol, and more protein than the chylomicron. Excess of VLDL particles in plasma makes the plasma diffusely turbid. The activity of lipoprotein lipase removes VLDL particles from plasma, with triglyceride breakdown. This process generates LDL via an intermediate density lipoprotein (IDL). VLDL remnants may be removed from the circulation by the liver and the receptor pathway (Fig. 19–1); the remaining VLDL remnants generate most of the LDL in plasma.

IDL

Compared with VLDL, IDL is enriched in the proportion of cholesterol relative to triglyceride (see Table 19–2). Atherogenic diets may give rise to the related beta-VLDL particle. Beta-VLDL is cholesterol-rich, contains apo-B and apo-E, and interacts with both the LDL receptor and the chylomicron (and VLDL) remnant receptor.

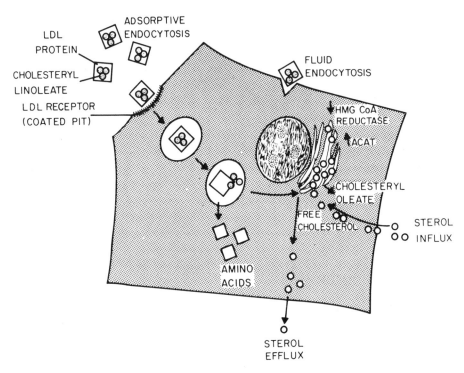

Figure 19-2. The LDL receptor pathway. (From Feldman, E.B.: Familial hypercholesterolemia—predecessor of coronary heart disease. Resident and Staff Physician 00:71, 1978, with permission.)

LDL

LDL is about 50 percent cholesterol, with more protein and less triglyceride than VLDL. LDL is taken up by a specific cell surface lipoprotein receptor in the liver and (to a lesser extent) in peripheral tissues (Fig. 19–2). It is the most atherogenic of the lipoproteins via a mechanism that remains unclear. A variant of LDL, Lpa, normally present in small amounts in blood, may be increased in patients with cerebrovascular disease.

HDL

A small particle that is generated both in the intestine and the liver, HDL is about half protein and half lipid. It is produced when lipoprotein lipase transfers surface lipids from other triglyceride-rich lipoprotein particles. The predominant lipid component is phospholipid (see Table 19–2). Protein and cholesterol contents vary in the HDL subfractions. The cholesterol-to-triglyceride ratio in HDL increases as dietary cholesterol increases. Feeding cholesterol results in the production of specific HDL particles that are larger, float at a lower density, and are enriched in cholesterol esters and apo-E.

HYPERLIPIDEMIAS AND HYPERLIPOPROTEINEMIAS

Hypercholesterolemia can either be due to a single gene or be polygenic, resulting from the effects of multiple genes and the diet. Elevated cholesterol levels in plasma may result from the increased synthesis and/or delayed or defective clearance of cholesterol and its lipoprotein transporter LDL. Mild to moderate hypertriglyceridemia may occur in subjects with no external signs. It is unclear whether hypertriglyceridemic individuals have increased risk of atherosclerosis solely on the basis of elevated triglycerides, i.e., that triglycerides are an independent risk factor. However, these individuals often are obese, with glucose intolerance or frank hyperglycemia, and therefore are at increased risk for vascular disease. Elevated triglyceride levels may occur in association with hypercholesterolemia and can result from genetic defects or diet or both.

The primary hyperlipoproteinemias are metabolic disorders characterized by an excess of one or more lipoproteins in the circulation. They may be diagnosed after at least three measurements of plasma lipids with the patient in a fasting state; the lipoproteins are fractionated to determine the type of hyperlipoproteinemia (Table 19-5).

Table 19-5. KEY FEATURES
DIFFERENTIATING THE
HYPERLIPOPROTEINEMIAS

Type	Feature
1	Increased exogenous triglycerides in the form of chylomicrons
2a	Hypercholesterolemia (increase in LDL) with normal triglyceride levels
2b	Hypercholesterolemia combined with mild hypertriglyceridemia (overproduction of apo-B)
3	Hypercholesterolemia with hypertriglyceridemia and increase in IDL
4	Mild to moderate hypertriglyceridemia (250–700 mg/dl) with increased VLDL
5	Moderate to severe hypertriglyceridemia (1000+ mg/dl) with mixed VLDL and chylomicrons

Type 1 Hyperlipoproteinemia

Exogenous triglycerides in the form of chylomicrons may be the only lipoprotein increased (type 1 hyperlipoproteinemia), but this condition is rare. It may result from a genetic defect in the clearance of chylomicrons from the blood that involves the removal mechanism, e.g., lipoprotein lipase or its apo-C-II apoprotein activator.

Hypercholesterolemia
(Types 2a and 2b Hyperlipoproteinemias)

Hypercholesterolemia is characteristic of types 2 and 3 hyperlipoproteinemias. In type 2a, the level of plasma triglycerides is normal; there is an increased level of cholesterol and its lipoprotein transporter LDL. Type 2b, however, combines hypercholesterolemia and hypertriglyceridemia, with increases in LDL and VLDL, and overproduction of apo-B.

Familial Hypercholesterolemia

Familial hypercholesterolemia (FH) is a single gene defect in the cell receptor that binds or internalizes circulating LDL (see Fig. 19-2). One in 500 individuals is heterozygous for the FH gene, while the homozygous state is seen in 1 in 1,000,000. To date, multiple mutations have been identified involving the synthesis, processing, binding, and clustering of the cell surface receptor. The homozygous phenotype also may be the result of a compound heterozygote with two genetic defects.

Mechanism

The specific cell surface receptor affected by FH serves to deliver cholesterol to cells (see Fig. 19-2). Cholesterol freed from the lipoprotein within the cell regulates endogenous cholesterol synthesis by suppressing the activity of hydroxymethylglutaryl CoA reductase (see Fig. 1-6), stimulates re-esterification and subsequent storage of cholesteryl ester within the cell, and suppresses the synthesis of the LDL receptor. In the FH heterozygote, the number of these receptors is about half normal, the LDL level doubles in the circulation and LDL occupies a normal number of receptor sites. The fractional catabolic rate of LDL is halved. With no receptors (the FH homozygote) there is a great increase in LDL synthesis and decrease in its removal, with a marked decrease in the fractional catabolic rate of LDL.

Clinical Manifestations

The patient with FH manifests hypercholesterolemia from birth. Cholesterol levels average 350 mg per dl in heterozygotes and 740 mg per dl in homozygotes. In patients with heterozygous FH, corneal arcus (Fig. 19-3) and tendon xanthomas (Fig. 19-4) may be seen in the latter part of the second

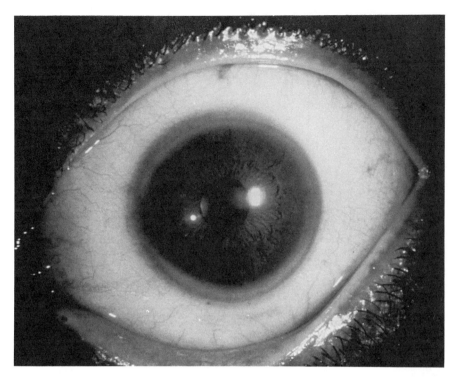

Figure 19-3. Corneal arcus characteristic of heterozygous familial hypercholesterolemia (see Case 19a).

decade of life, and by the third decade these stigmata appear in half the patients. Tendon xanthomas seldom occur without hypercholesterolemia and typically involve extensor tendons (e.g., Achilles, digits). As many as 80 percent of FH patients have tendon xanthomas before death. Homozygotes by age 4 have unique cutaneous xanthomas on the buttocks, the creases of the hands, and over the kneecaps.

Eyelid xanthelasma (Fig. 19-5) are a form of planar xanthomas also seen in patients with hypercholesterolemia. They are associated with normal cholesterol levels in about half the patients; recent studies have indicated that these normocholesterolemic patients have abnormal isoforms of apo-E (E phenotypes).

FH patients have an incidence of coronary heart disease 25 times that of persons unaffected by the gene, occurring at a mean age 15 years earlier than in the general population. The chance of first heart attack in men with heterozygous FH is 51 percent by age 50 and 85 percent by 60, and in women with FH 12 and 58 percent, respectively. The mean age of death of homozygotes is 21 years, with heart attacks occurring in infancy and early childhood.

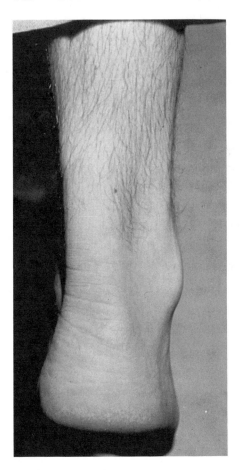

Figure 19–4. Achilles tendon xanthomas characteristic of heterozygous familial hypercholesterolemia (see Case 19a).

CASE 19a: FAMILIAL HYPERCHOLESTEROLEMIA

A 45-year-old man was referred for treatment of type 2a hyperlipoproteinemia. At age 30 he had a myocardial infarction. Hypercholesterolemia had been known since age 24. Cholesterol levels, untreated, ranged from 300 to 470 mg/dl. Triglyceride values consistently were normal. His management included diet, and at various times nicotinic acid (up to 2.5 g/day), clofibrate, d-thyroxine, and cholestyramine, including combined drug regimens. His compliance was generally poor. His three children, ages 15, 13, and 8, were also evaluated. One brother was known to have hypercholesterolemia and tendon xanthomas (see further on). His father was alive at age 81, but his mother had died at age 56 after gynecologic surgery. Her brother and mother had sustained myocardial infarctions. His stress test and coronary angiography were both positive.

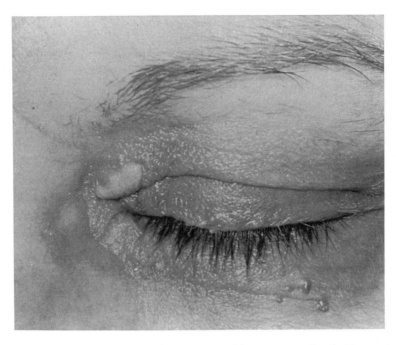

Figure 19–5. Eyelid xanthelasma characteristic of heterozygous familial hypercholesterolemia.

He weighed 83.6 kg and his height was 182 cm. He had bilateral corneal arcus (see Fig. 19–3), Achilles tendon xanthomas (see Fig. 19–4), and xanthomas of the extensor tendons of his hands. (He said these had been stable for about 10 years.) His plasma cholesterol values were: total 391, LDL 327, and HDL 48 mg/dl; triglycerides were 116 mg/dl. At his request he was counseled on a vegetarian diet containing 100 mg cholesterol per day. He was tried on a regimen of clofibrate and cholestyramine, but again compliance was poor and cholesterol values decreased only to 320 mg/dl; on diet alone, however, they increased to 360 mg/dl. At his last visit he was advised to try probucol. One year later he reported undergoing 4-vessel coronary bypass surgery.

The patient's 15-year-old son was observed to have corneal arcus and possible Achilles tendon xanthomas and an otherwise normal examination. His cholesterol values were: total 237, LDL 189, and HDL 47 mg/dl with triglycerides 59 mg/dl. He was counseled on a cholesterol-lowering diet; compliance was judged as moderate. One year later his cholesterol values were: total 327, LDL 289, and HDL 35 mg/dl, with triglycerides 84 mg/dl. He was advised to start cholestyramine with multivitamin supplements and twice weekly vitamin K. The patient's

13-year-old son's physical examination was normal. His cholesterol levels were: total 246, LDL 203, and HDL 49 mg/dl, with triglycerides 53 mg/dl. They were approximately the same one year later following a cholesterol-lowering diet. The 8-year-old son's cholesterol values were: total 137, LDL 90, and HDL 41 mg/dl.

The patient's 49-year-old brother had known of hypercholesterolemia since age 24, when a tendon xanthoma was removed from his elbow. Bilateral corneal arcus was present. Despite attention to diet and exercise, a stress test was positive 2 years earlier, and he underwent 2-vessel coronary bypass 1 year before. His cholesterol levels had been as high as 430 mg/dl. Generally they were maintained at about 280 mg/dl on a combination of diet and medication (clofibrate and cholestyramine). He weighed 79 kg and his height was 180 cm. He showed corneal arcus, eyelid xanthelasma, and tendon xanthomas of the extensor tendons of the hands and the Achilles tendons. His cholesterol levels were: total 306, LDL 253, and HDL 41 mg/dl, with triglycerides 114 mg/dl. He was counseled on a cholesterol-lowering diet, his cholestyramine dosage was doubled, and clofibrate was continued. His cholesterol levels subsequently were: total 270, LDL 195, and HDL 60 mg/dl, with triglycerides 45 mg/dl.

LESSON:

This family is a classic example of the disorder heterozygous familial hypercholesterolemia. Typical are the mode of inheritance, clinical stigmata of hypercholesterolemia and premature coronary heart disease, and resistance of the elevated levels of LDL cholesterol to a prudent diet, even combined with one or more cholesterol-lowering drugs. Family screening and early and aggressive therapy are mandatory preventive measures. For adults with FH the new class of drugs that inhibit cholesterol synthesis appear promising.

Type 3 Hyperlipoproteinemia

In type 3 hyperlipoproteinemia, also known as dysbetalipoproteinemia or broad beta disease, hypercholesterolemia and hypertriglyceridemia are due to an increase in IDL. This disorder may be suspected when levels of cholesterol and triglyceride in plasma are increased similarly. Type 3 is characterized by planar xanthomas in the creases of the palms of the hands and fingers (Fig. 19–6). Tuberous xanthomas over elbows and knees also may appear (Fig. 19–7). The condition commonly becomes manifest in the third decade of life and may be secondary to an endocrine abnormality such as hypothyroidism or hypopituitarism. Patients also may have premature peripheral vascular disease along with coronary heart disease. Confirmation

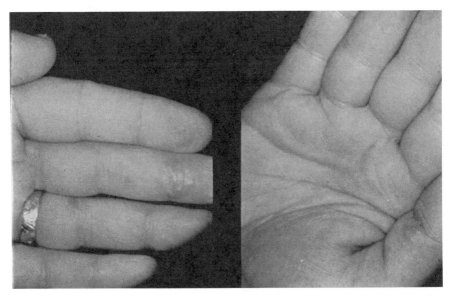

Figure 19-6. Planar xanthomas of middle finger and thumb, type 3 (see Case 19b).

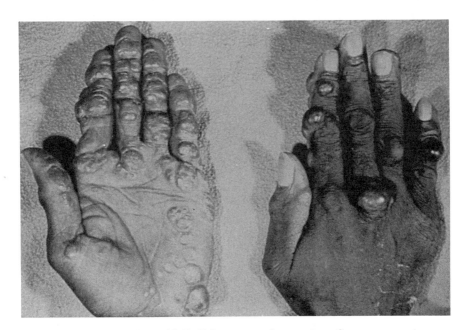

Figure 19-7. Tuberous xanthomas, type 3.

of this disorder requires preparative ultracentrifugation to demonstrate increased amounts of cholesterol in the lipoprotein fraction floating at d < 1.006 (VLDL). Electrophoresis of this fraction shows beta-lipoprotein, or LDL, which normally should sediment at this density, which accounts for the other name for type 3, "floating beta disease." Type 3 is characterized by a genetic defect with abnormal E isoforms (E_2 rather than E_3).

CASE 19b: TYPE 3 HYPERLIPOPROTEINEMIA

A 38-year-old hospital employee was referred for cardiac catheterization. He had a history of intermittent claudication and angina for 2 years, and had sustained a myocardial infarction 3 months earlier. He was a heavy smoker with a history of alcohol abuse and a family history of myocardial infarction (father at age 60 and uncle at age 46). Physical examination showed decreased arterial pulses in the lower extremities. There were several yellowish streaks (2 ×10 mm linear plaques) visible in the creases of the palm of his hands (see Fig. 19–6 for more advanced lesions in another patient with the same lipid disorder). His pulses were diminished in both popliteal regions. Plasma lipids were ordered. Values were: total cholesterol 526 mg/dl, triglycerides 1173 mg/dl. Ultracentrifugation of plasma obtained after the patient had received diet counseling yielded: total cholesterol 410 mg/dl, VLDL 279, LDL 106, and HDL 25 mg/dl, with triglycerides 573 mg/dl. Electrophoresis showed a broad beta pattern in whole plasma and a "floating beta" band in the VLDL fraction, confirming the diagnosis of type 3 hyperlipoproteinemia.

LESSON:

The patient illustrates that even in the presence of premature coronary heart disease the patient's serum lipids may not be measured. His type 3 disorder showed the classic manifestations of peripheral vascular disease and planar xanthomas of the hands along with elevated levels of cholesterol with approximately similar levels of triglycerides. The patient died 2 years later; he had not reported for follow-up treatment.

Types 4 and 5 Hyperlipoproteinemias

Mildly elevated triglyceride values (250 to 700 mg per dl) with increased VLDL characterize type 4 hyperlipoproteinemia (endogenous hypertriglyceridemia). The defect may involve excessive production and delayed removal of VLDL triglycerides. This type of hyperlipoproteinemia is associated with a probable increased risk of atherosclerosis.

Moderate to severe increases in triglyceride values (exceeding 1000 mg per dl) are found in type 5 hyperlipoproteinemia. Occasionally triglyceride levels may rise as high as 20,000 mg per dl. Chylomicrons appear along with

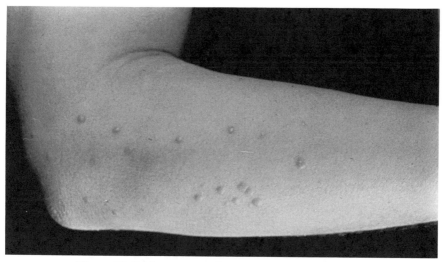

Figure 19–8. Eruptive xanthoma over forearm, type 5.

elevated levels of VLDL. The chylomicronemia syndrome is characterized by eruptive xanthomas (Fig. 19–8), typically found in the skin over the back of the neck or the buttocks. When the triglyceride level exceeds 3000 mg per dl, lipemia retinalis (Fig. 19–9) may be present. Patients with these high triglyceride levels are at increased risk for pancreatitis (although they may have abdominal pain without proof of that condition) and for atherosclerosis. More than half these patients have diabetes mellitus. Alcohol intake sometimes will convert a type 4 patient to a type 5.

CASE 19c: TYPE 5 HYPERLIPOPROTEINEMIA

An 18-year-old woman was diagnosed as having type 5 hyperlipoproteinemia. She had recurrent abdominal pain since age 6. Seven days after an episode of abdominal pain, nausea, and vomiting, examination of her blood showed a cholesterol level of 392 mg/dl and triglycerides of 4300 mg/dl. Three days later a serum amylase level was 290 mU/ml. On examination she had lipemia retinalis (Fig. 19–9). Her body weight was normal (56 kg, height 165 cm). She was treated with a type 5 diet and clofibrate with control of the abdominal pain and maintenance of triglyceride levels at about 600 mg/dl.

She became pregnant and triglyceride levels were 2000 mg/dl. Clofibrate was discontinued and the patient was controlled with a 20 g fat diet until the ninth month of gestation, when cholesterol rose to more than 500 mg/dl and triglycerides to 2400 mg/dl. She had an uneventful term vaginal delivery of a normal baby. She became pregnant a second time 13 months later. During this pregnancy, triglycerides increased in

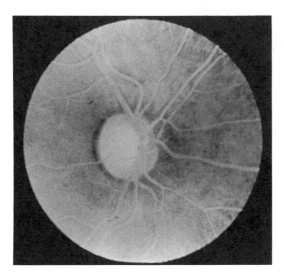

Figure 19-9. Lipemia retinalis, type 5 (see Case 19c).

the middle trimester and reached 3700 mg/dl at 35 weeks. She was hospitalized and placed on a 20 g fat, 1200 kcal diet for 2 weeks before
delivery. Triglycerides decreased to 1700 mg/dl. She delivered another
normal infant.

LESSON:

This patient illustrates the association of recurrent abdominal pain with
chylomicronemia. Her type 5 hyperlipoproteinemia was not associated
with diabetes mellitus. Pregnancy is associated with worsening of hyperlipidemia, which should be treated vigorously.

DIET, LIPIDS, AND RISK OF
CORONARY HEART DISEASE

There is a relationship between plasma cholesterol levels and the incidence of coronary heart disease. Increasing atherosclerosis has been shown to
be correlated with the absolute levels of plasma cholesterol and LDL cholesterol, and to be inversely correlated with the level of HDL cholesterol and the
ratio of HDL to total cholesterol or HDL to LDL cholesterol. The major risk
factors associated with coronary heart disease in addition to elevated plasma
cholesterol are hypertension and cigarette smoking. Serum cholesterol levels
also are influenced by nondietary factors such as heredity. Clinical trials,
however, have demonstrated that changing dietary intake, or combining dietary change with drug intervention, reduces serum cholesterol, and hypertension, and decreases the symptoms and signs of coronary heart disease.

Both prospective and retrospective epidemiologic studies have implicated the following dietary factors in the pathogenesis of atherosclerosis (and hence of symptomatic coronary heart disease):

- total fat
- saturated fat
- cholesterol
- trace minerals (such as selenium)
- meat
- animal protein

Possible mechanisms include an increase in the concentrations of plasma cholesterol, LDL cholesterol, or VLDL cholesterol; or a decrease in HDL cholesterol. Levels of total cholesterol and LDL cholesterol have been shown to increase with high intakes of saturated fatty acid and cholesterol, and with excess calories in the obese.

Control of Plasma Cholesterol

The levels of plasma cholesterol associated with an increased risk of coronary heart disease exceed 200 mg per dl (or perhaps 180 mg per dl). As an alternative to making dietary recommendations for the American public, the current emphasis is on a "cholesterol awareness" program, much like the blood pressure education program. The thrust of the cholesterol health promotion/disease prevention program is the concept that each individual should know his or her cholesterol level and thereby his or her individual risk of cardiovascular disease. With this knowledge, appropriate dietary modifications may be undertaken. Certain levels of plasma cholesterol, stratified for age and gender, are associated with "moderate" and "high" risk of atherosclerosis (Table 19–6). The recommendations derived from the results of multiple intervention and prevention trials are that individuals with cholesterol levels in the upper 10 percent of the population (above the 90th percentile), who are at high risk, merit at least intensive dietary treatment. If the diet is not successful, appropriate drug therapy should be instituted. Additionally, it is recommended that those above the 75th percentile, at moderate risk, receive dietary counseling to reduce plasma cholesterol levels. The presence of additional risk factors, such as cigarette smoking, hypertension, and diabetes, may make these people candidates for added drug treatment, as does already having coronary heart disease.

A simplified version of recommended and "risky" cholesterol levels is provided in Table 19–7. A recommendation for desirable LDL cholesterol levels is less than 130 mg per dl for prevention in those without coronary heart disease and less than 110 mg per dl for those who are already afflicted

Table 19-6. INTERVENTION LEVELS FOR SERUM
CHOLESTEROL BY SEX AND AGE*

Males			Females		
	Percentile			Percentile	
Age, yr	75th	90th	Age, yr	75th	90th
0-19	170 (4.40)	185 (4.80)	0-19	175 (4.50)	190 (4.90)
20-24	185 (4.80)	205 (5.30)	20-24	190 (4.90)	215 (5.55)
25-29	200 (5.15)	225 (5.80)	25-34	195 (5.05)	220 (5.70)
30-34	215 (5.55)	240 (6.20)	35-39	205 (5.30)	230 (5.95)
35-39	225 (5.80)	250 (6.45)	40-44	215 (5.55)	235 (6.05)
40-44	230 (5.95)	250 (6.45)	45-49	225 (5.80)	250 (6.45)
45-69	235 (6.05)	260 (6.70)	50-54	240 (6.20)	265 (6.85)
70+	230 (5.95)	250 (6.45)	55+	250 (6.45)	275 (7.10)

*From the Lipid Research Clinics Data. Values are given in mg/dl (millimoles per liter).

in order to reverse the disease. A simply way to calculate LDL cholesterol is to use the formula:

LDL cholesterol =
    Total cholesterol − HDL cholesterol − Triglyceride × 0.16

The data from multiple primary and secondary prevention trials indicates that roughly for each 1 percent reduction in serum cholesterol level, there is a 2 percent reduction in cardiovascular risk. Identification of elevated total or LDL cholesterol levels is especially important in people with other risk factors (hypertension, cigarette smoking), or with a family history of coronary heart disease, especially when occurring before age 60.

There is less consensus concerning the levels of plasma triglyceride warranting diet intervention, or additional drug therapy. Triglycerides may or may not be an independent risk factor for cardiovascular disease. Since ele-

Table 19-7. BLOOD CHOLESTEROL LEVELS
AS RISK FACTORS

	Blood Cholesterol Levels		
Age	Recommended	Moderate Risk	High Risk
20-29	<180 mg/dl	200-220 mg/dl	220+ mg/dl
30-39	<200 mg/dl	220-240 mg/dl	240+ mg/dl
40+	<200 mg/dl	240-260 mg/dl	260+ mg/dl

(From National Institutes of Health Cholesterol Consensus Conference.)

vated triglyceride levels often accompany glucose intolerance or diabetes, or obesity, treatment of these disorders, especially by weight reduction, may have a favorable effect on lowering triglyceride levels. Dietary measures are warranted when triglyceride levels exceed the 90th or 95th percentile, with drug treatment indicated when triglyceride levels in patients already prescribed an appropriate diet persist above 400 mg per dl, in order to prevent pancreatitis.

Dietary Fat

The hypercholesterolemic effect of saturated fat in humans was documented in studies published by Ahrens in 1957. Diets high in fat—especially saturated fat—are atherogenic for many animal species, particularly when cholesterol intake also is increased (Fig. 19–10). Dietary saturated long chain fatty acids, whether of vegetable origin (coconut oil, palm oil) or animal origin (butter, lard, beef tallow), raise plasma cholesterol levels. These fats tend to be solid at room temperature. The more unsaturated fats tend to be liquid; they may be either of vegetable origin (corn, safflower, soybean, and olive oils) or animal origin (fish oils). It has not yet been shown whether hydrogenation of unsaturated fats producing *trans* fatty acids is atherogenic, since the metabolic fate of such fatty acids has not been elucidated. Eicosapentaenoic acid, and other omega-3 fatty acids found in fish oils, may have a hypocholesterolemic effect and have demonstrated significant hypotriglyceridemic effects. Rather than consuming fish oil capsules, however, eating more cold water fish is recommended since these foods do not contain potentially toxic levels of vitamins A and D present in fish liver oils.

Dietary Cholesterol

The usual American daily diet for men contains about 450 mg cholesterol. Reducing the intake to 300 mg or less (100 mg per 1000 kcal) may decrease plasma cholesterol levels. Cholesterol is synthesized by all animal cells and therefore is present in all animal products (Table 19–8). Cholesterol is absent from any plant products, including all vegetable oils.

Protein

It has been suggested from results of studies in vegetarians and in animal models that some types of animal protein (e.g., casein) may be hypercholesterolemic and some kinds of vegetable protein (e.g., soy) are cholesterol-lowering.

SOURCE   COMPOSITION

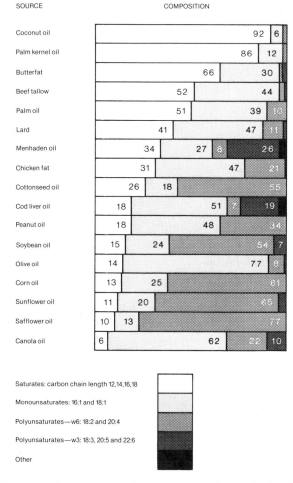

Saturates: carbon chain length 12,14,16,18	
Monounsaturates: 16:1 and 18:1	
Polyunsaturates—w6: 18:2 and 20:4	
Polyunsaturates—w3: 18:3, 20:5 and 22:6	
Other	

Figure 19–10. Fatty acid composition of some common fats and oils. The length of the bar is 100 percent and the numbers in the bars indicate the percent of total fat; values 5 percent or less are not so indicated.

Fiber

High fiber diets (see Chapters 1 and 4) have been proposed as protective against atherosclerosis; addition of some forms of fiber to diets may lower cholesterol levels and reduce hyperglycemia in diabetics. Partially digestible noncellulose pectin, in the "zest" of fruit, and other gums and mucilages may have a lipid-lowering effect. Wheat bran does not lower cholesterol, for example, but oat bran and barley do.

Table 19–8. CHOLESTEROL
CONTENT OF SOME FOODS*

Food	Cholesterol	
Fruits, grains, vegetables	0 mg	LOW
Scallops (cooked, about 3½ oz)	53 mg	
Oysters (cooked, about 3½ oz)	45 mg	
Clams (cooked, about 3½ oz)	65 mg	
Fish, lean (cooked, about 3½ oz)	65 mg	
Chicken/turkey, light meat (without skin) (cooked, about 3½ oz)	80 mg	
Lobster (cooked, about 3½ oz)	85 mg	
Beef, lean (cooked, about 3½ oz)	90 mg	
Chicken/turkey, dark meat (without skin) (cooked, about 3½ oz)	95 mg	
Crab (cooked, about 3½ oz)	100 mg	
Shrimp (cooked, about 3½ oz)	150 mg	
Egg yolk, 1	270 mg	
Beef liver (cooked, about 3½ oz)	440 mg	
Beef kidney (cooked, about 3½ oz)	700 mg	HIGH

*From National Heart, Lung and Blood Institute, NIH Publication No. 85-2696, January 1985.

Sterols

Large doses of plant sterols produce a hypocholesterolemic effect when given at or before mealtime. Marine sterols from clams or oysters may also be hypocholesterolemic. These sterols presumably inhibit intestinal absorption of cholesterol.

Calories

Restriction of calories in the obese patient is helpful in the management of any hyperlipoproteinemia, and diet modifications are indicated at least up to age 70.

Dietary Recommendations

In summary, to reduce hypercholesterolemia the dietary intake of saturated fat, total fat, calories, cholesterol, and animal protein should be decreased, while corresponding increases may be made in consumption of complex carbohydrates, and the proportion of polyunsaturated or monounsaturated fats, and vegetable protein (see Chapter 10 for more information on therapeutic diets). Diet counseling should be continued for several months in the treatment of any hyperlipidemia, with repeated measurements made of plasma lipids. Continued dietary control after this time is necessary for most patients.

It is interesting that there have been significant decreases in mortality from cardiovascular disease in several Western countries, including the United States, Finland, and Belgium. These reductions have been attributed to dietary changes and have been associated with decreases in serum cholesterol in these populations.

Hypertriglyceridemia

The dietary management of hypertriglyceridemia depends upon whether the triglycerides are of exogenous (dietary fat) or endogenous (dietary carbohydrate) origin. To lower chylomicron triglycerides (type 1 hyperlipoproteinemia), the total amount of fat in the diet should be restricted to less than 20 percent of calories, or less than 50 g. In cases of endogenous hypertriglyceridemia (elevated VLDL, as in type 4 or type 5 hyperlipoproteinemia), carbohydrate intake should be restricted. The specific effects of different monosaccharides and disaccharides in altering plasma lipids and in inducing atherosclerosis varies among species, and their role in atherogenesis in humans is uncertain.

Drugs

If dietary modifications are not adequate to control blood lipid levels, then the physician must add appropriate lipid-lowering drugs, alone or in combination. Some medications (e.g., thiazides, propranolol, estrogens, oral contraceptives) may raise plasma lipids and should be avoided in the patient with hyperlipidemia. Newer diuretics, antihypertensives, and adrenergic blockers have been developed without these adverse effects. Parenteral routes of estrogen administration may also have different effects on lipids and lipoproteins.

Other Risk Factors in Coronary Heart Disease

HDL Cholesterol Levels

Plasma levels of HDL cholesterol, which have been found to be inversely associated with atherogenesis, are affected by a variety of factors, as shown in Table 19-9. Lipid-lowering drugs may have variable effects on HDL cholesterol levels.

Table 19-9. DIETARY AND
OTHER FACTORS AFFECTING
HDL CHOLESTEROL LEVELS

Increased Levels	Decreased Levels
↑Saturated fats	Simple sugars/high
↑Dietary cholesterol	carbohydrate diet
Alcohol (≤2 drinks daily)	(short period)
Long-term aerobic	↑Polyunsaturated fat
exercise program	Androgens
Estrogens	

Vitamins

Despite intriguing evidence from individuals with inborn errors of metabolism or findings in animal models, there is no practical reduction in the risk of atherosclerosis from administering vitamins (pyridoxine, ascorbic acid, vitamin E). The lipid-lowering effect of nicotinic acid is pharmacologic. There also is no evidence that the xanthine oxidase in milk influences atherogenesis.

Minerals

Water softness has been suggested as an etiologic agent in atherosclerosis, implying that mineral deficiency may be a factor in atherogenesis. Metabolic processes may be adversely affected by deficiencies in several trace minerals, thereby contributing to atherogenesis. There is no direct proof, however, that mineral deficiency or imbalance of minerals such as sodium, magnesium, zinc, copper, vanadium, chromium, iron, or iodine causes atherosclerosis, and no practical benefit has been found in administering them.

DIET AND HYPERTENSION

Hypertension affects 20 percent of the adult population in the United States. Nutrients implicated in its etiology include excess calories, sodium, and alcohol, and deficits in potassium, calcium and other minerals, and polyunsaturated fats.

Weight Control

Calories are the single most important nutrient in the etiology of hypertension, since a rise in blood pressure is proportional to weight gain. A reduction to ideal body weight lowers blood pressure and thereby decreases the risk of coronary heart disease and mortality from cardiovascular disease. Severe or morbid obesity (more than 50 percent overweight) also results in an increase in cardiac output, oxygen consumption, blood volume, and heart weight, and results in heart failure. The accumulation of carbon dioxide in the blood causes drowsiness and even cessation of breathing during sleep (sleep apnea) (see Chapter 16).

Sodium

Excessive salt intake is correlated with the prevalence of essential hypertension in populations. It particularly has been shown to be a factor in raising blood pressure in older individuals and blacks. With sodium restriction alone, a reduction of blood pressure averaging about 8 mm Hg can be achieved, and diuretics that deplete body sodium and contract the extracellular fluid volume are effective antihypertensive agents. It has been suggested that salt intake be limited to less than 3 g per day, or about 40 percent of the usual intake in the American diet. (See Chapter 4 for further discussion of sodium in the diet.)

Potassium

Not only excess sodium but also insufficient potassium in relation to sodium is implicated in the etiology of hypertension. The blood pressure increment produced by ingesting too much sodium can be partially negated by increasing the potassium intake. (Dietary sources of potassium are tabulated in Chapter 2.)

Calcium and Other Minerals

Recently, calcium deficiency has been advocated as an important factor in hypertension, and may explain its association with soft water. An increased calcium intake has been associated with a lowering of blood pressure. Deficiencies of magnesium, chromium, and selenium have been implicated in the etiology of both hypertension and atherosclerosis.

Polyunsaturated Fats

Polyunsaturated fats in the diet (see Fig. 19–8) also have a blood pressure–lowering effect, and deficiency of essential fatty acids has raised blood pressure in experimental animals. Blood pressure may be lowered through the mechanism of synthesizing prostaglandins, particularly prostacyclins, that cause dilatation of blood vessels and decreased resistance to blood flow. Besides producing vasodilatation, prostacyclins also inhibit platelet aggregation, reducing thrombotic tendencies. (Saturated fatty acids, on the other hand, increase the tendency to thrombosis.)

DIET AND CARDIOMYOPATHY

Alcohol

A variety of cardiomyopathies can be attributed to dietary excesses or deficiencies. One of the most common in the United States is a restrictive alcoholic cardiomyopathy (see Chapter 17). The blood pressure is raised and the heart enlarges, with low output heart failure and arrhythmia (atrial fibrillation). The patient may experience chest pain similar to that of coronary heart disease. Alcohol itself is toxic to the heart and may also make the heart more susceptible to the effects of viral infection. The only management of this disorder is abstention from alcohol.

Weight Reduction Diets

Some popular low protein, low calorie weight reducing diets have been associated with either cardiomyopathy or sudden death. This effect was first reported in the case of liquid protein diets in which the protein was not complete and did not contain all of the essential amino acids.

There has also been an increased incidence of abnormal cardiac rhythms with use of the protein-sparing modified fast, in which calories are restricted but high quality protein is provided, sometimes as the only source of calories. These diets can be very effective in causing rapid and sustained weight loss and relief of right heart failure, but they should be reserved for the morbidly obese patient (Chapter 16) and should be administered only under the supervision of a physician, often while the patient is hospitalized. (Chapter 16 gives more information on the treatment of obesity.)

Vitamins and Minerals (see Chapter 14)

Cobalt, which was used as an additive in some beer in the 1960s, caused a fatal cardiomyopathy observed in Canada and the midwest.

Heart disease caused by vitamin deficiency is rare in this country. In Southeast Asia, India, Brazil, and Africa, however, beriberi heart disease still occurs as a result of inadequate thiamin.

In China, Keshan's disease, a serious cardiomyopathy leading to heart failure and death, occurred in children because of selenium deficiency. However, it now has been eradicated by the supplementation of salt with selenium (similar to iodizing of salt here).

CHAPTER 20

Oral and Dental Diseases

RALPH V. McKINNEY, JR., D.D.S., Ph.D.

A diamond is not as precious as a tooth.

Cervantes, "Don Quixote"

As the organ responsible for the introduction of food to the alimentary canal, the oral cavity represents the beginning of many nutrition-related problems and diseases. The complexity of the oral cavity is increased by its involvement with the functions of speaking, chewing, swallowing, secretion, and absorption. It affects our psychic well-being, as when it is deformed by cleft palate or lip and when teeth are irregular or misshapen. The cavity is associated with certain needs for gratification, as in the acts of eating, drinking, smoking, sucking, fingernail biting, and kissing. These factors make the mouth and its associated structures a microcosm that reflects nutrition-related health and disease processes in the body.

The teeth have been significant elements in medicine and folklore through the centuries. The above quotation from "Don Quixote" epitomizes our concern with having a healthy mouth, with dentition a key ingredient for a happy life. So dreaded are the diseases and malformations of teeth and the oral tissues that there is a patron saint of toothache, St. Appolonia, who suffered martyrdom in Alexandria, circa 248 A.D.

THE REQUIREMENT FOR NUTRITIONAL COMPONENTS AND THE INTEGRITY OF THE NORMAL ORAL TISSUES

The teeth and oral cavity require adequate nutrition for their health. The oral cavity also has irritating factors that contribute to the initiation of disease. Figure 20–1 depicts the overlap of the intrinsic nutritional needs in the oral cavity with extrinsic functional and local irritational problems.

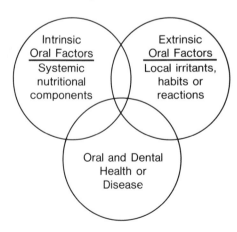

Intrinsic
Oral Factors
Systemic
nutritional
components

Extrinsic
Oral Factors
Local irritants,
habits or
reactions

Oral and Dental
Health or
Disease

Figure 20–1. Interplay of intrinsic and extrinsic factors that contribute to oral health or disease states. (Modified from Clark, J.W., Cheraskin, E., and Ringsdorf, W.M., Jr.: Diet and the Periodontal Patient. CC Thomas, Springfield, IL, 1970.)

Because specific nutritional deficiencies that contribute to disease manifestations in the oral cavity are difficult to identify, the health practitioner must search for multifactorial causes and treat these in their broadest aspect.

Nutritional Needs for Development of Teeth

Calcium

The Food and Nutrition Board of the National Academy of Sciences, National Research Council, recommends for proper calcification of teeth and bone a daily calcium intake (Table 20-1) of:

- 360 mg for children under 6 months of age
- 540 mg for children up to age 1 year
- 800 mg for children up to age 10

The recommended daily dietary allowance for adolescents is 1200 mg, gradually dropping to 800 mg for adults over 18 years. Pregnant and lactating mothers require 1200 mg of calcium per day. Teeth in the fetus begin to calcify in utero at the end of the first trimester of pregnancy, continuing until the child reaches age 18 to 20. Third molars do not complete full development until the early 20s in many individuals; thus, there is a real need for calcium through the early decades of life.

Phosphorus

Phosphorus is intimately associated with calcium in the metabolism of teeth and is utilized in the phosphorylation activities of cells (see Chapter 2). Phosphorus requirements are shown in Table 20-1. Phosphate deficiency in humans is relatively unusual, occurring with long-term use of antacids, which prevent absorption of phosphate from the gut. Experimental deficiency of calcium and phosphorus in laboratory animals reflects problems associated with long bones, but no deficiencies in teeth have been reported.

Vitamin D

Vitamin D, another requirement for dental development, is needed to activate the calcium-binding protein requisite to all calcification in developing teeth. Any interference with the vitamin D–calcium–phosphorus sequence results in incomplete calcification of the teeth, as well as rickets or osteomalacia (see Chapter 14). The need for vitamin D to activate this mechanism was dramatically shown in the early years of this century in urban areas where poor nutrition and inadequate dietary calcium and vitamin D were common. European case studies following World War II attributed de-

Table 20-1. DAILY DIETARY REQUIREMENTS FOR PROPER
DEVELOPMENT AND CALCIFICATION OF TEETH

Age	Protein (g)	Calcium (mg)	Phosphorus (mg)	Vitamin D (IU)
Birth to 6 mo	kg × 2.2	360	240	400
6 mo–1 yr	kg × 2.0	540	400	400
1–3 yr	23	800	800	400
4–6 yr	30	800	800	400
7–10 yr	36	800	800	400
11–14 yr	44	1200	1200	400
15–18 yr	54 (M) 48 (F)	1200	1200	400
19–22 yr	54 (M) 46 (F)	800	800	400
Pregnant	Additional 30	1200	1200	400
Lactating	Additional 20	1200	1200	400

M = male; F = female.

formed and misshapen teeth found in young children to inadequate vitamin D nutrition.

Vitamin D deficiency affects the calcification process of both dentin and tooth enamel, producing inadequately calcified teeth, developmental tooth anomalies, delayed eruption, and eventual misalignment of teeth in the jaws. In addition, children and adolescents who have had periods of hypovitaminosis D are more susceptible to dental caries. The latter phenomenon occurs even when an adequate daily vitamin allowance and the normal calcium–phosphate–vitamin D mechanisms have been restored.

Teeth also show defects of improper calcification and development in vitamin D–resistant rickets, a familial inherited X-linked dominant genetic trait.

Protein

The protein matrix of teeth, predominantly collagen, is laid down long before hydroxyapatite crystals are deposited on the collagen. Adequate protein nutrition, especially essential amino acids, is thus a direct requirement for the development of normal teeth. Large quantities of hydroxyproline are required for collagen production by ameloblasts and odontoblasts during early formation and remodeling. The calcification front of teeth occurs some distance behind development of the collagen matrix. When a swirling, irregular pattern (commonly called globular dentin) is seen in histologic sections of teeth, it is probable that the infant or child suffered impaired protein nutrition when dentition was developing.

Nutritional Needs for Development of Oral Epithelium and Connective Tissue

Protein

Proteins are a major component of cells and tissues, membranes, and various secretory products of cells. In the oral cavity this includes the secretion saliva, composed of proteins, carbohydrates, and some minerals.

Together with daily vitamin and mineral requirements, proteins are the major dietary requirement for adequate development of the oral epithelium, specialized tongue structures, and connective tissues in the fetus and growing child. Recommended dietary allowances of protein for infants, children, and adults are presented in Table 20–1. The rough estimate for body maintenance of 1 g of protein for each kilogram of body weight should be doubled or tripled during periods of rapid growth in the infant and during pregnancy and lactation. Requirements for development and calcification of the bones of the face and jaws are similar to those for teeth.

Carbohydrates

Carbohydrates, especially the glycosaminoglycans (GAGS) and proteoglycans (groups of GAGS with a central protein core) are essential in the development of the oral tissues. These hexosamine carbohydrate compounds serve as interlocking building blocks for the creation of basic tissue interrelationships. The acid properties of many of the GAGS allow them to engage in ion binding and basic hydrogen bridging activities associated with the "cementing" together of various connective tissues. Because they are seen throughout the body and have an important function in binding together the protein fiber of many tissues, the GAGS are often referred to as "ground" or "cementing" substances.

Carbohydrates are also essential for the production of salivary secretion, both serous and mucous. Saliva is rich in GAGS and proteoglycans, which function to lubricate food and aid in swallowing and speech. By providing a protective, moist coating to the surface layer of nonkeratinized oral stratified squamous epithelium, saliva contributes to the maintenance of oral tissue integrity.

Little is known about the possible effects of carbohydrate-deficient diets on the development of oral structures. The mucopolysaccharidoses, genetic carbohydrate deficiency diseases, affect development of connective tissues but are not nutritional disorders.

Nutritional Needs for Maintenance of the Integrity of Teeth and Oral Tissues

Information about the levels of various nutrients needed to maintain the functional integrity of the oral tissues is scanty. The National Research Council has recommended daily dietary allowances of proteins, vitamins, and minerals for maintaining good health, and deficient intake of some of these nutrients will produce adverse effects or disease in teeth or the oral cavity.

Both teeth and the oral cavity are subject to heavy wear and tear, and some clinicians believe that the level of nutrients needed to maintain oral health may be higher than that required for the rest of the body.

Conditions such as orthodontic treatment or periodontal disease may increase nutritional requirements for tissue repair. Other conditions, such as substance abuse—smoking and alcohol—increase nutrient needs for maintenance of good oral health.

Many elderly patients risk deficiencies in daily intake of proteins, vitamins, and minerals. Patients with ill-fitting dentures or missing teeth are often unable to masticate appropriate foods to maintain adequate nutrition and thus may become candidates for subclinical nutritional deficiencies (see Chapter 9).

Quality of Food in the Diet

Additional problems affecting the nutritional status of the oral cavity are related to the quality of food in the American diet (see Chapter 4). Many Americans derive considerable calories from sugars, fats, and alcohol, which provide no protein and inadequate vitamin or mineral content for oral tissue maintenance.

Calcium and Phosphorus

Calcium is essential to maintain healthy teeth and bones; deficiency is first recognized as osteoporosis, rather than as resorption of calcified teeth (see Chapter 14). Decreased calcium absorption from the gut may be an important factor in maintaining bone integrity in the elderly. Common foods usually contain adequate phosphorus.

Iron

An early subclinical manifestation of iron deficiency is a tongue that is sore, burning, or denuded of filiform papillae—signs that often indicate underlying nutritional deficiency disease. Insufficient dietary intake in the elderly, coupled with poor mastication, may produce iron deficiency.

Zinc

Trace amounts of zinc (15 mg per day) are essential for maintaining keratin production by epithelial cells during normal turnover of epithelium. (Both keratinized and parakeratinized epithelia are found within the oral cavity.) Oral diseases located exclusively in the epithelium (e.g., lichen planus, desquamative gingivitis) may respond to zinc supplements. Although the mechanism is not understood, zinc deficiency also may result in loss of the tongue's taste sensation (see Chapters 2 and 14). Zinc status should be evaluated in the older patient whose oral cavity has been subjected to years of wear and tear and who may be taking in marginal levels of zinc (the average zinc intake of the elderly in the United States is only 7 to 13 mg per day).

Vitamin A

Vitamin A is required to maintain the oral cavity's epithelial tissues and to differentiate epithelial cells from the basal layer to the more specialized surface-stratified layer. Deficiency of the vitamin leads to inadequate differentiation of the cells and early keratinization of the mucosa; in addition, the intercellular bridging and hemidesmosome cell contacts of the oral epithelium are disrupted. Early explorers who had periods of insufficient food intake noted that the mucosa of their oral cavity would peel off following weeks of vitamin A deprivation.

Effects on Developing Teeth. Lack of adequate vitamin A affects development of the teeth in the infant or child. The deficiency either disturbs or arrests the ameloblasts, which are of epithelial origin, and the enamel matrix formed is deficient, resulting in poor or absent enamel calcification and enamel hypoplasia in the mature tooth. In more severe cases of vitamin A deficiency, dentin may also be affected, leading to irregular tubular dentin formation. A high incidence of caries following tooth eruption usually is seen when there has been vitamin A deficiency during development of the teeth.

Vitamin C

Vitamin C is required for maintenance of adequate connective tissue integrity. The first signs of scurvy (avitaminosis C) often are gingival bleeding, periodontal destruction, and soft tissue ulceration (see Chapter 14). These signs are followed by capillary fragility, seen intraorally and elsewhere in the body.

In scurvy, oral tissue involvement may become severe since the periodontal ligament that holds the tooth within its bony crypt is composed of collagen fibers, and collagen usually shows early signs of vitamin C deficiency. The loss of collagen integrity in scurvy results in loosening and mobility of teeth, and, with continued deficiency, actual exfoliation of teeth may occur during mastication.

The role of mild nutritional deficiency of vitamin C as a major etiologic factor in the onset of generalized periodontal disease, however, remains unclear. Recent epidemiologic studies suggest that administering large doses of vitamin C for prevention or treatment of periodontal disease is not as significant a factor as the necessity for control of dental plaque. The recommended dietary allowance of ascorbic acid is adequate for good periodontal health.

Effects on Bone. Bone also is affected by chronic avitaminosis C. This is more evident in the infant, in whom developing bone is incomplete and osteoblasts fail to form adequate collagen matrix. The calcification process is unaffected by vitamin C deficiency because bone apatite crystals continue to be deposited in the cartilage matrix or the already cross-linked collagen matrix.

Effects on Developing Teeth. Vitamin C is important in the development of teeth. Avitaminosis C affects odontoblasts, which are of mesenchymal origin and are responsible for the laying down of dentin. Injury may vary from total failure of odontoblasts to produce dentin, to production of disorganized and poorly calcified dentin, resulting in malformed or shell-like teeth with normal enamel but inadequate dentin. This latter defect allows the enamel to fracture after teeth have erupted. (Because the ameloblast, which is responsible for producing tooth enamel, is of epithelial origin, it is unaffected by vitamin C deficiency.) In addition, the rate of caries is higher in poorly developed teeth.

NUTRITIONAL NEEDS DURING ORAL CAVITY WOUND HEALING AND ORAL DISEASES

Wound Healing and Surgical Procedures

Nutritional requirements for oral and dental tissues are highest in times of wound healing. Surgical procedures in the oral cavity increase metabolic requirements, and proper nutrition is needed to ensure rapid healing and tissue renewal (see Chapter 25).

Orthodontic Treatment

Orthodontic treatment produces considerable changes in the formation of the dental arches with resorption and deposition of new bone and connective tissue as the teeth are moved. Active bone remodeling is thus a period of strong demand for adequate nutrition.

Dentures

Improperly fitting dentures may be a source of constant irritation and may produce ulceration of oral tissues in the elderly patient. Areas of ulceration alternate between periods of inflammation and healing, thus periodically increasing nutritional needs. Such chronic problems may be further compounded when uncomfortable dentures result in inadequate mastication and lack of desire for food. Minor denture irritation sustained over a long period may develop into a significant disease problem, and for this reason all those suffering denture maladies require good nutritional intake to maintain oral tissue integrity.

Protein and Vitamin C

Protein and vitamin C are required immediately following surgery or extensive restorative dental treatment because demand for formation of new cellular structures is high at those times. Amino acid building blocks are needed because 70 percent or more of oral soft and hard tissues are composed of collagen and GAGS. Vitamin C is needed to assist in the cross-linking of collagen fibers produced by the fibroblast. Thus, to ensure adequate intake for early collagen formation, many clinicians favor supplementation with vitamin C and protein for several days following surgical treatment.

Vitamin A and Zinc

Also essential in adequate amounts following treatment stress are vitamin A, which assists in the keratinization patterns of the oral epithelium, and zinc, needed as a cofactor in periods of wound healing.

Levels of Supplementation

What is adequate supplementation? How much supplementation should be given in periods of stress such as surgery or restorative dentistry? These questions remain controversial, since methods to assess the needs of individual patients for proteins, vitamins, and minerals are inadequate. Two formulas for nutritional supplementation following dental surgery, disease, or stress are provided in Table 20–2. In some instances, doses are in the megavitamin range (see Chapters 2 and 6).

Table 20-2. VITAMIN-MINERAL SUPPLEMENTATION
FORMULAS USED IN ORAL AND DENTAL THERAPY:
COMPARISON OF TWO FORMULATIONS
WITH THE USRDA AND THE RDA

Nutrients	USRDA for Adults and Children Over Age 4	Williams' "Nutritional Insurance" Formula	Formula Range of Cheraskin, Ringsdorf, and Brecher
Vitamin A (1000 USP units)	5	7.5	10-25[‡]
Vitamin D (100 USP units)	4	4	10-25[‡]
Vitamin E (IU)	30	40	100-800
Riboflavin (mg)	1.7	2	10-25
Thiamin (mg)	1.5	2	10-25
Pyridoxine (mg)	2.0	3	10-25
Niacin (mg)	20	20	75-150
Panthothenic acid (mg)	10	15	50-200
Cobalamin (μg)	6	9	20-100
Folacin (mg)	0.4	0.4	0.075-0.1
Ascorbic acid (mg)	60	250	300-1500
Bioflavinoids (mg)*		200	50-300
Phosphorus (mg)	1000	250	100-200
Calcium (mg)	1000	250	250-1000
Magnesium (mg)	400	200	20-300
Iron (mg)	18	15	10-25
Zinc (mg)	15	15	2-20
Copper (mg)	2	2	0.5-2
Potassium (mg)[†]	1875-5625		20-40
Fluoride (mg)[†]	1.5-4.0		
Manganese (mg)[†]	2.5-5.0	5	2-20
Cobalt (mg)		0.1	
Molybdenum (mg)[†]	0.15-0.5	0.1	
Iodine (μg)[†]	0.15	0.15	0.15
Chromium (mg)[†]	0.05-0.2	1.0	0.02-1.0
Selenium (mg)[†]	0.05-0.2	0.02	0.05-2.0
Inositol (mg)*		250	100-500
Choline (mg)*		250	100-500
PABA (mg)*		30	25-50
Biotin (mg)	0.3	0.3	0.25-0.50

* Not essential nutrients in humans.
[†] Estimated safe and adequate intake for adults in Recommended Dietary Allowances (RDA).
[‡] Potentially toxic.
(*Editor's Note:* These formulations are controversial because of their overly large doses of most vitamins.)
(Adapted from Clark, J.W.: Nutrition in dental therapy. In Clark, J.W. (ed.): Clinical Dentistry, Vol. 1. Harper and Row, Hagerstown, 1983.)

DISEASES OF THE ORAL CAVITY

Dental Caries

Dental caries is a disease characterized by the localized destruction of tooth enamel and dentin, occurring with the highest incidence in teenagers and young adults (Fig. 20–2). The severity of the disease and the ensuing destruction of tooth structure stem from a combination of etiologic factors in the oral cavity:

- Dental plaque and Streptococcus mutans plus an adequate supply of fermentable carbohydrates must be present.
- Bacteria are present in the plaque, which attaches to the tooth; fermentable carbohydrate from the diet is acted upon by the bacteria, creating a lower pH, or acidic, environment.
- Demineralization of tooth enamel occurs when the pH falls below 5.5.
- The amount of demineralization is governed by the developmental structure of the tooth enamel, in particular whether fluoride ions have been incorporated into the enamel apatite crystals.

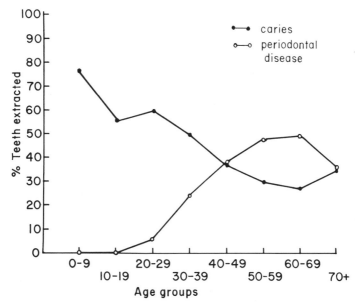

Figure 20–2. Graph of caries incidence and periodontal disease for various age groups in modern civilized populations. Note that the incidence of tooth loss due to dental caries decreases dramatically after age 25. However, there is an upswing in carious tooth loss after age 60 because of increasing incidence of root caries. Tooth loss because of destructive periodontal disease increases significantly after age 25. (From Feldman, E.B. (ed): Nutrition in the Middle and Later Years. John Wright, PSG, Inc., Littleton, MA, 1983, with permission.)

The complex pathogenesis of dental caries is depicted in the equation shown in Figure 20–3, and specific major factors are outlined in Table 20–3.

Sugars

The role of sugars in dental caries is supported by numerous controlled human studies, animal experimentation, and epidemiologic surveys. These studies conclude that the absence of sugars in the diet almost invariably results in a low or negative incidence of caries. Primitive tribes never exposed to refined carbohydrates have negligible caries rates, and in those instances when such populations became exposed to refined carbohydrates, caries incidence rose sharply. The classic example is the exposure of the American Eskimos to refined sugars.

Although all carbohydrates are potentially cariogenic, simple sugars—especially sucrose—are the most important substrate for bacterial colonization and fermentation. However, reduction of sucrose intake alone will not necessarily reduce caries incidence. Other factors also influence the complex pathogenesis of caries:

- amount of time sugars remain in the mouth
- frequency of sugar intake
- form of sugar consumed
- length of time between each sugar exposure
- "stickiness" of the sugar-containing foods
- whether the sugar is consumed alone or with other foods
- availability of the fermenting organisms

Many studies have validated the theory that the longer the teeth are exposed to an acid environment, the greater the incidence of dental caries.

Saliva

Saliva production is an additional significant factor in the caries equation (see Fig. 20–3). The composition of saliva is important because high content of GAGS in the saliva promotes higher caries rates. But the role of saliva is complex; for example, noncarious adults who experience dry mouth

$$
\begin{array}{c}
\text{Tooth} \\
\text{Morphology} \\
\text{and Structure}
\end{array}
\times
\begin{array}{c}
\text{Dental} \\
\text{Plaque}
\end{array}
\times
\begin{array}{c}
\overline{\text{Sugar Intake}} \\
\text{Frequency} \\
\times \text{ amount} \\
\times \text{ type}
\end{array}
\times
\begin{array}{c}
\text{Strep} \\
\text{Mutans}
\end{array}
\times
\begin{array}{c}
\overline{\text{Saliva}} \\
\text{Quantity} \\
\times \text{ Quality}
\end{array}
$$

$$= \text{Dental Caries}$$

Figure 20–3. Etiologic equation necessary to produce the disease dental caries. Breaking the chain or blocking any one of the terms of the equation does not always reduce the disease process to zero.

or decreased saliva production owing to certain diseases such as Sjögren's syndrome, or irradiation to salivary glands, experience rapid and severe carious destruction of their teeth. Obviously bathing of the teeth with normal saliva flow provides a protective washing or removal of potential plaque substrate and fermentable carbohydrates.

Therapeutic Regimens

Currently only two therapeutic regimens—scrupulous oral hygiene and adequate fluoride exposure—have conclusively been shown to alter or reduce caries rates in the individual.

Oral Hygiene. Application of scrupulous oral hygiene procedures, including periodic professional teeth cleaning, aims to prevent adherence of dental plaque, apparently the indispensable element in the dental caries equation (see Fig. 20–3).

Table 20–3. FACTORS IN PATHOGENESIS OF DENTAL CARIES

Factor	Level of Significance
Dental plaque	++++
Microorganisms	
Streptococcus mutans	++++
Lactobacillus acidophilus	+
Carbohydrates	
Monosaccharides	+++
Disaccharides	+++
Polysaccharides	+
Teeth	
Low levels of Ca, P, Mg, CO_3	+++
Low fluoride content in enamel and dentin	+++
Pits, fissures, developmental faults in tooth morphology	++++
Malocclusion	+++
Exposed dentin	+
Saliva	
Decreased saliva production	+++
High GAGS content	+
Heredity	++
Diet	
Low fiber/roughage content	++
High citric acid content	±
Between meal snacks	+++
Oral hygiene	
Inadequate brushing immediately following food ingestion	+++

Fluoride. The second therapeutic modality is exposure of teeth to fluoride in drinking water, oral supplementation, vitamin supplements containing fluoride, toothpaste, gel applications, or mouthwashes. The fluoride ion combines with the hydroxyapatite enamel crystal to make it more resistant to the demineralization process characteristic of an acid environment. This combination takes place both during tooth development and in the mature tooth where initial demineralization or actual caries has attacked the crystalline structure.

Fluoride Excess

Fluoride is the only mineral that, when taken in excess, dramatically affects the dentition. "Mottled enamel" is the phrase used to describe maldeveloped teeth caused by excessive fluoride ingestion (Fig. 20–4). This disease entity was first recognized in 1916 by G.V. Black and F. S. McKay, who noted its geographic distribution but did not conclude that fluoride was the etiologic agent.

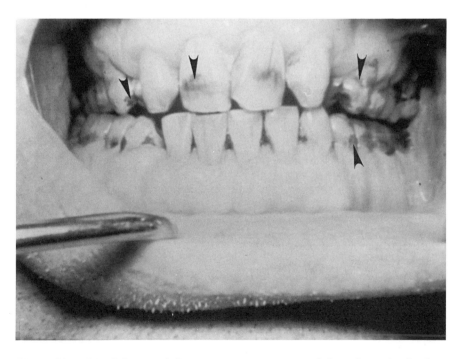

Figure 20–4. Mottled enamel due to excessive ingestion of fluoride in the drinking water supply.

Appearance of Lesions

While the precise nature of fluoride ion injury to developing teeth is unclear, histologic evidence suggests that the ameloblast is disturbed during its formation of the enamel matrix. There is a wide range in the distribution and pathologic appearance of fluoride-mottled teeth.

- Fluoride-induced hypoplasia may be as minimal as occasional white flecks or spotting of the enamel.
- Moderate lesions appear as white opaque areas on the enamel surface or as a brownish stain or slight pitting.
- Severe lesions show extensive irregularities in enamel development, with globular appearance, deep pitting, and brown staining.

These last lesions are disfiguring, with great psychologic impact on the patient, who usually is a candidate for prosthetic and cosmetic dental treatment.

Fluoride Concentration in Water

Mottled enamel is found in areas where fluoride concentration in the natural water supply exceeds 1.5 ppm. The malformations of tooth enamel found in regions with higher levels of concentration led to the selection of 1.0 ppm as the ideal concentration in drinking water—a public health measure directed toward prevention of dental caries; mottled enamel is extremely rare at this level. Some public health dentists have recommended raising the level to 1.2 ppm.

Mottled enamel is not limited to the United States; it has been described in Asia, Africa, and Europe. Four hundred areas in the United States have been targeted as communities having more fluoride in the drinking water than is recommended for normal tooth development. Most of these are located west of the Mississippi River, with a large number in Texas.

Periodontal Disease

Periodontal disease is a major factor causing loss of adult teeth throughout the world (see Fig. 20–2). Unlike dental caries—a modern disease— periodontal disease has existed for centuries. Evidence of chronic periodontal disease has been found even in skulls of ancient cave dwellers and other early populations. However, other mammals rarely display periodontal problems, an anomaly that has hampered scientific research of this phenomenon.

Periodontal disease is a collective designation for a number of problems that affect the periodontal structure of the oral cavity called the periodontium. The periodontium consists of the periodontal ligament, the cementum on the tooth root surface where periodontal ligament fibers embed, the bone where the other end of the periodontal ligament collagen fibers embed, and the free and attached gingiva. Destruction of any or all of these structures is considered within the spectrum of periodontal disease.

Pathogenesis

Periodontal disease usually begins as a marginal gingivitis that is without clinical symptoms and shows minimal clinical signs. If untreated, the initial inflammatory process continues to expand until it becomes full-blown chronic periodontitis, resulting in destruction of the periodontal ligament, the gingival mucosa, and—most importantly—the alveolar bony process. These factors together may result in loss of teeth owing to the irreparable breakdown of the periodontium.

Etiology

The etiology of periodontal disease is poorly understood. Both local and systemic factors usually must be present to generate periodontal disease (Table 20–4). Current therapeutic regimens are designed to interrupt this relationship, with the aim of modifying or partially controlling the severity of the disorder (Fig. 20–5).

Table 20–4. FACTORS IN PATHOGENESIS
OF PERIODONTAL DISEASE

Factor	Level of Significance
Increasing age	+++
Poor oral hygiene	++++
Malocclusion	+++
Tooth deposits	
Plaque	++++
Calculus	++++
Salivary pellicle	++
Bacteria	
Asaccharolytic organisms	+++
Saccharolytic organisms	±
Diet	
Lack of sound, normal diet	+++
Low vitamin C levels	+++
High sugar diet	+
Compromised immunologic status	++

Figure 20–5. Equation showing the interrelationship of the etiologic factors combined to create periodontal disease. (Modified from Clark, J.W., Cheraskin, E., and Ringsdorf, W.M., Jr.: Diet and the Periodontal Patient. CC Thomas, Springfield, IL, 1970.)

$$\frac{Aging}{Periodontium} \times \frac{Plaque}{Calculus} \times Diet \times Bacteria$$

$$\times \frac{Immunologic}{Status} = \frac{Periodontal\ Disease}{Oral\ Hygiene\ Status} =$$

$$Severity\ of\ Periodontal\ Disease$$

Relationship of Diet

The relationship of diet to periodontal disease is unclear. However, vitamin C in particular, as well as a generally adequate diet, appear to be important.

Vitamin C. In a number of studies, the lack of adequate vitamin C has been associated with periodontal disease. In the 1700s, British sailors who were deprived of fruits and vegetables over long periods developed bleeding gums and loose teeth, the syndrome of scurvy (see Chapter 14). From such evidence, researchers have proposed a relationship between avitaminosis C and gingival health and periodontal disease, but the connection has been difficult to study because of animals' and humans' differing requirements for ascorbic acid. Even the oxidative catabolism of vitamin C in animals and humans differs. More recent studies suggest that avitaminosis C may be an exacerbating factor but not a primary etiologic agent in periodontal disease.

Dietary Guidelines. Because adequate diet is an important factor in the management of periodontal disease, the following guidelines should be observed:

- adequate daily diet containing recommended dietary allowances and the appropriate amount of protein for body mass
- sufficient fiber and fiber-like food to stimulate adequate masticatory exercise in each 24-hour period
- fresh fruits and vegetables for adequate vitamin C
- consideration of the need for multivitamin supplementation in the aging patient, orthodontic patient, patient undergoing extensive dental restorative/oral surgical procedures, and patients who may be debilitated because of other disease or treatment procedures

Benign Migratory Glossitis

Benign migratory glossitis, or geographic tongue (Fig. 20–6), is a common oral disease with an incidence ranging as high as 1.4 to 2.4 percent of the

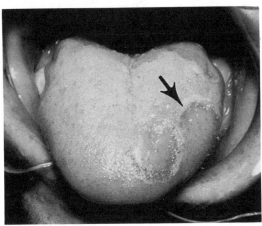

Figure 20-6. Geographic tongue (benign migratory glossitis). The smooth areas are denuded of filiform papillae.

population. Females are affected twice as often as males, with no apparent racial differences. Of unknown etiology, this condition is commonly seen in young adults during periods of heavy stress such as final examinations.

The nonpainful condition consists of multiple focal denuded areas of filiform papillae on the tongue dorsal surface that appear in circular patterns, often bordered by a thin, yellowish-white band of inflammatory reaction. The filiform papillae regenerate, but denuded areas then appear in other locations on the dorsal tongue. This migratory feature tends to alarm patients, stimulating them to seek professional help. Therapy has consisted of brushing the tongue and ingesting supplements of B complex vitamins. Although there is no evidence that the vitamin therapy is in fact beneficial, many patients show signs of improvement. The disease is self-limiting, although it may involve the buccal mucosa and may be associated with oral lichen planus.

Oral Lichen Planus

Lichen planus is primarily a dermatologic disease, but it often appears in the oral cavity, with or without skin lesions (Fig. 20-7). Patients with skin lesions usually have oral lesions, while only a minority of patients with oral lesions have associated skin lesions. The oral disease pattern is seen in several forms:

- generalized or nonerosive
- hypertrophic
- erosive
- bullous

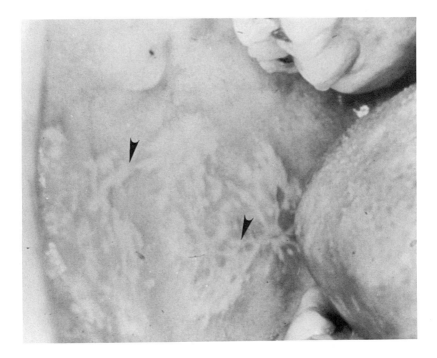

Figure 20-7. Lichen planus appearing as a whitish raised lesion on the cheek mucosa.

The buccal mucosa and tongue are the most frequent sites of occurrence. Tiny, white, elevated lines of the disease pattern often are referred to as "striae of Wickham." The disorder is most prevalent in middle-aged and elderly women.

Etiology

The etiology of lichen planus is unknown, but improper nutrition and stress may be activating factors. Dietary counseling and relief of stressful situations may alleviate symptoms and bring marked improvement in this generally painful, benign soft tissue condition. Because it may be masked by other conditions such as candidiasis or benign migratory glossitis, the disease may be difficult to diagnose clinically. Histology is diagnostic and oral biopsy usually will confirm the clinical suspicion.

Therapy

Although vitamin therapy has been advocated for treatment of lichen planus, it probably provides no more benefit than adequate nutritional counseling. Topical steroid cream may be used to assist in relief of pain and discomfort. Erosive lichen planus is an especially painful form of the disease, usually heralded by formation of fluid-filled vesicles and bullae on the oral mucous membrane that quickly burst, leaving erosive lesions. Erosive lichen planus is difficult to treat, usually requiring steroid therapy for pain relief. Occasionally xylocaine gel must be used so that patients can chew and swallow food. Empirical use of zinc sulfate (220 mg per day) as a trace nutrient supplement has been suggested to promote healing of the painful lesions.

Desquamative Gingivitis

Desquamative gingivitis, also known as gingivosis, is a chronic inflammatory problem of the gingiva of unknown etiology (Fig. 20–8). The disease, primarily affecting 40- to 60-year-old women, causes red, painful areas of the gingiva. The basic defect occurs immediately beneath the basilar cell layer of the oral epithelium. When pressure is applied to the oral epithelium by finger, the epithelium will slide and strip from the supporting connective tissue stroma (Nikolsky's sign).

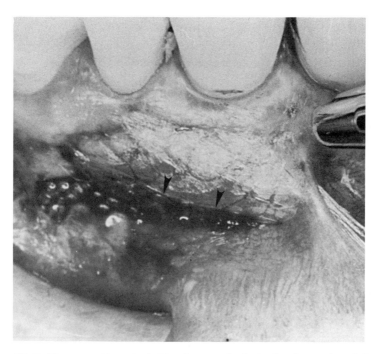

Figure 20–8. Desquamative gingivitis; the attached gingiva has stripped from the underlying connective tissue leaving a raw denuded area.

Differential Diagnosis

Benign mucous membrane pemphigoid (BMMP; see further on) and pemphigus vulgaris are diseases that must be ruled out when Nikolsky's sign is present on the gingiva. An oral biopsy should be performed and immunofluorescence diagnostic studies completed. The positive Nikolsky's sign helps in differential diagnoses among lichen planus, aphthous ulcers, herpangina, herpetic gingivostomatitis, and desquamative gingivitis.

Treatment

Treatment consists of nutritional and psychologic counseling and evaluation of hormonal status. Good oral hygiene must be instituted. Patients usually are sensitive to hot and spicy foods and find it difficult to eat. Palliative treatment with anesthetic topical gels (xylocaine), topical steroids in an emollient base (betamethasone cream), and, in very refractory cases, systemic steroids in decreasing doses to help patients with mastication and for general comfort. In addition, zinc sulfate, 220 mg per day, may be used to enhance epithelial integrity. Desquamative gingivitis lesions usually cycle and spontaneously regress. Attention to the problem and assurance that the disorder is non-neoplastic are supportive to the patient.

Benign Mucous Membrane Pemphigoid

Sometimes called cicatrical pemphigoid, BMMP is a vesiculobullous disease of unknown etiology. Added to oral mucous membrane lesions is involvement of the conjunctiva. Lesions may also be seen on the skin, nose, esophagus, pharynx, larynx, vagina, penis, and anus. Differential diagnoses include erosive lichen planus and pemphigus vulgaris. Histologic findings are specific, and direct immunofluorescence should be employed. The disease has no direct connection with nutritional patterns, but good nutritional counseling and therapeutic vitamins are helpful in treatment because of inadequate food intake.

Angular Cheilitis

Nonspecific cracking or fissuring occurring at the corners of the mouth is termed angular cheilitis, or perleche (Fig. 20–9). The condition may occur in any age group but is seen more often in the older adult. It begins with the patient noting dryness and a burning sensation at the corners of the mouth. The epithelium eventually becomes macerated, and fissures and cracks appear in surface epithelium. While these ulcerated areas are superficial and do

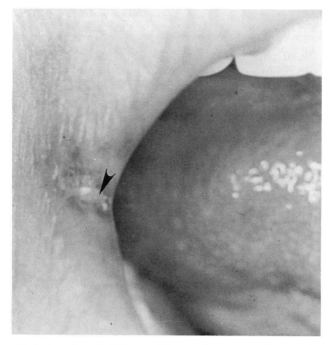

Figure 20–9. Angular cheilitis; cracking or fissuring at the mouth corner.

not bleed, they are painful, especially when salt or spicy foods are ingested. Patients usually self-treat the lesions with applications of Vaseline or some other over-the-counter salve.

Etiology

The etiology of cheilitis is complex. It has been suggested that the condition reflects ribloflavin deficiency (see Chapter 14), with potential superimposed fungal or bacterial infection, and many patients do respond well to therapeutic doses of B complex vitamins. In the older patient who has lost numerous teeth, the cause often is a decrease in the vertical dimension between the upper and lower jaws. A fold developing at the corners of the mouth where saliva tends to collect leads to maceration and fissuring of the epithelium. Many of these lesions develop secondary Candida albicans infections.

Treatment

The first step in treatment is a smear or culture for Candida. Next, the patient should be examined by a dentist to determine whether missing teeth or improperly fitting dentures have caused loss of vertical dimension. New dentures or crown and bridge prostheses may be indicated. Finally, there should be nutritional counseling, and if deficiencies are suspected, therapeutic use of B complex vitamins should be considered (see Chapter 14). All three factors may be involved in complex cases of this benign but aggravating disorder.

Other Perleche Problems

Other perleche problems may be seen in older patients who are not producing sufficient saliva (xerostomia), perhaps because of irradiation or Sjögren's syndrome. Other patients may exhibit such problems resulting from habitual licking of lips and corners of the mouth or, in the case of some handicapped patients, from saliva flowing from the mouth's corners. Some cases may be refractory and unresponsive to any form of treatment. However, some measure of relief in such cases may be obtained with use of a steroid ointment preparation.

Generalized Mucositis

The oral mucous membrane often reflects generalized systemic disorders such as Crohn's disease or chronic peptic ulcer disease. The membrane may also reflect the body's nutritional imbalances. Especially in older, postmenopausal females, the mucosa may develop a beefy red appearance or a generalized burning or itching. No specific disease can be diagnosed in these patients; nutritional or hormonal imbalances, or both, may be identified as contributing causes. Nutritional counseling and use of appropriate vitamins may help to eliminate or reduce symptoms. Endocrinologic consultation should be employed when indicated. The status of zinc in the diets of these patients should be evaluated, as this mineral enhances epithelial integrity.

Burning Tongue

Glossodynia, or burning tongue, is frequently seen in postmenopausal women, although men are not immune. Burning tongue may reflect local or systemic problems, including nutritional deficiencies (especially B complex and iron), pernicious anemia, pellagra, diabetes mellitus, hyperthyroidism, gastric hyperacidity, or xerostomia. Local factors include excessive use of tobacco, particular spices, ill-fitting dentures, excessive use of antibiotics, or poor oral hygiene with presence of calculus, plaque, and/or malopposed teeth. Biopsy usually is nonspecific.

Evaluation and Treatment

Clinicians tend to ignore middle-aged or older women's complaints of burning tongue. However, since this symptom may be the harbinger of more serious underlying disease, it merits attention and appropriate evaluation. Blood and hormonal assays are in order especially to rule out anemia and diabetes mellitus, and dentures should be examined and treated as needed in edentulous patients. Consideration should be given to therapeutic vitamin (especially B complex) and iron supplementation to bolster integrity of the epithelial tissues of the tongue (see Chapter 14). Nutritional counseling by a qualified professional and an appropriate vitamin regimen often are helpful.

Candidiasis must be ruled out since denuded or burning tongue lesions often are signs of this fungal infection. Not all Candida infections in the oral cavity appear white or "thrush-like."

Loss of Tongue Filiform Papillae

Loss of filiform papillae in scattered areas of the tongue is another disturbing nonspecific lesion. The loss may occur at any age, but is more commonly seen in the young child and the older adult. The young person usually is experiencing some degree of tooth eruption or has oral hygiene problems, while the older person may present with periodontal disease, ill-fitting dentures or missing teeth, lack of proper oral hygiene, and nutritional inadequacy, especially iron. Patients usually complain of loss of taste or a woody taste sensation. The filiform papillae generally are atrophied, leaving small, bald, reddish spots on the tongue (not to be confused with geographic tongue). These areas usually clear spontaneously. This problem is not always directly attributable to nutrition, but dietary components may contribute to discomfort and iron supplementation often is helpful.

Osteoporosis of the Jaw

Osteoporosis affects the jaw just as it does other bone. Recent studies indicate that the disease may result from long-term negative calcium balance. Generally the condition will be suggested during routine radiographic examination by the dentist. The trabeculation pattern of the bone will appear thin and somewhat radiolucent. Confirming the diagnosis requires a complete workup of the patient's calcium and phosphorus status. (Osteoporosis and requirements for calcium and phosphate are covered in Chapters 2, 9, and 14).

Osteoporotic Bone Marrow

A common condition in the jaw is osteoporotic bone marrow defect, which presents as thinned areas of trabecular bone. Its localized, well-delineated radiographic appearance should not be confused with osteoporosis. At times oral bone biopsy must be performed to rule out other bone diseases.

Dystrophic Calcification

Dystrophic calcification is the deposition of calcium salts, usually in dead or dying tissues. Abnormally placed calcium is a common occurrence in the oral cavity, especially in the gingiva, buccal mucosa, and tongue. In addition, dystrophic calcification may be found in the pulp of the teeth, sometimes referred to as "pulp stones." The oral cavity is subject to many forms of local trauma and inflammation, such as cheek and lip biting, plaque and calculus deposits, food impaction, and improper oral hygiene and brushing habits. Many of these irritants cause reactive lesions such as benign fibromas and overgrowth of connective tissue (hypertrophy, hyperplasia) in the oral cavity. Areas of focal dystrophic calcification are centrally located in many of these latter lesions. The benign reactive lesion found on the attached gingiva around teeth is so common that it is known as "peripheral odontogenic ossifying fibroma." It is in fact nothing more than a benign reactive fibroma or pyogenic granuloma with dystrophic calcification.

Etiology

Dystrophic calcification is not related to the level of calcium in circulating blood. It seems to occur because of a local increase in pH in diseased tissue (compared with adjacent normal tissue) that causes precipitation of calcium salts in the area. Following an initial nidus of calcium deposition, dystrophic hard tissue usually grows concentrically. Layering concentric rings may be seen on these structures, even though their complete outline may be irregular.

Epulis Fissuratum

Dystrophic calcification is found in other reactive areas of the oral cavity. For example, epulis fissuratum, a specific reactive hyperplasia-hypertrophy of connective tissue in the vestibular sulci of the jaws owing to denture irritation, may show deposits of salt in the connective tissue stroma (Fig. 20–10). These deposits generally do not elicit an inflammatory or foreign body response; they are benign and of no significance.

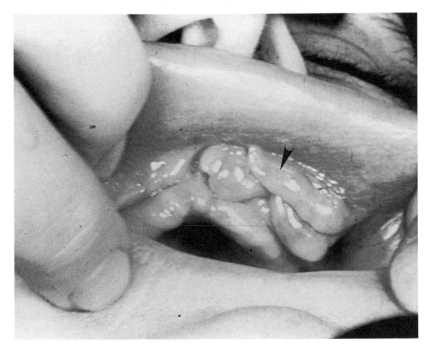

Figure 20-10. Epulis fissuration or denture hypertrophy due to an ill-fitting denture. Note the extensive soft tissue overgrowth in the maxillary vestibule.

Nonspecific Disorders

A number of nonspecific oral mucosa problems may be related to nutrition, including bleeding gums, painful gingiva or oral mucosa, overt burning sensation, and inability to masticate food properly. Eliminating local irritants and initiating a good oral hygiene protocol will assist in the differential diagnosis of these difficult clinical problems. If the patient continues to have problems after local factors have been eliminated, nutritional aspects must be considered. Usually a diet survey is made and recommendations for appropriate nutritional supplements are given to these patients (see Chapter 3). Clark, Cheraskin, and Ringsdorf have documented instances of improved health of the oral mucosa accompanying better nutrition.

CHAPTER 21

Gastrointestinal Diseases and Malabsorption

The gastrointestinal tract and nutrition are interrelated in various ways: components of the diet or their delivery may induce some gastrointestinal diseases; some gastrointestinal disorders are managed by diet modifications; and because of the vital role of the gastrointestinal tract in the handling of food, damage to its structure and/or function is likely to result in impaired nutritional status. In turn, malnutrition impairs the structure and function of the intestine (see Chapter 13). (Some diseases of the oral cavity and pharynx are reviewed in Chapter 20.)

Table 21-1. MAJOR GASTROINTESTINAL HORMONES

Hormone	Produced	Stimulus	Action
Gastrin	Antrum Duodenum	Protein	↑Gastric acid
Secretin	Small intestine	Acid in duodenum	↑Pancreas and liver
CCK	Duodenum Jejunum	Fat in duodenum	↑Pancreatic enzymes ↑Gallbladder contraction
Glucagon	Stomach fundus Intestine	CHO, fat in duodenum	↑Hepatic glycogenolysis ↓Motility
	Pancreatic islets		
Insulin	Pancreatic islets		

*Adapted from Floch, M.H.: Nutrition and Diet Therapy in Gastrointestinal Disease. New York, Plenum Publishing, 1981, pp. 16, 17.

A peristaltic wave moves the bolus of food that is swallowed down the esophagus. This temporarily releases the lower esophageal sphincter. The bolus of food then enters the stomach and is acted upon by acid and pepsinogen secreted by the stomach in response to gastrin. The chyme enters the duodenum and its acid and protein content stimulates secretion of cholecystokinin (CCK). The latter hormone stimulates secretion by the liver and pancreas (see Chapter 22) as well as intestinal fluid, thereby promoting digestion and absorption. CCK acts as a satiety agent, while glucagon and insulin regulate gut motility. The gut hormones (Table 21-1) interact with the central nervous system in addition to affecting metabolic functions. The roles of particular foods in stimulating secretion of gastrointestinal hormones and other fluids have not been clarified.

THE ESOPHAGUS

Diseases of the esophagus include

- disorders of motility (achalasia, stroke) involving the neuromuscular mechanism controlling the lower esophageal sphincter
- hiatal hernia and reflux
- inflammation
- infiltration or stricture or both
- neoplasm
- foreign bodies
- diverticula

Dysphagia

Difficulty in swallowing characterizes diseases of the esophagus and may be associated with chest pain. Patients also may have anorexia and weight loss. Swallowing difficulty may be intermittent and aggravated by drinking very hot or cold liquids, or dysphagia for solids or liquids may be more prominent. Progressive dysphagia is suggestive of narrowing of the esophagus from neoplasm, stricture, or infiltrative disease. It may be difficult to differentiate esophageal chest pain from that due to coronary heart disease (angina).

Reflux Esophagitis and Hiatal Hernia

Reflux esophagitis and hiatal hernia produce mucosal damage from regurgitation of acid chyme from the stomach. Dysphagia is common along with heartburn precipitated by heavy meals or change in posture. Episodes of vomiting may lead to distal esophageal stricture. The condition is more common in the obese. Diagnosis of this and other esophageal disease is by endoscopy with visualization and biopsy. Manometric measurements may be necessary. Radiographs of the esophagus using radiopaque material may be helpful.

Treatment

The "antireflux regimen" involves the exclusion of smoking, coffee, alcohol, citrus fruits, and chocolate. In addition, patients may react adversely to some nuts and numerous spices. Patients are advised to raise the head of the bed 6 to 8 inches using shock blocks. Weight reduction for the obese, small frequent meals, and adequate chewing of food are encouraged. No food should be eaten within 3 hours of going to bed, or when lying down. Heartburn may be relieved by antacids. In addition, antacids and cimetidine, especially at night, are helpful in reducing gastric acid secretion, and bethanecol and metoclopramide may improve gastric emptying.

Esophageal stricture is treated by dilatation and may require surgical correction. These patients may need a liquid diet, or enteral or parenteral feeding (see Chapters 11 and 12).

Cancer

Esophageal cancer causes symptoms similar to those of stricture—namely, progressive dysphagia. Because of weight loss as a consequence of dysphagia, many patients present with malnutrition at the time of diagnosis.

Correction by a regimen of nasogastric tube feeding, by gastrostomy or jejunostomy (see Chapter 11), or by parenteral feeding (see Chapter 12) may improve the patient's response to specific treatment with surgical resection or radiotherapy. Esophagectomy, esophagogastrectomy, and/or irradiation may result in continued anorexia and persistent malnutrition. (Dietary factors in the etiology of esophageal cancer are reviewed in Chapters 17 and 24.)

THE STOMACH

Disorders of the stomach include

- gastritis
- peptic ulcer disease
- gastric outlet obstruction and gastric atony
- gastrectomy and dumping
- cancer

Gastritis

Gastritis, or inflammation of the gastric mucosa, may be acute or chronic. Acute gastritis occurs following ingestion of an irritant or corrosive substance. Ethanol probably is the most frequently precipitating cause of gastritis, along with anti-inflammatory drugs, especially aspirin and phenylbutazone. Symptoms of the condition include epigastric pain, anorexia, nausea, heartburn, vomiting, hematemesis, and fever. Diarrhea is a symptom of associated enteritis. Treatment may require parenteral fluids, with provision of a light diet when the patient can tolerate food. Chronic atrophic gastritis may be due to an autoimmune reaction and is associated with pernicious anemia and iron deficiency anemia (see Chapter 15).

Peptic Ulcer Disease

Both gastric and duodenal ulcer will be discussed here since both disorders result from inability of the mucosal epithelium to resist autodigestion by gastric acid and pepsin. The reasons for this susceptibility are unknown. Duodenal ulcer may manifest as burning epigastric pain relieved by meals and antacids, or predominantly with symptoms of weight loss, anorexia, and anemia from bleeding. Perforation or intractable pain may complicate the disease. Gastric ulcer is more common than duodenal ulcer after age 50 and may present with epigastric discomfort after meals, dysphagia, weight loss, and symptoms of chronic blood loss (melena). Susceptibility to gastric ulcer is increased by aspirin and corticosteroids. With a large hemorrhage, hematemesis of "coffee ground" material is usual. Endoscopy—with biopsy in the case of gastric ulcer—assists in diagnosis, together with upper gastrointestinal radiographs with contrast.

Medical Treatment

Antacid therapy and cimetidine are effective symptomatic treatment. However, magnesium-containing antacids may cause diarrhea, while aluminum-containing antacids may cause hypophosphatemia and constipation. Current management of peptic ulcer disease no longer calls for bland diets; instead, patients are advised to avoid foods such as spices, coffee, and alcohol that cause epigastric discomfort. Rather than decreasing gastric acid, milk may actually induce gastric secretion due to its calcium content. While patients with acute significant upper gastrointestinal bleeding are fed, patients with perforated peptic ulcer or pyloric obstruction are managed with parenteral nutrition and continuous gastric suction with appropriate replacement of electrolyte and fluid losses (see Chapters 2 and 12).

Surgery for Peptic Ulcer

Indications for emergency surgery in peptic ulcer disease are massive recurrent bleeding or perforation. Elective surgery may be performed for persistent or recurrent gastric ulcer, in pyloric obstruction, or when there is intractable pain or suspicion of malignancy. The principal operations are partial gastrectomy with anastomoses to the duodenum (Billroth I) or the jejunum (Billroth II), the vagotomies (selective, truncal, proximal gastric), pyloroplasty, and gastroenterostomy.

Complications of Surgical Treatment. Gastric surgery often results in permanent gastrointestinal malfunction, with diarrhea occurring in about half of patients. About 20 percent of patients develop malabsorption of protein, fat, iron, folate, vitamin B_{12}, and lactose following gastrojejunostomy. Osteopenia with malabsorption of vitamin D and calcium occurs in 25 to 40 percent of patients after Billroth II anastomosis; therefore, supplementation with these nutrients may be necessary.

The dumping syndrome also occurs after Billroth II gastrojejunostomy and gastrectomy, with delivery of large volumes of hyperosmolar fluid into the jejunum. Diarrhea, abdominal pain, and vomiting are seen 30 to 60 minutes after eating because of the distention of the jejunum with hyperosmolar fluid. Palpitations, sweating, weakness, drowsiness, and dyspnea may occur. Hypoglycemia, due to insulin release 1 to 4 hours after eating, may also be present; its symptoms include sweating, palpitations, lightheadedness, confusion, and—rarely—stupor. Patients should be managed with frequent small, dry meals high in protein with restriction of refined carbohydrates and concentrated sweets. Fluids should be taken not less than 30 minutes before nor 60 minutes after meals. There may be reflux of bile into the stomach, accompanied by nausea and vomiting. Since recumbency may slow gastric emptying following gastric surgery, patients should be advised to lie down for 30 minutes after eating.

Weight loss is invariable following total gastrectomy and may occur in one third of patients after Billroth I partial gastrectomy and even more often after the Billroth II procedure. Permanent effects of the various vagotomy procedures have not been as well defined. Weight loss after gastric surgery is caused by the combination of malabsorption and inadequate food intake. On average, the postgastrectomy patient takes in only 75 percent of the calories needed for maintenance. Dietary counseling may improve food intake (see Chapter 10).

Anemia occurs in about half of patients following gastric surgery, usually due to iron deficiency resulting from a combination of prior bleeding, decreased absorption, reduced intake, and, occasionally, continued blood loss from gastritis, erosions, or recurrent ulcer disease. Megaloblastic anemia due to cobalamin deficiency may occur 1 to 5 years after total gastrectomy. There may be cobalamin deficiency due to loss of intrinsic factor in a small number of patients following partial gastrectomy. Patients postgastrectomy should thus be followed with yearly measurement of serum cobalamin levels. Deficient patients should be given cobalamin parenterally (see Chapter 15).

Bezoars

Gastric bezoars form in the stomach from concretion of undigested foods such as plant fibers, hair, or other foreign bodies. Masses also may form following gastric surgery or with gastroparesis secondary to visceral neuropathy in diabetes mellitus. Symptoms include fullness of the stomach, nausea, and vomiting. Large bezoars may become palpable and cause ulceration with bleeding. The bezoar may be disrupted under endoscopic control or by surgery. The patient's diet should be modified to avoid excessive consumption of fresh fruits and vegetables.

SMALL INTESTINE

Water, sodium, chloride, and potassium secreted into the gut (see Chapters 1 and 2) are reabsorbed into the duodenum and jejunum, largely by solvent drag, along with elements of the diet. Sodium is absorbed and bicarbonate secreted in the ileum via the active sodium pump. In the distal ileum,

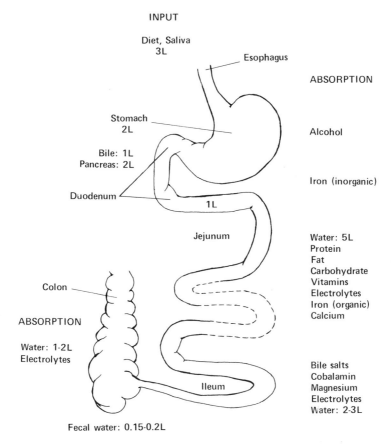

Figure 21-1. Nutrient handling in the gastrointestinal tract. Input includes the diet, saliva, bile, and gastric, pancreatic, and intestinal secretions. Absorption of various nutrients occurs at various sites along the gastrointestinal tract. The final output is the feces.

the concentrations of sodium, potassium, chloride, and bicarbonate are, respectively, 125, 9, 60, and 74 mEq per liter. Approximately 600 ml of ileal fluid passes into the colon, containing 75, 5, 36, and 44 mEq of the respective electrolytes. Water, sodium, and chloride are absorbed, and potassium and bicarbonate are excreted. Ultimately, 4 to 8 mEq of sodium and 9 to 18 mEq of potassium are excreted in the feces, with 2 and 3 mEq of Cl$^-$ and HCO$_3^-$ and about 100 ml of water. With abnormalities in absorption of fluid and electrolytes, and in the presence of diarrhea, there may be serious losses of these nutrients (see Chapter 2 and Fig. 21-1).

Diarrhea

Diarrheas are classified as

- simple
- osmotic
- secretory
- motility and transit
- exudative
- drug-induced
- complex (malabsorptive, metabolic)

Treatment for the various types of diarrhea is symptomatic, and appropriate management requires understanding the underlying mechanisms. For examples, see sections on Bile Acid Diarrhea (p. 497), and on Fatty Acid Diarrhea (pp. 497–498). Acute and chronic infectious diarrheas are described in Chapter 8.

The Malabsorption Syndromes

A result of various abnormalities of the small intestine, the malabsorption syndrome has multiple etiologies (Table 21–2). Causes include

- disorders of the intestinal wall resulting from intolerance to one or another dietary component, including alcohol (see Chapter 17)
- inflammation, infection, or infiltration
- parasitic infestation
- circulatory disorders
- resection, bypass, stricture, fistula
- effects of irradiation

(Absorption problems relating to pancreatic exocrine insufficiency or bile salts are discussed in Chapter 22.)

Diagnosis

Malabsorption due to small intestinal disease results in symptoms of diarrhea, weakness, and weight loss, accompanied by signs of vitamin deficiency, anemia (often megaloblastic), moderate steatorrhea, hypocalcemia, and hypomagnesemia.

The quantitative chemical analysis of fat excreted over a period of 72 hours is the most sensitive test for malassimilation of fat and is the most important test to identify maldigestion or malabsorption (Table 21–3). Ninety-five percent or more of ingested fat normally is absorbed, and thus a useful screening test is a qualitative test for fat in the stool. A stool sample on a glass slide is stained with Sudan III and examined for neutral fat (triglyceride). A

Table 21-2. CAUSES OF
MALABSORPTION

Atrophic gastritis
Gastrectomy
Pancreatic insufficiency
Bilary deficiency
Celiac disease (gluten enteropathy)
Tropical sprue
Food intolerance
Small bowel resection
Small bowel bypass
Small bowel infiltration
Small bowel resection
Crohn's disease (inflammatory bowel disease)
Immune deficiency
Parasitic infestation
Vascular
Endocrine
Drugs

second sample is treated with acetic acid (36 percent), stained, and heated. Split fats will appear and may be quantitated by size. Globules normally are small and difficult to count. One hundred or more globules of 1 to 8 microns in size indicate possible fat malabsorption, while those of 6 to 75 microns indicates probable malabsorption.

Following ingestion of 25 g xylose, normal individuals excrete more than 4 g in the urine in 5 hours; plasma xylose should be 10 to 20 mg per dl per 1.73 m^2 after 60 to 75 minutes. (The Schilling test for absorption of vitamin B_{12} is described in Chapter 15.) The bile acid breath test is appropriate for patients suspected of bacterial overgrowth or ileal dysfunction. This test indicates de-

Table 21-3. DIAGNOSTIC
PROCEDURES
FOR MALABSORPTION   .

Fecal fat analysis
Xylose absorption
Bile acid breath test
Jejunal biopsy
Small intestine radiography
Schilling test
Small intestine aspiration culture

conjugation of radiolabeled glycine-conjugated bile acid with subsequent metabolism and absorption of the radiolabeled glycine and subsequent excretion of radiolabeled CO_2 by the lungs.

The small intestinal perioral biopsy yields a histologic picture of the intestinal mucosa. A flat biopsy may be observed in celiac disease and other forms of sprue, in protein-energy malnutrition, in the presence of parasitic disease (giardiasis), or drug or radiation damage. Small intestine radiographs assist in the diagnosis.

Lactose Intolerance

Lactose intolerance, caused by a deficiency of the small intestinal enzyme lactase, is believed to affect 30 million people in the United States. Lactase hydrolyzes the milk sugar lactose into galactose and glucose. Lactase deficiency may be congenital or secondary to disorders of the small intestine such as celiac disease, sprue, protein-energy malnutrition, or Crohn's disease. Enzyme deficiency may also be induced by some antibiotics, or result from damage to the intestinal wall by infection. Blacks, Orientals, and American Indians often are affected, and the incidence increases with age.

Deficiency of lactase results in abdominal cramps, flatulence, bloating, and/or diarrhea, occurring after eating foods containing lactose. Symptoms may appear after drinking only one glass of milk or, in less severe cases, after three or four glasses. Cold milk may bother some people more than warmer milk, while others can tolerate milk with a meal better than milk alone. Fermented dairy products such as yogurt may be better tolerated because of the conversion of lactose to lactic acid, or the production of lactase by the bacterial culture. A few ounces of cheese can be tolerated by many patients.

Enzyme activity may be detected by

- tests of the hydrogen exhaled after an oral dose of lactose (hydrogen breath test)
- stool culture for undigested lactose
- the appearance of galactose in the urine

Lactase activity is maximal at birth, remains high through early childhood, and declines to a residual level of 5 to 10 percent by age 5 or 6 in most individuals. A minority of adults, primarily from northern and western Europe, sustain high lactase activity. Lactase is the most sensitive of the intestinal disaccharidases to mucosal disease.

Lactase enzyme powder added to milk converts about 70 percent of the lactose into glucose and galactose, which are absorbed more easily. Low lactose milks are also now readily available. (Normally, 1 quart of milk contains 50 g lactose.)

Other Intolerances

Other intestinal enzyme disorders leading to food intolerance include sucrase isomaltase deficiency (Eskimos) and starch intolerance.

Celiac Disease

Celiac disease (gluten enteropathy, nontropical sprue) results from sensitivity to gluten in wheat flour, rye, oats, and barley. The small intestinal lesion impairs absorption of all nutrients and therefore results in multiple deficiencies if left untreated. Prominent signs and symptoms include

- diarrhea
- weakness
- flatulence
- weight loss
- anorexia
- nausea
- vomiting
- bone pain
- glossitis
- abdominal pain
- tetany
- abdominal distention
- edema

Treatment is strict elimination of gluten from the diet. Many foods can be thickened with wheat flour, including soups, sauces, processed cheese, creamed dishes, salad dressing, ice cream, candies, instant coffee, ale and beer, mustard, soy sauce, and horseradish. Average gluten intake for the adult American has been estimated at 8 to 13 g. The small intestinal mucosa will appear normal and symptoms will be controlled following 3 to 6 months of a gluten-free diet.

Tropical Sprue

Tropical sprue is believed by many to be an infectious disease caused by persistent contamination of the small bowel by an enteric pathogen. Symptoms are glossitis, diarrhea and steatorrhea, and malnutrition. Clinical improvement follows treatment with folic acid (5 mg daily) or antibiotics (tetracycline). Heavy infestation with Giardia may cause diarrhea and malabsorption of fat, d-xylose, and vitamin B_{12}, which are corrected with eradication of the parasite.

Short Bowel Syndrome

This syndrome is caused by inflammatory disorders of the small intestine such as Crohn's disease, infarction or trauma requiring surgical resection involving 50 percent or more of the small intestine, or radiation enteritis compromising intestinal absorptive function. The patients are at high risk of developing nutritional deficiencies.

- Duodenal resection results in deficient iron absorption and anemia.
- Resection of large segments of the jejunum results in malabsorption of glucose, fats, amino acids, calcium, water- and fat-soluble vitamins.
- Resection of the terminal ileum is associated with vitamin B_{12} deficiency and bile acid malabsorption with diarrhea (cholerrheic enteropathy). With ileal resection there is a tendency to increased absorption of oxalates in the colon and increased incidence of oxalate renal stones (see further on).
- Small bowel resection may cause watery diarrhea of 3 to 6 liters daily. The diarrhea will subside as the small intestine adapts and increases its absorptive capacity, usually in about 6 months.

Patients with short bowel syndrome are initially managed with nutritional supplements, often elemental (Table 21–4; see also Chapter 11). Small, low fat meals may be tolerated with supplements of medium chain triglycerides. Parenteral alimentation may be necessary when massive resection has left only a few feet of small intestine (see Chapter 12). Patients with less than 2 feet of small intestine may require some degree of intravenous feeding for the remainder of their life; this is a major indication for home TPN. Vitamin

Table 21–4. VITAMIN/MINERAL
SUPPLEMENTS IN
SEVERE MALABSORPTION*

Vitamins A	100,000 units daily[†]
D	50,000 units 3 times weekly
K	10 mg daily
Folic acid	5 mg daily
Vitamin B_{12}	1000 μg daily intramuscular[‡]
B complex	Multivitamin 2 times daily
Minerals	
Calcium	500 mg elemental 2–3 times daily
Magnesium	25 mg 4 times daily
Iron	65 mg elemental 3 times daily

*Route is oral unless specified.
[†]5000–50,000 daily maintenance.
[‡]Monthly maintenance.

and mineral supplements should be provided (Table 21–4), and antibiotic therapy is helpful. Diarrhea associated with bile acid malabsorption can be controlled with bile acid–binding resins. Increased bacterial breakdown of carbohydrates in the intestine may lead to increased lactic acid absorption and acidosis.

CASE 21a: SHORT BOWEL SYNDROME

A 38-year-old nurse was referred for management of short bowel syndrome. Five years earlier, because of infarction of the intestine, she underwent removal of more than 10 feet of necrotic distal small intestine. Since that time she had had diarrhea with 8 to 10 bowel movements daily and her weight had varied between about 112 and 118 pounds (51 and 54 kg) (her height was 5 feet 8 inches [173 cm]), so she was at about 80 percent of desirable weight. She had been maintained on multiple nutritional supplements, a low fat diet and her diarrhea when severe was controlled with paregoric. She is essentially intolerant to raw fruit and fruit juices, fried foods, legumes, corn, and some other raw vegetables.

On examination, the patient was thin with somewhat dry skin. The physical examination was otherwise within normal limits.

The patient was followed for a year and a half and has maintained her weight. She follows a 50 g fat diet and continues to take multiple vitamin and mineral supplements. Her main complaints are of hypothermia and insomnia. She continues to menstruate regularly with normal hormone levels. Her bone density is within normal limits. She alternates between one and two bowel movements daily versus up to 5 to 15 watery bowel movements, which she continues to control with paregoric. A major problem is with changes in drinking water.

Her laboratory values were all within normal limits, including vitamin A and zinc, which are included in her supplements. She has been maintained on her vitamin/mineral supplements and has followed a low fat diet with addition of MCT oil.

Bile Acid Diarrhea. When inadequate reabsorption of bile acids in the ileum permits their excretion into the colon, bile acid diarrhea follows. Water and electrolyte secretion is stimulated, with resultant diarrhea. Administration of cholestyramine or colestipol will bring improvement.

Fatty Acid Diarrhea and Oxaluria. Hydroxy fatty acids formed in the colon by bacteria in the presence of inadequate bile salts and fat malabsorption produce fatty acid diarrhea. Decreasing fat intake is indicated in these patients, and feeding medium chain triglycerides as an energy source may bring improvement in nutritional status. Oxaluria predisposing to oxalate stones correlates with steatorrhea. Excess unabsorbed free fatty acids in the intestinal lumen bind calcium, which is rendered unavailable to form a salt with oxalic acid. Sodium oxalate—which is more soluble—is formed and ab-

Table 21–5. OXALATE CONTENT
OF FOOD (PER 100 G)

>100 mg	70–100 mg	40–70 mg
Beets	Collards	Blackberries
Cocoa butter	Leeks	Celery
Parsley	Okra	Sweet potatoes
Peanuts		
Rhubarb		
Spinach		
Swiss chard		
Tea		
Wheat germ		

sorbed by the colon in the presence of bile acids not absorbed in the ileum. Trial of a low oxalate diet (Table 21–5) may not be effective, since only about 10 percent of the body's oxalate pool is derived from the diet. Calcium supplements are also prescribed.

Bacterial Overgrowth and Blind Loop Syndrome

The bacterial overgrowth syndrome reflects a combination of malabsorption and increased bacteria in the small intestine. Following surgical procedures such as Billroth II partial gastrectomy, the blind loop syndrome can result from luminal stasis or increased access of bacteria to the small intestine. Symptoms of bacterial overgrowth are weight loss with steatorrhea and vitamin B_{12} deficiency with megaloblastic anemia. Normal intestinal flora is less than 10^4 organisms per cc intestinal fluid in the jejunum, increasing to twice that amount in the distal ileum. The number of organisms in the colon increased markedly. In bacterial overgrowth, 10^6 to 10^{11} organisms per cc are found in the upper small intestine, with enteric coliform organisms and strict anaerobes predominating.

Bacterial overgrowth is a consequence of

- anatomic changes resulting from various surgical procedures on the stomach and small and large intestine
- structural and motility disorders of the gastrointestinal tract
- malnutrition
- immune deficiency states

Damage to the intestinal mucosa may result in decreased amounts of intestinal enzymes with malabsorption of sugars and amino acids. The effects of bile acids and hydroxy fatty acids in inducing diarrhea have been discussed previously. Vitamin B_{12} deficiency may result from tight binding of the vitamin B_{12}–intrinsic factor complexes to the cell surfaces of anaerobic bacteria, making the complexes unavailable for absorption. Inactive metabolites of vitamin B_{12} are produced by the abnormal intestinal bacteria, blocking attachment of vitamin B_{12} to intrinsic factors and the vitamin B_{12}–intrinsic factor complex to the ileal receptor.

Diagnosis is made by intestinal intubation with aspiration and culture of duodenal contents. The bile acid breath test is usually performed. Broad spectrum antibiotics are used, commonly tetracycline given for 10 days. At times a therapeutic trial of antibiotics follows an abnormal Schilling test of vitamin B_{12} absorption; if vitamin B_{12} absorption improves, this is presumptive of bacterial overgrowth.

Radiation Enteritis

Radiation therapy of 5000 rads or more to the small intestine produces nausea, diarrhea, and malabsorption in 10 to 20 days following exposure. Effects of radiation may be delayed months or years with development of ischemic endarteritis, fibrosis, and stricture.

Crohn's Disease

Any part of the gastrointestinal tract may become inflamed as a result of Crohn's disease (inflammatory bowel disease). Features of the chronic disease, the cause of which is unknown, are diarrhea, malabsorption, bleeding, obstruction from stricture, and fistulas. Anorexia is common, in association with cramping abdominal pain on eating. Decreased food intake along with malabsorption and excessive losses via the gastrointestinal tract may lead to serious malnutrition characterized by weight loss and multiple nutritional deficiencies. Corticosteroid therapy often results in severe bone demineralization. Extensive surgical resection results in the short bowel syndrome.

Treatment includes low residue and elemental diets with appropriate supplements to meet energy, protein, essential fatty acid, vitamin, and mineral needs. Many patients are intolerant of lactose and caffeine. Parenteral feeding is indicated in more severely malnourished patients or those with intractable pain, diarrhea, extensive fistulas, or prior to surgery. Zinc may be needed in addition to the usual vitamin or mineral supplements because of excessive gastrointestinal losses.

CASE 21b: CROHN'S DISEASE

A 49-year-old white woman was diagnosed as having Crohn's disease at age 30. Her terminal ileum and right colon were resected. Her current complaints were 4 to 6 weeks of increasing diarrhea with loose, watery, brown, large volume stools immediately after eating, occurring three to four times a day; and a 10 to 12 pound (4.5 to 5.5 kg) weight loss. She has noted fatigue and weakness, but no abdominal pain, nausea, or vomiting. Her appetite has remained good. Her long-term treatment has included cholestyramine, prednisone, and imodium.

Tuberculosis was treated with INH for 1 year; a left upper lobe coin lesion has been stable over the past 3 years. She became amenorrheic at the age of 34 and has a history of vertebral compression fractures.

Her height is 5 feet, 4½ inches and weight 92.5 pounds (75 percent IBW). The abdominal exam showed visible peristalsis and active bowel sounds. The stool was strongly positive for occult blood.

She was hospitalized to evaluate possible exacerbation of Crohn's disease and protein-calorie malnutrition and vitamin deficiencies. Spinal radiographs showed a compression fracture at T8 and loss of height in T9 and T5. This was attributed to probable osteoporosis, secondary to chronic glucocorticoid therapy. Bone densitometry showed the patient to be 2.6 standard deviations below the norm. Recommendation for therapy was to increase daily exercise and decrease the prednisone if possible. The patient was to continue on estrogen therapy.

Colonoscopy and gastrointestinal radiographs showed what was considered reactivation of Crohn's disease through a strictured area just proximal to the surgical anastomosis.

Abnormal low laboratory values were a hemoglobin of 9.1 g%, serum iron of 11 mg/dl, and a serum ferritin of 10 mg/dl. Levels of serum carotene was 25 μg/dl. Serum and RBC folate, vitamin B_{12}, vitamins A and E, prealbumin and retinal binding protein, zinc, 1,25-dihydroxy and 25-hydroxy vitamin D were within normal limits. Transferrin was increased to 449 mg/dl.

The patient received supplemental peripheral hyperalimentation and was placed on oral iron. The prednisone was continued for treatment of what was considered reactivation of her Crohn's disease. In follow-up, her hemoglobin had increased and her diarrhea was better controlled. She was given MCT supplements and protein supplements to a low fat, lactose-free, caffeine-free, low residue diet. She gained 7 lb (3 kg) in 3 months despite continued diarrhea. Her serum iron was 59 mg/dl.

LESSON:

This patient illustrates the symptomatic improvement achieved by bettering the nutritional status of the patient with Crohn's disease.

COLON

Diseases of the colon influencing nutritional status and/or managed by nutritional intervention include

- ulcerative colitis
- diverticular disease

- irritable bowel syndrome
- constipation

Colon cancer also may be related to antecedent dietary habits, and its treatment can have an impact on the patient's nutritional status (see Chapter 24).

Ulcerative Colitis

In contrast with Crohn's disease, ulcerative colitis involves only the colon and rectum in an inflammatory process of unknown etiology. The chief symptoms are diarrhea and rectal bleeding; abdominal pain is not prominent. Patients may have mild disease involving only the rectosigmoid with minimal systemic manifestations, or may be acutely ill. Weight loss occurs when severe disease induces anorexia. While malabsorption is not characteristic, lactose intolerance results from lactase deficiency as a side effect of active disease. Toxic megacolon may occur with a severe attack, in which case oral feeding should be withheld and the patient fed via the parenteral route. Those with mild or moderate symptoms may be managed with a high protein, low residue, lactose-free diet. Long chain fat may not be tolerated and the patient may require medium chain triglycerides. Patients with chronic ulcerative colitis may require nutritional support and/or vitamin and mineral supplementation; however, oral iron supplementation may not be well tolerated. The disease itself is currently treated with corticosteroids and salazosulfpyrine.

Patients with an ileostomy and subtotal colectomy must maintain adequate intake of water and sodium, normally reabsorbed in the colon. Their fluid intake should be about 2 liters per day, and more during hot weather.

Diverticulosis

Diverticulosis of the colon usually involves the sigmoid colon and may be asymptomatic or be complicated by acute inflammation, or diverticulitis. Hemorrhage, abscess formation, and/or perforation may ensue. Diverticula are more common in older individuals and occur only in people who ingest diets relatively low in fiber (less than 15 g per day). Diverticular disease is thus managed by a high fiber intake (more than 15 to 20 g per 1000 kcal) with increased stool bulk. Fiber should be increased gradually. (Fiber in the diet and its sources are discussed in Chapter 1. Adverse and therapeutic effects of a high fiber diet are also reviewed in Chapters 16, 18, and 19.) Remedies include bran (cellulose and hemicellulose), psyllium, (1 tsp two or three times daily), methylcellulose, and polycarbophil. The bulk laxative effect of fiber is due in part to its capacity to absorb and retain water, increase fecal weight, and promote peristalsis. Fiber also may influence intestinal and colonic ultrastructure. Patients may be advised to avoid ingesting small seeds of fruits, which may contribute to the development of diverticulitis.

Irritable Bowel Syndrome and Constipation

The high fiber diet also is used to treat the irritable bowel syndrome, with its symptoms of alternating diarrhea and constipation and intermittent abdominal pain. The symptoms generally do not occur at night, and weight loss is minimal. Intestinal gas with bloating and abdominal distention is common. In addition to fiber supplements, the diet should contain whole grains, fresh fruits, and green vegetables, while avoiding legumes, lentils, and certain fibrous fruits that are not digested and undergo bacterial fermentation.

Constipation alone should also be treated with stool softeners in addition to a diet containing bran, fruits, and vegetables; laxatives may be needed, but there is much abuse of these agents, especially among the elderly (see Chapter 9). Increasing physical activity and attention to hydration may be beneficial. It is important to investigate constipation of recent onset, which may be evidence of colon cancer.

CHAPTER 22

Hepatic and Pancreatic Disease

Because the liver has a vital role in the handling of nutrients, hepatic diseases influence nutritional status and are significant causes of malnutrition. In turn, nutritional deficiencies such as protein-energy malnutrition affect liver function adversely. Alcohol induces malnutrition directly by its effects on liver function and indirectly as a major cause of liver disease (see Chapter 17). Indeed, malnutrition is almost universal in patients with severe alcoholic liver disease. Finally, nutritional intervention is required in managing the patient with liver disease, especially in cases of encephalopathy.

Similarly, the pancreas is essential for digestion of complex macronutrients, and maldigestion resulting from pancreatic malfunction induces multiple nutritional deficiencies. Not only does alcohol-induced pancreatic disease result in impaired function, but also management of the disorder, especially with pseudocyst formation, may require aggressive nutritional support (see Chapter 12). Abnormalities of the endocrine function of the pancreas produce diabetes mellitus (see Chapter 18) and hypoglycemia (islet cell adenoma). (Liver and pancreatic neoplasms are discussed in Chapter 24, cystic fibrosis in Chapter 8.)

THE LIVER'S ROLE IN METABOLISM

Carbohydrate Metabolism

The liver plays an important biochemical role in carbohydrate, fat, and protein metabolism. Both glycogen synthesis and breakdown and gluconeogenesis are thus important metabolic functions of the liver (see Chapters 1 and 13). Diseases that impair these processes include the various forms of inherited glycogen storage disease (see Chapter 8), as well as the impaired glucose tolerance or hypoglycemia of liver disease. Hepatic disease results in hyperinsulinemia because of impaired insulin degradation; high insulin levels often are accompanied by increased circulating glucagon. Effects on glucose metabolism are determined by the absolute and relative amounts of these hormones. An excess of glucagon in relation to insulin results in a catabolic state.

Fat Metabolism

Increased fat in the liver (fatty liver) may result from excessive carbohydrate, fat, or alcohol intake, or the latter two combined, or it may occur in diabetes mellitus (see Chapters 17 and 18). There may be increased mobilization of fatty acid from adipose tissue; increased serum free fatty acids may increase the amount of unbound tryptophan by displacing tryptophan from albumin, thereby causing sleepiness. Fatty liver also results from increased fatty acid synthesis in the liver, or decreased fatty acid oxidation. The liver may be unable to effectively secrete triglyceride in triglyceride-rich lipoproteins (see Chapter 19). There may be impairment of lecithin-cholesterol acyltransferase activity in liver disease that results in low levels of circulating cholesterol esters.

Protein Metabolism

The liver synthesizes many important proteins, including albumin, fibrinogen, prothrombin and other clotting factors, haptoglobin, transferrin, and ceruloplasmin. Albumin functions to regulate osmotic pressure and is an important carrier protein. The body pool of albumin is about 500 g, distributed approximately 40 percent in the plasma, with 60 percent extravascular in skin, muscle, gut, and liver, and small amounts in bile, feces, sweat, and other secretions. The amount of albumin is determined by synthesis versus degradation, and the level in circulation also reflects its distribution. Six to 10 percent of plasma albumin is replaced daily, and 150 to 200 mg per kg, or about 12 g, is synthesized daily.

Albumin synthesis is rapid (15 to 20 minutes) and requires adequate protein intake. Its intravascular equilibration occurs within two or three circulations; equilibration in extravascular sites is much slower, requiring 7 to 10 days. Administration of intravenous albumin is indicated only when there is need for a transient rise in oncotic pressure, or preoperatively or postoperatively as a colloid vascular volume expander. Otherwise, albumin is best increased by correcting protein-energy malnutrition.

Vitamin-Mineral Metabolism

The role of the liver in vitamin and mineral metabolism is covered in Chapters 2, 14, and 17. Specific mineral metabolic disorders—Wilson's disease (copper) and hemochromatosis (iron)—cause liver disease (cirrhosis). Copper levels are also increased in cholestatic liver disorders.

Wilson's Disease

Copper accumulates in patients with Wilson's disease because of a genetic defect (see Chapter 14) that results in gross reductions in the rate of copper incorporation into ceruloplasmin and in the biliary secretion of copper. Nonceruloplasmin copper increases in plasma. This defect results in increased deposition of copper in the liver, impairing its function. Overflow from the liver results in copper deposits in the brain and kidney. Treatment of Wilson's disease is by chelation; some physicians also prescribe a low copper diet (see Chapters 2 and 14 for foods high in copper). Wilson's disease is the most frequent cause of chronic liver disease in American children.

Hemochromatosis

Iron storage disease (hemochromatosis) results in fibrosis of the liver, pancreas, endocrine glands, and the heart. Idiopathic hemochromatosis is treated by phlebotomy. Hemolytic anemias and transfusion may result in increased iron accumulation. Iron overload may result from increased dietary intake, especially in the presence of alcohol, which enhances iron absorption.

Amino Acid Metabolism

The role of the liver in amino acid metabolism is described in Chapters 1 and 13. In liver disease, amino acids normally metabolized by the liver may accumulate in the blood and cross the blood-brain barrier to influence brain function adversely (see discussion of hepatic encephalopathy further on). The diseased liver manifests decreased urea synthesis from ammonia, with resultant increase in blood ammonia levels.

Malnutrition

Liver disease results in malnutrition primarily because of poor dietary intake. Absorption of nutrients may be decreased, especially those requiring adequate bile secretion, and there may be abnormal metabolism of nutrients. Liver pathology may thus induce deficiencies of calcium, phosphorus, magnesium, or zinc as a consequence of diminished intake or excessive losses because the minerals are neither stored nor protein-bound. In chronic cholestatic liver disease, fat-soluble vitamin deficiencies occur along with hypercholesterolemia and steatorrhea; patients usually lose weight. Abnormalities in vitamin metabolism in liver disease include

- impaired phosphorylation of thiamin
- increased degradation of pyridoxal phosphate
- decrease in retinol-binding protein and defective transport of vitamin A (also related to low zinc levels)
- decreased 25-hydroxylation of vitamin D

DIET AND LIVER DISEASE

Diseases of the liver include

- fatty liver
- acute and chronic hepatitis and cirrhosis
- obstructive disease, either intrahepatic (cholestatic) or extrahepatic

The prevalence of the clinical features of alcohol-induced fatty liver, hepatitis, and cirrhosis is presented in Table 22–1.

- Fatty liver is relatively benign, reversible with removal of the inciting cause, and represents the earliest stage of alcoholic liver disease.

Table 22-1. CLINICAL FEATURES OF HOSPITALIZED
PATIENTS WITH ALCOHOLIC LIVER DISEASE

	Fatty Liver	Hepatitis	Cirrhosis
Hepatomegaly	75%	81%	Many
Jaundice	15%	46%	67%
Abdominal tenderness, pain	18%	46%	—
Ascites	—	35%	Common
Encephalopathy	—	11%	Variable
Spider nevi	8%	—	Common
Biochemical tests	Minimal ↑	Frequent ↑	Common ↑
Treatment	Abstinence from alcohol; regular diet	Abstinence; fluids; electrolytes; parenteral alimentation	Abstinence; if encephalopathic: 20–35 g protein → 70 g ?Vegetable protein ?BCAA*

*Branched chain amino acids.

- Hepatitis (inflammation of the liver) reflects liver necrosis and inflammation. Acute hepatitis may also be caused by viruses, drugs, and toxins. It also may resolve.
- Cirrhosis represents advanced fibrotic disease and is the least reversible liver disorder.

Hepatitis

Anorexia, nausea, and epigastric discomfort tend to reduce oral intake in hepatitis patients. Patients should be encouraged to eat a larger breakfast, since nausea usually is less in the morning. Viral hepatitis is self-limited. Patients generally can tolerate a relatively bland diet, avoiding very fatty foods; the aim should be to have the patient ingest 4 to 5 g carbohydrate per kg body weight. If oral intake is poor, glucose should be given intravenously. The patient with adequate hepatic function should be fed at least 25 kcal per kg, increasing to maintenance levels. Protein intake should be 70 to 80 g per day with the aim of producing positive nitrogen balance. Protein restriction (0.5 g per kg body weight) is needed only in patients with severe hepatic dysfunction and encephalopathy.

Encephalopathy

Symptoms and Diagnosis. Hepatic encephalopathy is characterized by

- personality change

- irritability
- weakness
- apathy
- confusion and somnolence

These symptoms may progress to coma. Patients may have apraxia, hypothermia, and asterixis and may show Babinski's response, rigidity, and/or spasticity. Encephalopathy may be provoked by increased protein intake or gastrointestinal hemorrhage. The electroencephalogram is abnormal. Blood ammonia levels are increased. In chronic liver disease the plasma amino acid pattern shows increased levels of methionine, the aromatic amino acids, glutamic and aspartic acids, and histidine, with decreased levels of branched chain amino acids.

Management. Management of the patient with hepatic encephalopathy requires the following steps:

1. Restricted but adequate protein intake
2. Adequate calories and carbohydrate
3. Restricted water and sodium
4. No sedation
5. Correction of electrolyte imbalance, especially low potassium
6. Control of infection with broad spectrum antibiotics, if necessary
7. Neomycin 3 to 4 g per day in divided doses and/or lactulose 20 to 30 g three times daily
8. Laxatives or enemas

Steps 7 and 8 serve to reduce ammonia levels. Bacteria in the colon produce ammonia that is absorbed and that the diseased liver cannot detoxify. With this regimen, improvement should be observed in 80 percent of patients within 1 or 2 days.

Management of Pre-Encephalopathic Patients. Patients with severe liver disease who are in a pre-encephalopathic state may be managed by providing protein adequate to maintain nitrogen balance (intake greater than 40 g) in the form of an amino acid formulation enriched in branched chain amino acids (up to 50 percent of total) and with decreased methionine and aromatic amino acids (see Chapters 1, 11, and 12). Foods high in ammonia content should be avoided, including salami, lima beans, egg yolk, bacon, and blue and cheddar cheeses. Vegetable protein may be better tolerated than animal protein because of its amino acid content (see Chapter 1).

Cirrhosis

Cirrhotic patients are evaluated and classified as stable or as having edema, ascites, and/or encephalopathy. Stable cirrhotics tolerate a good protein intake but should avoid excessive sodium and should take a multivitamin supplement daily.

Cirrhotics develop edema and ascites with increases in total body water secondary to sodium retention. Diminished free water clearance due to increased levels of antidiuretic hormone may be observed in end-stage cirrhosis. These patients retain sodium because of increased renal tubular reabsorption of sodium due to secondary hyperaldosteronism resulting from renal vasoconstriction. Hyponatremia is common, with serum sodium less than 130 mEq per liter, and normal or low serum potassium levels. If alkalosis should develop, encephalopathy may be precipitated by the facilitated conversion of ammonium ion to ammonia, which crosses the blood-brain barrier.

Management of edematous patients includes these steps:

1. Reducing sodium intake to 500 to 1000 mg, depending on the degree of edema.
2. Decreasing fluid intake to less than 1 liter per day if serum sodium is low.

And for increasing severity:

3. Use of aldosterone antagonists.
4. Use of sodium-excreting diuretics.
5. Administering albumin and/or performing paracentesis.

Steps 3 to 5 are added for management of the patient with ascites, a condition suspected in those with weight gain and increased abdominal girth who may also manifest symptoms of shortness of breath and ankle edema. These patients commonly have mild steatorrhea due to decreased bile salt secretion. They also have portal hypertension, hypoalbuminemia, alterations in renal and endocrine functions, and abnormal lymph flow. Many have hypokalemia from vomiting and diarrhea, and may manifest muscle wasting and renal tubular acidosis. Serum levels of zinc, calcium, and magnesium are low. One fourth to one half of these patients do not survive the year.

Chronic Cholestatic Liver Disease

Obstruction of bile canaliculi within the liver produces cholestatic jaundice, often due to hypersensitivity to drugs. These patients should be given fat-soluble vitamins monthly by the parenteral route, including vitamins A and D, 100,000 units, and vitamin K, 15 mg. Their diet should be reduced in long chain fats, and medium chain triglycerides should be used. Calcium supplements should be provided, and copper-containing foods avoided (see Chapter 2).

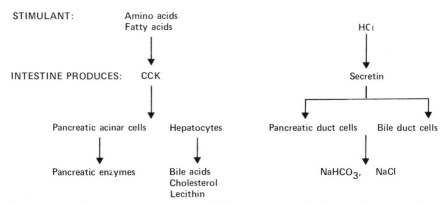

Figure 22-1. Control of pancreatic and biliary secretion by diet and intestinal hormones. (Adapted from Floch, M.H.: Nutrition and Diet Therapy in Gastrointestinal Disease. Plenum Publishing, New York, 1981, pp 19, 21.)

SECRETION OF BILE AND PANCREATIC JUICE

Both biliary and pancreatic secretions are stimulated by the products of digestion (amino acids and fatty acids) and by gastric acid (Fig. 22-1). Cholecystokinin stimulates the hepatocytes to secrete bile constituents (bile acids, cholesterol, lecithin) and pancreatic acinar cells to secrete pancreatic enzymes (trypsin, chymotrypsin, peptidases and other proteolytic enzymes, amylase, and lipase). Secretin stimulates the bile and pancreatic duct cells to produce bicarbonate, sodium, and chloride.

Defects

- Defective biliary secretion induces gallstone formation when lithogenic bile is produced.
- Absence of bile salts impairs fat absorption and eliminates cholesterol absorption.
- Defective pancreatic enzyme production produces maldigestion of fat and protein and vitamin B_{12} malabsorption due to defective binding.

Steatorrhea will thus result from hepatic or pancreatic insufficiency.

PANCREATITIS

Recurrent or chronic pancreatitis results early in increased secretion and later in diminished secretion. Patients with the disorder may have protein malnutrition and resulting malabsorption (see Chapters 13, 17, and 21), as well as maldigestion. Chronic, excessive use of ethanol is the most common cause of pancreatitis (up to 75 percent). Biliary tract disease (gallstones) is present in 10 to 70 percent of pancreatitis patients. In one third of patients, causes of acute or chronic pancreatitis may include

- associated trauma
- use of steroids, thiazides, or estrogens
- viral infection
- vasculitis
- pregnancy
- hereditary or metabolic factors

Acute Pancreatitis

Patients with acute pancreatitis develop severe epigastric or periumbilical pain radiating to the back 12 to 48 hours after a bout of drinking. There is associated nausea and vomiting, with increase in serum amylase. Various additional signs and symptoms may occur:

- Because glucose intolerance may be present, blood and urine glucose should be monitored.
- Patients may have hyperlipidemia (see section on Hyperlipidemia, further on).
- Serum calcium levels may decrease markedly in some patients.
- Maldigestion will occur with 90 percent loss of pancreatic function; this may develop with a single, severe bout of pancreatitis, or with recurrent episodes.

Management

Treatment is supportive, with nasogastric suction and intravenous fluids and electrolytes. Pain relief should be provided. Diet should be introduced slowly with subsidence of symptoms, starting with clear liquids or an elemental formula, and avoiding fatty foods.

Hyperlipidemia

Patients with acute pancreatitis may develop hyperlipidemia, with elevated cholesterol and triglycerides and chylomicronemia. Conversely, those with type 5 hyperlipoproteinemia may develop episodes of acute pancreatitis as triglyceride levels approach 1000 mg per dl (see Chapter 19). Chylomicronemia responds to withdrawal of long chain fat from the diet.

Table 22-2. SOME COMMERCIAL
PANCREATIC ENZYME PREPARATIONS

Product	Manufacturer	Type	Activity Per Capsule or Tablet, USP Units		
			Protease	*Amylase*	*Lipase*
Cotazym	Organon	C	30,000	30,000	8,000
Pancrease	McNeil	C	25,000	20,000	4,000
Pancreatin*	Vitaline	T	60,000 N.F.	60,000	12,000
Viokase	Viobin	T	30,000	30,000	8,000

T = tablet; C = capsule.
*N.F. units.

Chronic Pancreatitis

This condition is diagnosed by performing endoscopic retrograde cannulation of the pancreas (ERCP). With chronic pancreatitis, 25 percent of patients will have endocrine pancreatic insufficiency; the incidence rises to 75 percent in the presence of pancreatic calcification. In order to prevent diarrhea and steatorrhea, patients may require treatment with pancreatic enzymes (Table 22-2), which should be given with meals and snacks. Administration of vitamin B_{12} may be required to treat deficiency.

Patients with exocrine pancreatic insufficiency are managed on a low fat diet, using medium chain triglycerides as a source of fat. Triglycerides of fatty acids of 6 to 12 carbon chain length are hydrolyzed more readily than triglycerides containing long chain fatty acids, may be absorbed directly without digestion by pancreatic lipase, do not require bile salts for solubilization, and are transported via the portal vein directly to the liver. The diet should be adequate in protein.

Pseudocyst

Patients with chronic pancreatitis who develop pseudocyst may be placed on no oral intake and be maintained by total parenteral nutrition (see Chapter 12) until the pseudocyst matures. Treatment is by surgical excision if the pseudocyst does not resolve spontaneously. The process usually takes about 6 weeks. Management requires careful attention to blood glucose and lipid levels, with appropriate adjustment of the TPN regimen.

Acute and Chronic Renal Failure

The kidney functions as an organ of excretion through specific mechanisms of glomerular filtration and renal tubular secretion; it also serves to conserve substances by tubular reabsorption. The end products of protein metabolism—urea, creatinine, uric acid, ammonia, amino acids—are filtered and excreted (see Chapter 1). Extrarenal production of urea amounts to about 20 percent of the total produced, and yields ammonia and CO_2 from the action of bacteria in the gastrointestinal tract. The electrolytes (sodium, potassium, calcium, phosphate, magnesium) and the trace minerals (iron and zinc) are variously filtered, reabsorbed and/or secreted by the kidney, which is important in controlling their status in the body. The kidney also maintains fluid balance and pH by secretion of hydrogen ion, which is derived primarily from protein catabolism. Additional important functions of the kidney include

- blood pressure regulation (renin)
- erythropoiesis (erythropoietin)
- vitamin D activation by hydroxylation
- amino acid metabolism (glutamine catabolism, synthesis of alanine, production of serine from glycine)
- gluconeogenesis (see Chapters 1 and 13)
- destruction of peptide hormones (gastrin, insulin, parathormone, glucagon, thyrotropin)

This chapter describes the etiology, clinical manifestations, and pathophysiology of the syndromes of acute and chronic renal failure, then focuses on nutritional implications and management. Nutritional therapy for the patient undergoing dialysis also is discussed.

ACUTE RENAL FAILURE

Acute renal failure (ARF) is defined as a sudden fall or cessation of glomerular filtration. ARF is caused by acute tubular necrosis about 75 percent of the time. Two to 3 weeks are needed for recovery of renal function, provided the patient recovers from the underlying illness.

Causes

The important precipitating factors of ARF include

- post-trauma
- surgical shock with significant fall in blood pressure lasting more than 5 minutes
- pregnancy
- toxic metals
- organic compounds
- halogenated hydrocarbons (anesthetics)
- drugs (some antibiotics, analgesics)
- radiographic contrast media
- acute glomerulonephritis
- obstruction by renal stones or tumor
- occlusion of renal blood vessels
- renal papillary necrosis
- sepsis
- rhabdomyolysis

Sepsis, rhabdomyolysis, and shock produce catabolic states with nitrogen loss four times that of other causes of ARF. The marked net protein breakdown yields a sharp rise in plasma potassium, phosphorus, and nitrogen, together with a fall in pH.

Symptoms, Signs, and Laboratory Tests

The hallmark of ARF is the development of oliguria or anuria lasting from days to weeks. On average, recovery occurs in about 11 days, bringing an increase in urine volume of low specific gravity. Various associated symptoms may be present:

- Symptoms of anorexia, nausea, and vomiting are common, and many patients are unable to eat.
- Fluid retention will develop if the usual food and fluid intake persists.
- Many patients experience ileus.
- Gastrointestinal bleeding may occur due to elevated levels of gastrin and gastric acid, and patients may develop anemia.
- Patients are susceptible to infection.
- Excretion of nitrogenous metabolites decreases and plasma concentrations of urea, uric acid, and creatinine increase.
- Electrolyte abnormalities include decreases in serum sodium and calcium, and increases in potassium and phosphate. Hypertension and edema result.
- Hyperkalemia may result in cardiac arrhythmia and arrest (see Chapter 14).
- Acidosis may develop from impairment of sulfate and hydrogen ion excretion.
- There is an increase in hepatic gluconeogenesis, perhaps related to increased glucagon levels, with increased rates of transamination and increased activity of urea cycle enzymes (see Chapters 1 and 13). Patients are in a catabolic state.

Nutritional Therapy

Nutritional management of the ARF patient must provide adequate calories and protein and tailor intake of sodium, potassium, water, and alkali. Most patients undergo dialysis, permitting liberalization of nitrogen, energy, mineral, and fluid intake. The goals of nutritional therapy are

1. to diminish uremic toxicity and its associated metabolic derangements

2. to maintain or improve nutritional status with resultant favorable impact on wound healing, immune function, and resistance to infection
3. to facilitate repair of the kidney

Specific features of the nutritional management regimen include providing

- fluid daily in the amount of 400 to 500 ml plus the urine output and other measured sources of fluid loss
- calories to maintain body weight
- protein—the amount depending on the glomerular filtration rate (GFR) and whether the patient is dialyzed (see section on Chronic Renal Failure, further on)
- sodium intake to equal output

In addition, potassium is monitored, dietary potassium intake is minimized, and phosphorus and magnesium intakes are restricted to prevent accumulation.

Parenteral Alimentation With and Without Dialysis

Patients requiring parenteral alimentation who are not being dialyzed should receive 21 to 30 g essential amino acids (including histidine) daily. This is provided by administering 2 liters of a commercially available renal TPN formula (see Table 12–4). Nutritional therapy can be more aggressive in patients undergoing dialysis. Standard amino acid solutions (see Chapter 12) can be infused to provide protein in amounts of 1 to 1.5 g per kg body weight, providing a total of 12 g amino acid nitrogen or 70 to 100 g protein per day for the average male patient. This level of protein can be infused in 2 to 3 liters of fluid along with sufficient glucose to provide 35 to 50 kcal per kg per day. Electrolytes, vitamins, and insulin should be added to meet the recommended intake for uremic patients (Table 23–1).

Supplementation for Patients With Enteral Alimentation

The patient who is taking some nutrients by mouth can be given additional calories by providing lipid peripheral intravenous infusion (see Chapter 12). The tube-fed patient can be given a carbohydrate-rich formula supplemented with lipid by peripheral intravenous infusion. Essential amino acids may be supplied by the intravenous route or given in an enteral formula (Tables 23–2 and 23–3).

CHRONIC RENAL FAILURE (UREMIA)

Approximately 40,000 to 45,000 patients develop chronic renal failure (CRF) each year; about 20 percent enter a chronic dialysis program. CRF

Table 23-1. COMPOSITION OF
TPN SOLUTION FOR PATIENTS
WITH ACUTE OR CHRONIC
RENAL FAILURE

Volume (liters)	1.0
Dextrose (D-glucose) (g/l)	350
Essential and nonessential amino acids (g/l)	42.5–50
Energy (kcal/l)	1339–1365
Electrolytes, minerals	
Sodium (mEq/l)	50
Chloride (mEq/l)	25–35
Potassium (mEq/day)	40
Acetate (mEq/l)	35–40
Calcium (mEq/day)	10
Phosphorus (mEq/day)	20
Magnesium (mEq/day)	8
Iron (mEq/day)	2
Vitamins	
Vitamin A (USP units/day)	—
Vitamin K (mg/week)	4
Vitamin D (USP units/day)	Not established
Vitamin E (IU/day)	10
Niacin (mg/day)	20
Thiamin HCl (B_1) (mg/day)	2
Riboflavin (B_2) (mg/day)	2
Pantothenic acid (mg/day)	10
Pyridoxine HCl (B_6) (mg/day)	10
Ascorbic acid (C) (mg/day)	100
Biotin (μg/day)	200
Folic acid (mg/day)	1
Vitamin B_{12} (μg/day)	4

(Adapted from Fischer, J.E. (ed.): Surgical Nutrition. Little,
Brown, Boston, 1983, p. 583.)

develops with loss of 50 to 75 percent of renal function. In almost half of the
patients the cause of CRF is chronic glomerulonephritis; the remainder have
pyelonephritis, polycystic kidneys, renovascular disease (hypertension), diabetes, obstruction, or drug-induced disease. Azotemia, or nitrogen retention,
is symptomatic (nausea, vomiting, lethargy, and tremors) when elevations of
serum urea nitrogen exceed 150 mg per dl (see also section on Symptoms,
further on). Hypertension and congestive heart failure, with headache and
edema, indicate disordered volume regulation and accumulation of extracellular fluid. These symptoms occur when the glomerular filtration rate (GRF)
is less than 4 to 10 ml per minute.

Table 23–2. PROTEIN COMPOSITION
OF RENAL ENTERAL FORMULAS

Protein Composition	Amin-Aid (McGaw) 4 pkg/day	Travasorb Renal (Travenol) 6 pkg/day
Total Amino Acids, g	26.4	48
Total nitrogen, g	3.2	7.3
Essential Amino Acids, g		
Leucine	4.4	4.44
Isoleucine	2.8	3.72
Valine	3.2	5.52
Lysine	3.2	3.30
Methionine	4.4	4.20
Phenylalanine	4.4	3.60
Threonine	2.0	2.76
Tryptophan	1.0	1.20
Total	25.4	28.74
Nonessential Amino Acids, g		
Histidine	1.0	3.12
Arginine	—	3.84
Proline	—	2.76
Glycine	—	2.58
Alanine	—	4.08
Serine	—	2.58
Tyrosine	—	6.36
Total	1.0	25.32

Metabolic Derangements

Polydipsia, polyuria, and nocturnal frequency indicate failure of the kidney's concentrating ability (isosthenuria).

- As the GFR decreases to less than 40 ml per minute, patients develop hyperphosphatemia.
- Hypocalcemia and low vitamin D levels are attributed to secondary hyperparathyroidism, which develops with loss of 25 percent of renal function.
- Soft tissue calcinosis and renal osteodystrophy develop. These mineral metabolic derangements may increase at the rate of progression of renal failure.
- Bone demineralization occurs in 40 to 90 percent of patients with bone pain and pathologic fractures.

Table 23-3. RENAL ENTERAL FORMULAS

Characteristics	Amin-Aid (McGaw) 4 pkg/day	Travasorb Renal (Travenol) 6 pkg/day
Volume, ml	1360	2100
Water, ml	1000	1620
Total calories, kcal	2660	2800
Nonprotein calories, kcal	2552	2608
Protein, amino acids, g	26.4	48
Carbohydrate, g	497	568
Carbohydrate composition	Maltodextrins, sugar, citric acid	Glucose, oligosaccharides, sucrose
Fat, g	62.8	37.2
Fat, composition	Partially hydrogenated soy, lecithin, monoglycerides, diglycerides	MCT:sunflower oil 70:30
Nitrogen	4.2	7.7
Protein, % calories	4.0	6.9
Carbohydrate, % calories	74.8	81.1
Fat, % calories	21.2	12.0
Concentration, kcal/ml	2.0	1.35
Osmolarity, mOsm/l	850	470
Electrolytes/Other minerals	0	0
Vitamins, % USRDA	0	C 150, Folic acid 250, B_1 100, B_2 100, Niacin 100, B_6 500, Biotin 200, Pantothenic acid 100
Flavors	Lemon-lime, orange, berry, strawberry	Apricot, strawberry
Cost	$27.20	$34.20

- Serum magnesium levels may increase with ingestion of magnesium-containing antacids.
- Bicarbonate wastage occurs, contributing to the acidosis that results from retained hydrogen ions. The acidosis worsens bone resorption.

Fluid and Electrolytes

Postural hypotension and rales are clues to sodium and water status. Dilutional hyponatremia is common in patients with CRF. Some patients are sodium depleted with reduction in extracellular fluid and blood volumes, causing worsening of low levels of renal blood flow and GFR. Weight changes are indications of fluid status. Serum potassium levels may be increased because of excessive intake, acidosis, oliguria, hypoaldosteronism, or effect of catabolic stress. With tubular disease, potassium may be lost, with development of hypokalemia. Hypertension, edema, and features of water intoxication develop.

Micronutrients and Hormones

- Levels of retinol-binding protein and vitamin A are increased in CRF patients
- Vitamin B_6 clearance is enhanced.
- Trace mineral levels (iron, zinc, copper) are decreased, although aluminum levels may increase.
- Patients develop glucose intolerance or frank diabetes mellitus due to insulin resistance.
- Hyperuricemia may result in symptomatic gouty arthritis.
- Type 4 hyperlipidemia develops.
- Serum insulin, parathormone, glucagon, growth hormone, gastrin, prolactin, and LH levels are raised, while levels of somatostatin, erythropoietin, and 1,25-dihydroxy vitamin D decrease.
- Renin levels may be high or low.
- Serum protein levels decrease.
- Conversion of phenylalanine to tyrosine is impaired, so that tyrosine (as well as histidine and arginine) may be an essential amino acid in the uremic patient.
- There is decreased glutamine catabolism and diminished conversion of glycine to serine.
- Serum levels of leucine and valine are decreased, with increases in methionine, cystine, and citrulline.

Symptoms

Symptoms of CRF include anorexia, nausea, hiccups, fatigue, weakness, thirst, itching, chest pain and pericarditis, irritability, drowsiness, confusion, peripheral neuropathy, purpura, and normochromic, normocytic anemia. Vascular complications include ischemic heart disease and stroke. Uremic symptoms develop when the GFR is 10 to 15 ml per minute, creatinine clearance falls to 20 ml per minute, and serum urea nitrogen reaches 90 mg per dl.

The uremic patient is wasted and malnourished primarily because of poor intake. This is related in part to the restrictive diet; for example, potassium and phosphate restriction limits vitamin content. Blood loss and intercurrent illness also worsen nutritional status. The malnutrition causes greater susceptibility to infection and leads to poor wound healing and diminished strength.

Nutritional Therapy

The role of nutrition in the management of chronic renal failure is related to the stage of the disease. The patient who has lost 20 to 50 percent of renal function is in the predialysis stage, while one who has lost more than 50 percent requires dialysis. With 20 percent loss of renal function, the regimen may be varied. Dietary modifications can decrease uremic symptoms and delay progression of disease and the need for dialysis. In addition, adequate intake of dietary fiber (15 to 20 g per 1000 kcal) is recommended to optimize bowel function. A high protein intake, on the other hand, may hasten renal failure.

Protein and Calories

Protein intake is regulated in an attempt to keep serum urea nitrogen (SUN) below 80 mg per dl, or better, below 60 mg per dl. In the absence of dialysis, such regulation is accomplished by providing a graded level of protein intake in accordance with the GFR (Table 23–4). The patient with a GFR exceeding 25 ml per minute is allowed 1.3 g protein per kg body weight, or 60 to 90 g per day, while the patient with a GFR less than 10 ml per minute is limited to 0.55 to 0.6 g per kg, or about 40 g protein for men and 35 g for women (Table 23–5). Sixty percent of the protein should be of high biologic value and rich in essential amino acids (Table 23–6; see also Chapter 1). For the patient with a GFR less than 4 to 5 ml per minute who is not dialyzed, protein intake may be limited to the essential amino acids or to a combination of these and a very low protein diet (15 to 25 g). Calories are then provided in the form of a semisynthetic electrolyte- and nitrogen-free, oligosaccharide liquid or powder (see Chapter 11). For those patients unable to tolerate oral intake, the eight to nine essential amino acids may be infused intravenously (histidine is essential in uremic patients). A higher energy intake is needed with protein restriction (see Chapters 1 and 13). The keto acid analogues of the amino acids (except lysine and threonine) may be provided as calcium or ornithine salts. Such preparations are not yet available in the United States.

Table 23–4. PROTEIN INTAKE IN RENAL FAILURE

GFR (ml/min)	Protein	
	g/kg	Total, g
< 25	1.3	60–90
15–20	< 1	50–70
10–15	< 0.7	40–55
< 10	0.55–0.6	35–40
< 4–5	Dialysis	

Table 23–5. RECOMMENDED DIETARY INTAKES FOR
PATIENTS WITH CHRONIC RENAL FAILURE MANAGED
WITH OR WITHOUT MAINTENANCE DIALYSIS

Component	No Dialysis*	Hemodialysis (HD) or Peritoneal Dialysis (PD)
Water	Up to 3000 ml/day	Usually 750–1500 ml/day
Minerals	Range	
Sodium (mg/day)	1000–3000	750–1000
Potassium (mEq/day)	40–70	40–70
Phosphorus (mg/day)[‡]	600–1200	60–1200
Calcium (mg/day)	1000–2000[§]	1000–1500[§]
Magnesium (mg/day)	200–300	200–300
Iron (mg tid)	As needed	Ferrous sulfate, 320
Vitamins	Supplementation	
Thiamin (mg/day)	1.5	1.5
Riboflavin (mg/day)	1.8	1.8
Pantothenic acid (mg/day)	5	5
Niacin (mg/day)	20	20
Pyridoxine HCl (mg/day)[†]	5	10
B_{12} (μg/day)	3	3
C (mg/day)[†]	70–100	100
Folic acid (mg/day)[†]	1	1
A	None	None
D	Not established	Not established
E (IU/day)	15	15
Calories	≥ 35 kcal/kg/day unless patient is obese	> 35 kcal/kg/day
Protein	Men: ≥ 40 g/day (0.60 g/kg/day) (28 g of high biologic value) Women, small men: ≥ 35 g/day (25 g of high biologic value)	HD: 1.0 g/kg/day PD: 1.2–1.5 g/kg/day (> 50% of high biologic value)

(Adapted from Kopple, J.D.: Nutritional management of renal failure. Postgrad Med 64:135, 1978, and from Feldman, E.B.: Nutrition in the Middle and Later Years. Wright PSG, Littleton, MA, 1983, pp. 176–177.)
*Glomerular filtration rate > 4–5 ml/min but < 15–25 ml/min.
†Exceed RDA.
‡Phosphate binders (aluminum carbonate, aluminum hydroxide) usually needed as well.
§Dietary intake must be supplemented to provide these levels; 25 mg if SGOT < 10.

Table 23-6. PROTEIN QUALITY
OF FOODS

High Biologic Value Protein
7 g protein per ounce
  Eggs (1)
  Fish
  Fowl (chicken, duck, turkey)
  Meat (beef, lamb, liver, pork, veal)
Low Biologic Value Protein
1 to 2 g protein per 1/2 cup
  Cereals and bread
  Vegetables:
    Tubers and roots (potatoes, yams, sweet
    potatoes)
    Leaves (spinach, collard greens)
    Legumes (peas, beans)
  Nuts
  Yeast

(From Feldman, E.B.: Nutrition in the Middle and Later Years. Wright PSG, Littleton, MA, 1983, p. 179, with permission.)

Severe Protein Restriction. Before the wide availability of dialysis for patients with CRF, attempts were made to control uremic symptoms by diets severely restricted in protein. An example is the Giordano-Giovanetti diet, which provides 20 g per day of protein, primarily from two eggs. A sample low protein menu for a day is shown in Table 23–7. These patients need supplements of methionine and vitamins.

Aminogram Results. The plasma (or CSF) aminogram in the protein-restricted patient with CRF compared with normal levels (Fig. 23–1) shows decreased levels of valine, leucine, isoleucine, lysine and threonine, and serine; increased levels of methionine and cystine; and normal levels of phenylalanine and decreased tyrosine. Free tryptophan levels may be altered from normal.

Fluid and Electrolytes

Water intake is limited to 1.5 to 3 liters per day, or 500 ml plus urine output. Sodium intake is limited to 43 to 130 mmol per day, or 1 to 3 g, and is adjusted according to urinary sodium excretion. Patients with no edema, hypertension, or heart failure can tolerate more sodium, which can be cautiously increased. With dilutional hyponatremia, water should be restricted

Table 23-7. SAMPLE MENU FOR
PATIENT WITH CHRONIC
RENAL FAILURE PREDIALYSIS*

Breakfast
  1/2 broiled grapefruit*
  1 blueberry muffin*
  3/4 cup (180 cc) coffee or tea, sugar to taste
Lunch
  1 serving pizza*
  1 serving tossed green salad*
  1 slice low protein bread,* 1 tsp salt-free
    margarine
  1 slice (1/6) lemon pie*
  3/4 cup (180 cc) coffee or tea, sugar to taste
Snack
  2 chocolate chip cookies*
Dinner
  1 slice (1/8) honeydew melon or (1/4) cantaloupe
  1 serving omelet aux fines herbes*
  1/2 cup cooked rice, 1 tsp salt-free margarine
  2/3 cup cooked green beans (fresh or frozen) with
    dill, or 2/3 cup cooked asparagus (fresh or
    frozen)
  1 serving peppermint cream dessert*
Snack
  4 scotch shortbread cookies*
  1/2 cup (120 cc) coffee or tea, sugar to taste
Sample menu provides:

Protein	17.45 g
Calories	2471
Sodium	490 mg (21.3 mEq)
Potassium	1592 mg (40.8 mEq)
Fluid	1040 cc

*Specially designed recipes in Margie, J.D., Anderson, C.F.,
Nelson, R.A., and Hunt, J.C.: The Mayo Clinic Renal Diet
Cookbook. Golden Press, New York, 1974.

to 800 to 1000 ml per day. Body weight is monitored, and patients usually are
slightly edematous. Potassium intake should be limited to 70 mEq per day.

Serum phosphorus is maintained at a low normal level, 2 to 3 mg per dl,
with phosphorus intake limited to 600 to 1200 mg per day, or even as low as
300 to 700 mg. This is accomplished by eliminating milk and milk products.
Calcium is supplemented at 1 to 2 g per day in the form of calcium lactate or
carbonate. Acidotic patients with pH less than 7.35 should be given bicarbonate when CO_2 levels are less than 15 to 20 mEq per liter.

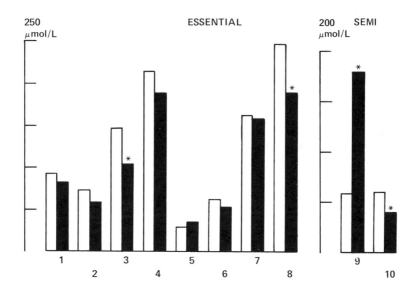

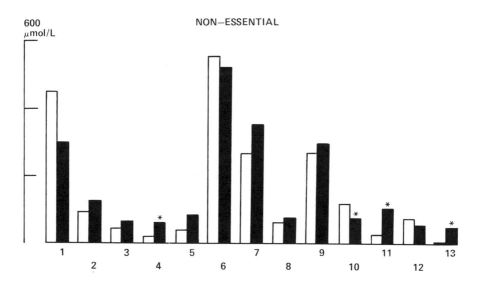

Figure 23-1. Levels of plasma amino acids in patients with chronic renal failure *(solid bars)* in comparison to the plasma amino acid pattern of healthy people *(clear bars)*. The essential amino acids are *(1)* histidine, *(2)* isoleucine, *(3)* leucine, *(4)* lysine, *(5)* methionine, *(6)* phenylalanine, *(7)* threonine, *(8)* valine. Semiessential amino acids are *(9)* cystine, *(10)* tyrosine. Nonessential amino acids are *(1)* alanine, *(2)* arginine, *(3)* asparagine, *(4)* aspartic acid, *(5)* glutamic acid, *(6)* glutamine, *(7)* glycine, *(8)* ornithine, *(9)* proline, *(10)* serine, *(11)* citrulline, *(12)* taurine, *(13)* N-methylhistidine. Values marked * differ significantly from normal.

Vitamins

Vitamin D may also be provided but is not recommended when serum phosphorus is increased or if the product of calcium and phosphorus concentration exceeds 55. The point at which vitamin D should be provided in renal failure is controversial. Because of the restricted diet, other vitamins—except vitamin A—are needed. A multivitamin supplement suggested for the CRF patient provides vitamin C 70 to 100 mg per day, vitamin B_6 5 mg, folate 1 mg, and other vitamins to meet the RDA (see Table 23-6). Nutritional status should be periodically assessed (see Chapter 3).

NUTRITIONAL THERAPY FOR THE DIALYSIS PATIENT

The patient maintained on dialysis has special nutritional requirements relating to intake of protein, calories, fluids and electrolytes, and vitamins and trace minerals. In addition, a "prudent" diet is recommended to control hyperlipidemia (see Chapter 19).

Protein and Calories

The hemodialysis patient routinely loses 20 g protein in a 6 to 8 hour treatment, or 6 to 7 g free amino acids over 4 hours. These treatments are typically done three times a week. Dietary protein is not rigorously restricted but is provided at about 1 to 1.2 g per kg per day, with one half to two thirds of high biologic value (see Table 23-5). Because protein losses in continuous ambulatory peritoneal dialysis are higher, with estimates of 9 to 22 g loss over 10 to 24 hours (equating to 1.5 to 5 g amino acids), protein intake should be further increased in such patients, to 1.2 to 1.5 g per kg per day.

Calories are provided at a level of 35 kcal per kg per day, with provision of adequate amounts of complex carbohydrates. Patients undergoing continuous ambulatory peritoneal dialysis receive about 180 g glucose per exchange and may become obese. Hemodialysis with glucose-free solution removes 20 to 50 g glucose over 4 to 6 hours.

Fluid and Electrolytes

Intake of sodium (1 to 1.5 g) and water (750 to 1500 ml) should be regulated to maintain body weight between dialysis treatments. Sodium should be decreased if blood pressure rises. The water content of food must be considered in addition to liquid intake. For example, fruits and vegetables are 85 to 90 percent water, cooked cereal 70 to 85 percent, and meat 45 to 60 percent.

From 30 to 70 mEq of potassium are provided daily in food. Serum calcium should be maintained at 10.5 to 11 mg per dl, with reduction of serum phosphorus achieved through use of aluminum antacids. Calcium 1 to 1.5 g per day should be provided.

Vitamins and Trace Minerals

With appropriate indications and monitoring of serum calcium, 1,25-dihydroxy vitamin D may be given, 0.25 to 0.5 μg per day. Other vitamins and trace minerals needed by the dialysis patient include vitamin C 100 mg per day, vitamin B_6 10 mg per day, zinc (220 mg zinc sulfate), and iron (300 mg three times per day ferrous sulfate). The last is required because of the blood loss in dialysis—from 5 to 20 ml per treatment.

Supplementation

Amino acids and glucose may be supplemented during hemodialysis to improve nutritional status. For example, 20 to 30 g essential amino acids may be infused near the end of dialysis, or 40 to 42 g of a mixture of essential and nonessential amino acids, with 150 to 200 g glucose infused at a constant rate into the blood leaving the dialyzer. In the latter case, the patient is fed a high carbohydrate snack 20 to 30 minutes before the end of the infusion to prevent rebound hypoglycemia.

Specific Nutritional Regimens

The specific of nutritional regimens for patients with chronic renal failure with and without dialysis are shown in Table 23–5, and characteristics of special renal enteral and parenteral formulations are shown in Tables 12–4 and 23–3.

OTHER RENAL DISEASES

Nutritional status is also affected by other renal diseases:

- In the nephrotic syndrome, there are excessive urinary protein losses and secondary hyperlipidemia, which are managed with provision of

2 g per kg protein daily and with restriction of fat to less than 30 percent of total caloric intake.

- The hepatorenal syndrome superimposes renal failure on hepatic failure (see Chapter 22). A form of prerenal azotemia, it may respond to appropriate increase in renal perfusion.
- Renal calculi may be managed with provision of high water intake and limited oxalate dietary intake (see Chapter 21).

CHAPTER 24

Cancer

Cancer is another significant chronic disorder in which diet may contribute to both the etiology and the treatment. In addition, the presence of a tumor profoundly affects the host's nutritional and metabolic status, and cancer treatment regimens unquestionably have an impact upon the patient's nutritional status. Cancer is a leading cause of death in the Western world, and is the primary cause of death in some gender and age groups. As mortality from other causes has declined, cancer deaths have become more frequent, with a current annual death rate in the United States of 500,000. Cancer incidence and mortality increase with advancing age.

DIET IN CANCER CAUSATION AND PREVENTION

With rare exception, the cause of cancer is unknown. Diet has been implicated in the cause and prevention of about one third of the cancers occurring in the United States, placing diet and cigarette smoking as major determinants. This assumption is based on varied evidence:

- large differences among cancer incidence in different countries
- correlation of cancer incidence with diet constituents
- laboratory studies showing effects of specific dietary components on tumor size, incidence, and mortality

A variety of mechanisms have been demonstrated or postulated:

- immune
- humoral
- enzymatic
- bacterial flora
- metabolic
- via antioxidants

Nutritional factors involved are

- fat
- low fiber
- low vitamin A
- low vitamin C
- low vitamin E
- low selenium
- alcohol
- pickled and smoked foods

Less conclusive data implicate saccharin, coffee or caffeine, aflatoxins, other food additives, and foodborne mutagens. These dietary components have been associated with the most common cancer sites: lung, breast, colon, and prostate (Table 24-1). It is thus becoming clear that what is eaten during a lifetime may strongly influence the probability of developing certain types of cancer.

Epidemiologic Evidence

United States rates for breast and colon cancer vary from five to eight times those of some other countries. The incidence of such cancers shows a close relationship with fat intake (Fig. 24-1), with correlation coefficients of 0.6 to 0.9. Studies of migrant populations show that cancer rates equal those of the new location in the first generation for some populations, and for oth-

Table 24-1. DIET AND INCREASED RATE OF CANCER
AT SPECIFIC SITES

Cancer Site	Dietary Constituent
Esophagus	*Alcohol*
	Low intake: lentils, green *vegetables*, fresh *fruit*, animal products, vitamins A, C, riboflavin, nicotinic acid, *trace elements* (Mo, Zn), fat, calcium, magnesium
	High intake: *pickles*, pickled vegetables, moldy food, *very hot beverages*, grain (wheat, corn)
Stomach	Spiced, pickled, smoked foods, iron deficiency, nitrate
	Low intake: milk, raw green or yellow vegetables (lettuce), vitamin C
Colon/Rectal	Fat (?saturated), meat, cholesterol, beer
	Low intake: fiber, cruciferous vegetables
Liver	Alcohol, aflatoxin
Pancreas	Alcohol, ?coffee, meat
Gallbladder	Calories
Lung	Low intake: vitamin A, β-carotene
Urinary Bladder	Coffee, non-nutritive sweetener
	Low intake: vitamin A
Kidney	Cadmium
Breast	Fat
	Milk (dairy products), eggs, calories, meat
Endometrial	Fat, calories
Ovary	Fat
Prostate	Fat, protein
	Low intake: vitamin A, vegetables

ers only in later generations. Large changes may be seen in rates for cancer within a stable population, as in recent decreases in gastric cancer in the United States.

Laboratory Evidence

Studies in laboratory animals have demonstrated the effects of various dietary components on tumor incidence, size, and mortality, occasionally providing evidence of the mechanism of cancer induction. Such studies may be performed in intact animals, may utilize cultured cells, or may determine mutagenicity in bacteria. The latter two may support a suspicion of carcinogenicity, but do not establish it as fact.

All three methods have shortcomings in terms of their applicability to humans. The high doses used in animal studies may not reflect the human

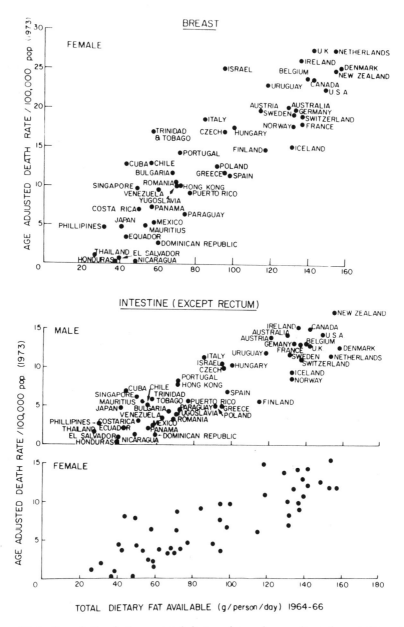

Figure 24–1. Correlation between total dietary fat and age-adjusted mortality rates from breast and colon cancers in various countries. (From Carroll, K.K.: Role of lipids in tumorigenesis. J Am Oil Chem Soc 61:1889, 1984, with permission.)

experience. Also, species differ; results cannot be extrapolated from rat or beagle to the human being. Testing in bacteria bypasses possible effects of the metabolism of dietary substances and the influence of processes of permeability, hormonal balance, or immune response.

Age and Immune Mechanisms

Age may predispose an individual to cancer for various reasons:

- The older person would have greater duration of exposure to environmental carcinogens.
- Deterioration in immune function may result from aging or nutritional imbalances, and such deterioration may permit uninhibited tumor growth. The immune system may function to prevent the multiplication of tumor cells or to eliminate new cells as they arise. Immunosuppressed hosts are more prone to cancer than those with normal immune status.
- Mature thymic or T lymphocytes are responsible for cell-mediated immunity, including delayed hypersensitivity reactions. The thymus also is involved in modulation of B lymphocytes (antibody-producing cells) and natural killer (cytolytic) cell activity. The latter may be responsible for the destruction of tumor cells. Decline in thymic function with age or through another cause may thus predispose individuals to tumor formation.

Protein Malnutrition

Protein malnutrition is associated with severe immune defects involving the thymus and T lymphocytes, with resultant lymphopenia, defect in T-cell maturation, and loss of reactivity to skin antigens (see Chapter 13). Such findings would interfere with effective treatment with anticancer agents (see pp. 540–541). On the other hand, experimental evidence in tumor-bearing mice shows that severe caloric restriction prolongs lifespan and reduces cancer incidence. One must be cautious in extrapolating these findings to mankind, but they may fit in with data correlating excessive calorie intake and obesity with increased cancer incidence.

Mineral Deficiencies

Immune defects may also be caused by mineral deficiencies—especially a deficiency in zinc, which may cause thymic and lymphocytic dysfunction (see Chapter 14). Whether zinc-induced immune deficits promote cancer is unknown.

Calories

Calorie excess or obesity may be related to many cancers. Marked increases in the incidence of cancer of the uterus, gallbladder, kidney, stomach, colon, and breast have been associated with obesity. Men and women more than 40 percent over ideal body weight have been found to have a 55 percent (women) and 33 percent (men) greater risk of cancer than persons of normal weight. Cancer incidence is reduced and life expectancy increased in animals maintained at ideal body weight or lower. Cancer of the uterus (endometrium) shows the strongest association between obesity and cancer.

Obesity may exert its tumor-enhancing effect by means of the altered distribution of specific nutrients in the diet that influence other processes (e.g., hormone secretion or metabolism). The ratio of fat to carbohydrate may be increased or the concentration of fiber decreased. Since both fat and fiber may affect carcinogenesis, it is difficult to gauge the independent effect of calories or energy excess over expenditure.

Fat

Excessive fat intake—saturated or unsaturated, from plant or animal sources—increases the risk of breast, prostate, and colon cancers. A high fat diet may act synergistically with low fiber intake to increase the risk of colon cancer. A strong association has been noted between the consumption of total fat, saturated fat, and cholesterol and the incidence of colon cancer. Meat intake may also be related to the risk of this type of cancer; in addition to a high meat intake, colon cancer patients in Greece also have low vegetable intake, thus contributing to lack of fiber or cruciferous vegetables (see p. 536).

Cholesterol

Confounding the colon cancer diet etiology is the observation that some persons with hypercholesterolemia treated with cholesterol-lowering drugs showed increased rates of colon cancer. Some reports noted that persons with lower serum cholesterol levels had increased colon cancer rates. It is hypothesized that increased turnover of cholesterol in the enterohepatic circulation may be associated with such higher rates or that those persons already had cancer. High levels of fat and cholesterol in the diet increase the excretion of bile acids and neutral sterols. Such diets may alter intestinal bacterial flora, which may then modify bile acids enzymatically to transform them into potential carcinogens. More studies of these mechanisms are needed, together with further evaluation of the possible relationship between low circulating cholesterol levels and increased cancer rates.

Fat-Hormone Relationships

It has been suggested that hormonal mechanisms mediate the effect of high fat diets on the rate of breast cancer. Increased estrogen levels may result from increased synthesis and reabsorption induced by adding fat to the diet. Fat may also affect the risk of breast cancer by altering prolactin secretion. Interaction between polyunsaturated fats and antioxidants may be associated with increase risk of breast and other cancers (see also effects of selenium, p. 537).

Dietary variables may be most significant relatively early in life. Prospective studies relating diet and cancer in women are needed to characterize the relation between breast cancer and fat intake, addressing specifically the role of various types and levels of fat. Studies planned or in progress are assessing the effects of a low fat diet (20 to 30 percent of calories) as an adjuvant to chemotherapy in women with stage II breast cancer (with axillary node metastases), or as prophylaxis in women at high risk for developing breast cancer (first-degree relatives of women with breast cancer, for example). Of all dietary components reviewed by the National Research Council, fat intake was most suggestively linked to the occurrence of cancer.

Fiber

The "fiber hypothesis" originates from the low colon cancer rates observed in Africans with high dietary fiber consumption and stool bulk. The latter may dilute potential carcinogens, speeding their transit through the colon. Substances that may have this protective effect include certain types of whole grains, fruits, and vegetables (see Chapter 1). The hypothesis has been complicated, however, by the finding that neither transit time nor bulk are consistently affected by the addition of fiber to the diet (see Chapter 21). Other possible explanations for the effect of fiber are that it may bind carcinogens, alter bacterial flora, or contain other compounds that reduce cancer incidence.

Vitamins

Vitamin A and Carotene

Foods rich in vitamin A and carotene (see Chapter 2) may reduce the risk of cancers of the lung, larynx, esophagus, urinary bladder, upper gastrointestinal tract, and breast. The mechanism of the antitumor effect may be associated with the function of vitamin A in controlling cell differentiation or influencing host immune defenses, while carotene may protect against oxidative damage. Individuals with overall highest cancer rates have been reported to have lower serum retinol levels than individuals with lower cancer rates; these studies need to be confirmed. Because of the known toxicity of vitamin A, supplementation is not recommended (see recommended diet further on). A current trial in American male physicians 40 to 85 years of age is comparing the effects on cancer incidence of beta carotene versus placebo administration.

Vitamin C

Diets high in fruits and vegetables, thereby rich in ascorbic acid, have been associated with a decreased incidence of cancer of the stomach and esophagus. Vitamin C may inhibit the formation of carcinogenic nitrosamines in the stomach (see Chapter 5). An important role for vitamin C in the prevention of cancer is not supported by current evidence, although neither is there strong evidence disproving such an association. The antioxidant activity of vitamin C (see Chapter 2) as well as its effects in maintaining the integrity of the intercellular matrix and enhancing immune mechanisms provides a theoretic basis for exploring a possible protective function against cancer. Such studies should determine the level of intake required, that is, usual dietary levels versus those found in large supplements.

Vitamin E

As an important antioxidant, vitamin E deserves study as a possible inhibitor of carcinogenesis. No data are now available, however, concerning this vitamin's relation to cancer risk or inhibition of neoplasia.

Other Dietary Factors

Cruciferous Vegetables

Epidemiologic studies have associated consumption of cruciferous vegetables (cabbage, broccoli, cauliflower, brussels sprouts) with reduction in cancer at several sites. The compounds in these vegetables that may have a protective function have not been identified, although indoles are a possibility.

Alcohol

Heavy drinkers of alcohol, especially those who also smoke cigarettes, are at high risk for cancers of the oral cavity, larynx, esophagus, and liver (see Chapter 22). Excessive beer consumption has been associated with increased risk of rectal cancer in the United States.

Selenium

There is a strong inverse correlation between selenium intake and the incidence of breast and colon cancer. Those with the highest serum selenium levels showed an overall cancer risk half that of those in the lowest quintile. Selenium has antioxidant activity, may favorably affect carcinogen metabolism, and may enhance immune defenses. However, it would be premature to recommend an increase in selenium intake, and medically unsupervised use of selenium as a supplement is unwarranted because of possible toxicity. Currently, clinical trials are under way testing selenium supplementation in the prevention of some skin cancers.

Smoked and Pickled Foods

Conventional smoked foods may absorb tars arising from incomplete combustion. The tars contain carcinogens similar to those in tobacco smoke. Conventional smoking of meats and fish and charcoal broiling also may deposit mutagenic and carcinogenic compounds on the surface of food. Stomach and esophageal cancers are common in those parts of the world where nitrates and nitrites are prevalent in food and water, or where cured and pickled foods are consumed.

Other Potential Carcinogens

- At high intake levels, saccharin causes cancer of the urinary bladder in rats. The long-term consequences of saccharin consumption—especially by children and pregnant women—are unknown.
- Data concerning coffee or caffeine as risk factors in human cancer are inconclusive.
- Aflatoxins are unavoidable contaminants, especially in peanut products and corn in the United States. It is unclear whether primary hepatocellular carcinoma, especially in Africa and Asia, is related to high levels of aflatoxin ingestion or to exposure to hepatitis B virus, or both. There is no current evidence that aflatoxin contamination of food is related to cancer risk in the United States.

The National Research Council has emphasized the need to minimize food contamination with carcinogens, to weigh the potential carcinogenicity of food additives prior to approval for their use, and to identify foodborne mutagens and determine their carcinogenic potential.

Diet to Prevent Cancer

The combined recommendations of the National Research Council and the American Cancer Society to prevent cancer include the following:

1. Reduce intake of saturated and unsaturated fats. It is suggested that the amount of fat consumed be decreased to 30 percent of total calo-

ries by moderating consumption of fats, oils, and foods rich in fats. This is also an effective way to reduce total calories and maintain ideal body weight.

2. Increase consumption of fruits (especially citrus), vegetables (especially carotene-rich and cruciferous), and whole-grain cereal products. A high fiber diet of fruits, vegetables, and whole grains offers a wholesome substitute for fatty foods, thereby decreasing fat and calorie intake. Consumption of cruciferous vegetables may reduce the risk of cancer of the gastrointestinal and respiratory tracts.

3. Minimize consumption of foods preserved by smoking or salt curing (including salt pickling).

4. Consume alcohol in moderation, if at all.

5. Avoid obesity.

6. Identify mutagens in food and remove or minimize their concentration unless the nutritive value of foods is jeopardized or other potential hazard introduced.

7. Minimize contamination of foods with carcinogens from any source.

NUTRITIONAL STATUS OF THE PATIENT WITH CANCER

Cachexia is frequently associated with advanced cancer; protein-energy malnutrition is virtually universal in hospitalized cancer patients. Patients nearer death (less than 70 days) are usually more severely malnourished than other hospitalized patients, as measured by the usual criteria of nutritional assessment (see Chapter 3). Weight loss is associated with reduced survival. The leading cause of death in cancer patients is malnutrition resulting from combined effects of the tumor and specific anticancer therapy. The patient's poor nutritional status may compromise response to therapy, while the resultant malnutrition itself leads to worsening of the nutritional status by its effects on the gastrointestinal tract (see Chapters 13 and 20).

Adverse Effects of Cancer

Direct Interference With Eating or Digestion

Patients with oral or gastrointestinal cancer often have direct interference with eating and digestion (as those with head and neck cancer, especially following surgical resection). Obstruction of esophagus, stomach, or intestine may interfere with the normal passage, digestion, and absorption of food. Gastrointestinal tumors may cause difficulty in swallowing, nausea, vomiting, diarrhea, fistula formation, or bacterial overgrowth. Obstruction of biliary or pancreatic secretions and malabsorption due to direct mucosal involvement may contribute to malnutrition, while obstruction of intestinal lymphatics may be associated with protein-losing enteropathy.

Indirect Effects on Eating

The cancer patient may be unwilling to eat, for a variety of reasons. Some metabolic abnormalities may cause anorexia. The sense of satiety often increases to the extent that the patient loses the sense of hunger and feels satisfied after eating grossly inadequate amounts of food. Discomfort, pain, and malaise, together with the psychologic distress produced by an awareness of the diagnosis and the unpleasant aspects of treatment, often contribute to depression, and hence to loss of appetite and weight. Cancer patients with food aversions have greater incidence of weight loss, anorexia, and early satiety than cancer patients without such aversions. The role of vitamin (niacin, vitamin A) and mineral (zinc, copper, nickel) deficiencies in food aversions is not clear.

In addition, there may be alterations in taste and smell (see Chapter 20). Such changes may be associated with aging (see Chapter 9), malnutrition, and/or the cancer itself. Zinc deficiency is also a possible cause of altered taste acuity and appetite change. Cancer patients tend to have an increased threshold for sweet and a decreased threshold for bitter, sensations that lead to meat aversion and low calorie intake.

Cancer Cachexia

The progressive wasting syndrome, cancer cachexia, differs from simple starvation in its carbohydrate, protein, and fat metabolism, with failure in compensatory decrease in oxygen consumption, the normal long-term adaptation to starvation (see Chapter 13). Changes in carbohydrate metabolism in cancer patients include increased gluconeogenesis, accelerated glucose turnover, decreased glycogen stores, and elevated levels of blood lactate. Tumors are efficient extractors of glucose, while the host displays insulin resistance. The main energy source for tumors is anaerobic glycolysis. The tumor metabolizes glucose to lactate, releasing lactate that is resynthesized to glucose in the liver (Cori cycle; see Chapter 13). However, this cycle is inefficient, possibly explaining why energy requirements are increased in the presence of cancer. The tumor gains two molecules of ATP while the liver expends six ATPs for each molecule of glucose cycled. Provision of more glucose to the host may result in lactic acidosis; elevated blood lactate may generate anorexia.

Nitrogen Balance

Negative nitrogen balance is virtually universal in cancer patients. Protein anabolism is impaired with decreased amino acid incorporation into protein. Catabolism of skeletal and visceral protein is accelerated, supplying energy via gluconeogenesis and nitrogen to the tumor. Protein restriction of the host will not be successful because the tumor competes for nitrogen at the host's expense.

Fat Stores

Fat stores are mobilized in the course of cancer cachexia. Free fatty acid mobilization persists in the fed state, unlike simple starvation. The mechanism underlying the maladaptation is unknown but may relate to the production of cachectin (tumor necrosis factor). Cachectin induces hypertriglyceridemia by inhibiting lipoprotein lipase.

Effects of Treatment

The treatment modalities used in cancer patients, including surgery, radiation, and chemotherapy, themselves contribute to nutritional problems.

Surgery

Surgery involving the gastrointestinal system may produce marked alterations in nutritional status, including the following:

- vagotomy—gastrointestinal stasis, hypochlorhydria, steatorrhea, diarrhea, altered appetite
- gastric resection—loss of intrinsic factor, dumping syndrome, malabsorption
- intestinal resection—malabsorption, hyperoxaluria, cholerrheic enteropathy, secretory diarrhea, disturbances of acid-base balance
- pancreatectomy—diabetes mellitus

Radiation Therapy

Radiation therapy may also have adverse effects on nutritional status.

- Head and neck irradiation may induce sore mouth and throat, dry mouth, altered taste and smell (see Chapter 20), or dysphagia, and may foster increased susceptibility to infection and to caries.
- Irradiation to the chest may produce esophagitis with dysphagia and susceptibility to infection. Fibrosis with esophageal stricture may result.

- Gastric irradiation may decrease gastric acidity or induce ulceration.
- Nausea, vomiting, and diarrhea are common sequelae of irradiation of the small intestine, with transient weight loss and malnutrition. Malabsorption, fistula and stricture formation, and mucosal ulceration are frequent. Less commonly, there is more serious radiation-induced enteritis, with chronic diarrhea or partial or complete intestinal obstruction.

Chemotherapeutic Drugs

The mucosal effects of chemotherapeutic drugs produce gastrointestinal symptoms, including nausea and vomiting, oral ulcers and stomatitis, diarrhea, abdominal pain, and altered taste (Table 24–2). Anorexia may result, in part from anticipating these symptoms. Gastrointestinal toxicity is almost universal with high-dose combination chemotherapy. Severe side effects may compromise the host's nutritional status, but fortunately symptoms usually subside spontaneously.

Adrenocortical steroids may produce fluid and electrolyte disturbances, with negative nitrogen, potassium, and calcium balances. However, steroids do stimulate appetite.

Additional adverse effects of chemotherapy may include hypoglycemia or hyperglycemia, hyperuricemia, hypercalcemia (often a feature of neoplastic disease itself), and inappropriate secretion of antidiuretic hormone.

Table 24–2. NUTRITIONAL ADVERSE EFFECTS OF
CANCER CHEMOTHERAPY

Drug Class	Vomiting	Stomatitis	Diarrhea	Hepato-toxic	Fluid Retention	Miscellaneous
Antibiotics	xxx	xxx	xx			Abdominal pain
Alkylating agents	xxx	xx	x	x		Abdominal pain Metallic taste
Antimetabolites	xx	xxx	xx	x		Abdominal pain
Vinca alkaloids	x	xx				Abdominal pain Constipation
Hormones	xx			xx	x	Dizziness
Other	xx	x		xx		

Nutritional Intervention

Feeding the Patient Versus Feeding the Tumor

An important question relating to the nutritional management of the cancer patient is whether in feeding the host, the tumor also is fed. Since tumors are successful metabolic parasites, the answer is yes; however, tumor growth apparently is not stimulated disproportionately to the host. The requirements, distribution, and utilization of nutrients may differ between tumor and host, and antitumor therapy based on "starving" or depleting the tumor exists (methotrexate, L-asparaginase). New modalities selectively nourishing the host may be developed. Such nutritional manipulations offer a promising avenue for reserach in cancer therapy.

Starving the host generally results in impaired immune function, adverse endocrine changes, skin breakdown, impaired wound healing, decreased response to hypoxia, and functional deterioration leading to increased morbidity and mortality with delay in treatment. However, it remains moot whether repletion of the malnourished patient can in fact be accomplished, and whether attempted vigorous nutritional support improves prognosis. Resolution of anergy with nutritional support may be associated with improved prognosis.

Effects of Nutritional Intervention

The most clear-cut benefits of nutritional intervention result from supportive regimens in relation to specific treatment of cancer with surgery, radiation, and/or chemotherapy. Thus, improvement of clinical status to allow surgery to be undertaken with less risk justifies perioperative nutritional support. Parenteral nutrition in conjunction with chemotherapy may not influence tolerance and response to therapy or limit bone marrow toxicity, although some studies suggest that nutritional support enhances response to chemotherapy. Disappointingly, nutritional intervention has not been demonstrated to improve survival; indeed a detrimental effect may be noted, especially with vigorous attempts at nutritional repletion. The specific needs of each patient in relation to his or her disease, treatment, and nutritional status must be considered in order to develop the optimal nutritional regimen.

Helpful Actions

A number of actions may help to improve the cancer patient's nutritional status:

- Assess nutritional status periodically, focusing on maintenance.
- Take conservative measures that aim to improve voluntary food in-

take, for example, encouraging patients to eat in a pleasant social setting, catering to food preferences, and providing companionship.

- Relieve pain with appropriate analgesics.
- Treat pain from mucositis with topical anesthetics such as viscous xylocaine (see Chapter 20).
- Prescribe antiemetics, antispasmodics, and antimotility agents when helpful.
- Use cholestyramine and cimetidine to relieve cholerheic diarrhea and hyperacidity, respectively.
- Try supplemental pancreatic enzymes to improve symptoms from exocrine pancreatic insufficiency (see Chapter 22).

Meals. Trying new foods and experimenting with seasonings may help the patient cope with unpleasant taste sensations. The cancer patient is most prone to aversions to meat (beef and pork) and chocolate. Specific foods or ways of preparing and serving foods may be helpful in many cases. (Table 24–3 lists specific foods recommended to increase calorie and protein intake.)

- Eggs and dairy products can serve as a substitute source of adequate protein provided that the patient has not developed lactose intolerance as a result of radiation therapy, intestinal resection or bypass, malnutrition, or intercurrent illness.
- Offer food in the form of multiple small feedings.
- Patients may prefer high protein, high calorie liquid supplements to solid foods (see Chapter 11); these may be commercial or home-prepared.
- Foods should have high nutrient density; modular supplements may be used to provide protein or calories.
- Patients with mucositis may prefer foods served at room temperature or slightly chilled.
- Foods moistened with gravies, sauces, or other high fat substances or foods that have been pureed may facilitate intake in patients with mucositis or dysphagia.
- Remember to consider the consequences of fat malabsorption and its management (see Chapter 21).
- Elemental diets may be useful in patients with compromised digestion or severe malnutrition (see Chapter 11).

Nutritional Support Options

When additional forms of cancer treatment are available, nutritional intervention should be aggressive. In patients without such hope, the benefits of nutritional regimens must be weighed against prolonging a life of poor quality. Nutritional support is indicated in the presence of moderate or severe

Table 24-3. FOODS RECOMMENDED TO INCREASE
CALORIE AND PROTEIN INTAKE OF THE
PATIENT WITH CANCER

Food Group	Recommendations
Fruits and vegetables	Fruit juice added to mashed or canned fruit; mashed or pureed fruit added to milk beverage, cereals, pudding, ice cream, jello made with fruit juice in place of water; tender, cooked vegetables such as mashed white or sweet potatoes, squash, spinach, carrots, beets; vegetables in soups and sauces; vegetables in cream or cheese sauce such as scalloped potatoes and cream-style corn.
Grain	Hot cereals prepared with milk instead of water; ready-to-eat cereals softened in milk; high protein noodles; noodles or rice in casseroles and soups; breaded or floured meats; bread or rice pudding.
Beverage	Milk beverages; shakes made with fruit juices and sherbet when milk is not tolerated.
Milk and calcium equivalents	Custards; milkshakes; ice cream; yogurt; cheeses; cheesecake; double strength milk (1 qt fluid milk mixed with 1 cup skim milk powder); cottage cheese; flavored milk; pudding; eggnog; cream soups; milk powder; skim milk powder added to casseroles and mixed dishes.
Meat and protein equivalents	Diced meat; casseroles; smooth peanut butter; cheese; egg and egg dishes; cut, diced, or pureed meat mixed with soups, sauces, and gravies; fish, poultry and vegetable protein meat substitutes; tuna, meat, or cheese in cream sauces.
Fat	Margarine or oil added to vegetables, hot cereals, and casseroles; cream used in place of milk or added to fruits and desserts; sour cream; salad dressings; mayonaise mixed with tuna, egg, chicken, or fruit salad.
Sweet	Desserts made with dry milk powder, peanut butter, or eggs.

malnutrition, or where the risk that it may develop is high (see Chapter 3). Enteral administration, using small bore tubes if necessary, is preferable to parenteral nutrition and can be carried out at home. (Parenteral alimentation using the peripheral or central vein route was discussed in Chapter 12.) Unfortunately, optimal nutrition for the cancer patient remains largely undefined.

CHAPTER 25

Trauma and Critical Care

This chapter discusses disorders that have in common the factor of stress, whether from trauma (surgical, thermal, or accidental), infection, or chronic disease. Patients with severe hypermetabolic and catabolic states, at a high level of stress, are often encountered in medical or surgical intensive care or critical care units. Their underlying disorders may be complicated with other diseases and with multiple organ failure (see Chapters 22 and 23) requiring administration of multiple forms of life support. Provision of nutrients to these patients may be life-saving and must be included in their management.

545

Providing appropriate nutritional support often taxes the knowledge and ingenuity of the physician and the team of health professionals because of the opposing needs of one or another malfunctioning organ system.

METABOLIC CHANGES IN STRESS

Stress is a catabolic state with an increase in the metabolic rate. It is characterized by

- erosion of the lean body mass manifested by muscle wasting
- excessive loss of nitrogen in the urine along with potassium
- reduced urinary output of water and sodium
- abnormal carbohydrate metabolism
- increased resting oxygen consumption

The catabolic response to injury and stress in women is less than that in men of the same age and weight. Protein loss and negative nitrogen balance become significant when a marked catabolic hypermetabolic state lasts 3 to 7 days. Anorexia usually is present. Recovery from this state of stress is followed by an anabolic phase when wound healing is established. This period lasts from 2 to 5 weeks, during which the patient usually can be repleted, will ingest more calories, and can achieve positive nitrogen balance. Finally, a fat gain phase occurs. A prolonged catabolic phase requires a prolonged period of anabolism to complete recovery.

Hormones

Many hormones are involved in the response to stress, with catecholamines assuming primary importance (Table 25–1). In severe trauma such as burns, nitrogen loss from skeletal muscle may rise as high as 40 g per day (Table 25–2). The metabolic reaction is characterized by increased oxidation

Table 25–1. NEUROHUMORAL METABOLIC EFFECTS IN STRESS

| | Metabolic Function | | | |
Hormone	Glycogenolysis	Gluconeogenesis	Lipolysis	Proteolysis
Cortisol	−	+++	++	+++
Catecholamine	++++	++	++++	+
Glucagon	++	+++	+++	+
Growth hormone	−	+	++	−

*Vasopressin secretion increases with a fall in urine volume and increase in osmolarity. Water retention results. Aldosterone and thyroxine also increase.

Table 25–2. METABOLIC VARIABLES IN STRESS

Example	Urinary Nitrogen Loss (g/day)	Plasma Lactate (μM/L)	Plasma Glucose (mg/dl)	Insulin Resistance	Glucagon to Insulin	Urinary 3-Methylhistidine Excretion (μM/24 hr)	O_2 Consumption Index (ml/M²)
Starvation	<5	10±5	100±20	—	2±0.5	<100	90±10
Elective surgery	5–10	1200±200	150±25	—	2.5±0.8	130±20	130±6
Polytrauma	10–15	1200±200	150±25	±	3±0.7	200±20	140±6
Sepsis	>15	2500±500	250±50	+	8±1.5	450±50	160±10

Table 25-3. PREFERENTIAL SUBSTRATE UTILIZATION

Organ	Energy Substrate					
	Lactate	Glucose	Fatty Acids	Ketone Bodies	Branched Chain Amino Acids	Nonbranched Chain Amino Acids
Heart	**		**	**		
Skeletal muscle		*	**	**	**	
Brain	***			*		
Liver		*	**			**

* Modest preference.
** Moderate preference.
*** High preference.

by muscle of branched chain amino acids, while the liver extracts alanine released from muscle, plus glycine and tyrosine for gluconeogenesis (Table 25-3). Relative insulin-to-glucose and insulin-to-glucagon ratios decrease in catabolic states. The rise in glucagon results in increased hepatic uptake of glucogenic amino acids, increased hepatic gluconeogenesis, and hyperglycemia (see Chapter 1).

TRAUMA AND SURGERY

The trauma associated with surgery increases the need for nutrients, while concomitantly food intake usually is restricted, if only temporarily. After injury or surgery, metabolism is higher, especially with fever and hemorrhage, exudate, fistulas, or sinuses may occur. Difficulty in feeding occurs with anorexia.

Metabolism

Additional characteristics of metabolism in trauma (Fig. 25-1) include the use of glucose by the wound to produce lactate. Nitrogen loss usually exceeds the increase in metabolic rate in injury; starvation accentuates this dissociation (see Chapter 13).

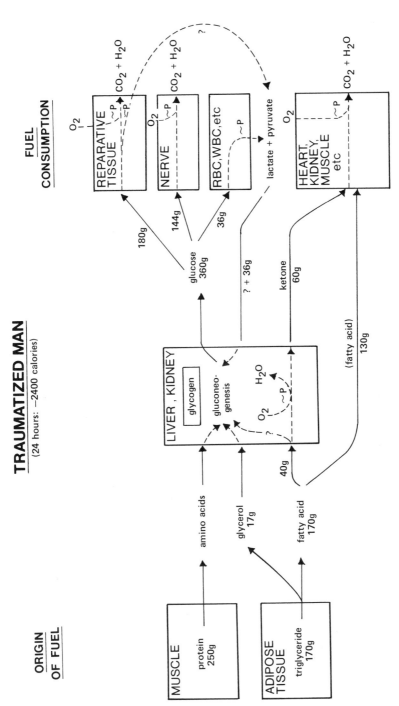

Figure 25–1. Pattern of fuel metabolism in traumatized man.

Nutritional Assessment and Basic Care

Nutritional assessment of such patients should include

- protein status
- anthropometrics
- immune function
- calorimetry and measurement of the RQ (if available)

The patient should be weighed daily, with daily estimates made of caloric intake and nitrogen balance. Keeping the patient warm and providing sufficient analgesia, attention to fluid balance, and appropriate antibiotic therapy are essential elements of care.

Nutritional Management

Management includes provision of increased calories and increased nitrogen (Table 25–4). The calorie-to-nitrogen ratio in the critically ill should be decreased from the normal value of 350:1 to 100:1, and even lower. Provision of glucose decreases protein breakdown and decreases the amino acid pool, with little effect on protein synthesis. Provision of protein stimulates protein synthesis with no effect on protein breakdown.

- The patient undergoing routine elective surgery who is able to progress rapidly to oral intake can be provisionally maintained with intravenous solutions of 5 to 10 percent dextrose with electrolytes.
- The patient with pre-existing malnutrition or a longer period without oral intake, or both, needs enteral or parenteral administration of glucose in larger quantities as well as nitrogen (see Chapters 11 and 12).
- With uncomplicated major surgery the patient can receive 25 to 50 percent of his or her total calories from fat.
- The critically ill patient needs calories provided as carbohydrate.
- It is important to provide 20 to 25 mEq phosphorus per 1000 kcal (see Chapters 2, 12, and 14).

THE BURNED PATIENT

The severely burned patient is at a high level of stress. The response to extensive third-degree burns is predictable; thus, the expected metabolic alterations and endocrine response must be met with appropriate nutritional support. Rapid weight loss in the burned patient increases the mortality rate. Infection is more likely in the presence of disturbed immunocompetence, while protein malnutrition and deficiency of other nutrients interfere with wound repair.

Table 25–4. METABOLIC NEEDS AND THEIR PROVISION
IN THE STRESSED PATIENT

		Stress Level		
	Starvation	Low	High Early	High Late
Protein				
Total body synthesis (net)	↓	↓	↓	↓
Hepatic synthesis	±	↑	↑ ↑	↓
Proteolysis	±	±	↑	↑ ↑
Metabolic regulation	Normal	Present, but higher threshold	Less responsive	Failed
Estimated calories	BEE	1.3 × BEE	1.5 × BEE	2.0 × BEE
Fraction of daily calories				
Glucose, %	60	50	40	70
Fat, %	25	30	35	—
Amino acids, %	15	20	25	30
Protein calorie needs				
Nonprotein calorie-to-nitrogen ratio, kcal/g N	160:1	100:1	90:1	80:1
Amino acids, g/kg/day	1	1.5	2	2.5+
Total nonprotein calories, kcal/kg/day	25	25	30	35
Total calories, kcal/kg/day	28	32	40	45

↑ Increased.
↓ Decreased.
± Little or no change.
BEE = Basal energy expenditure.
(Adapted from Cerra, F.B.: Pocket Manual of Surgical Nutrition. CV Mosby, St. Louis, 1984, p. 60.)

Initial Metabolic and Hormone Responses

Within minutes or days, usually over 3 to 5 days, the burned patient undergoes a decrease in metabolic rate and cardiac output. There is massive fluid loss and release of pyrogens. Hormonal responses include increases in cortisol, catecholamines, and antidiuretic hormone, with decreased response to insulin and decrease in the peripheral utilization of glucose. Hyperglycemia and increases in serum lactate and free fatty acids are characteristic. Provision of fluid and adequate resuscitation and oxygenation are of paramount importance in the early stage of critical care.

Later Metabolic and Hormonal Responses

A hypermetabolic state (increases of 50 to 150 percent) follows, with hyperthermia, increased pulse and respiratory rates, fluid losses, and accelerated losses of nitrogen, sulfur, phosphorus, and potassium. Hormonal mediators of this reaction include catecholamines, glucagon, and cortisol. There may be uncoupling of oxidative phosphorylation and substrate cycling (futile cycles). These changes are similar to those observed with severe nonthermal trauma and sepsis.

Muscle catabolism and anabolism are increased, with catabolism of branched chain amino acids, release of alanine to provide substrate for synthesis of nonessential amino acids and glucose, and production of glutamine. There are also a decrease in the utilization of free fatty acids and ketone bodies for energy and increases in serum levels of free fatty acids and triglycerides. In addition, there is increased excretion of 3-methylhistidine. Glucose production is increased and the Cori cycle is active.

Nutrition Support

Aggressive nutrition support is required for patients with

- burns exceeding 20 percent of the body surface area
- pre-existing malnutrition
- complicating sepsis or trauma
- weight loss exceeding 10 percent

This nutritional therapy should be started 3 to 4 days after injury. In massive burns involving more than 30 percent of the body surface, caloric requirements may more than double basal calories (based on ideal body weight). Such requirements may be estimated at 25 kcal per kg + 40 kcal per percent body surface burn.

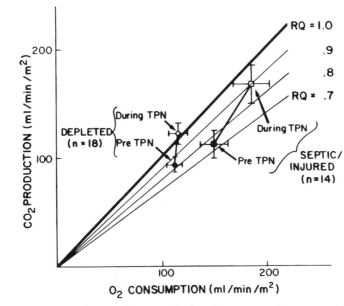

Figure 25-2. Patterns of gas exchange in depleted patients and trauma patients. Both groups increase CO₂ production during TPN. Trauma patients are hypermetabolic. (From Askanazi, J., et al.: Influence of total parenteral nutrition on fuel utilization in injury and sepsis. Ann Surg 191:42, 1980, with permission.)

Enteral Nutrition and Complications

Glucose should be infused at a rate of 5 mg per kg per min, protein provided at 2 to 3 g per kg with a calorie-to-nitrogen ratio of 100:1, and remaining calories provided as fat. The enteral route is preferred, although patients may have anorexia, altered taste, or facial burns that interfere with normal oral intake. Such patients may be tube-fed using continuous infusion via pump, with the usual precautions against aspiration (see Chapter 11). Metabolic complications of tube feeding include hyperglycemia, fluid overload, electrolyte imbalance, and/or CO_2 overproduction. Provision of excessive amounts of glucose may result in abnormal liver function with increases in serum levels of liver enzymes and bilirubin and development of cholestasis and fatty liver. Excessive production of CO_2 may result with excess carbohydrate calories (see section on Ventilatory Failure, further on, and Fig. 25-2).

Parenteral Nutrition

Patients with burns that exceed 40 percent require parenteral nutrition. This route may also be required

- in patients with ileus

- in addition to the enteral route
- in patients with gastrointestinal pathology

Complications of parenteral nutrition include

- technical (pneumothorax or hemothorax, thromboembolic)
- metabolic (hyperglycemia, amino acid or micronutrient imbalance, acidosis)
- septic (especially through burned skin and in the presence of impaired immunocompetence)

These problems are discussed in Chapter 12. Specific micronutrient needs of the stressed patient are unknown, but patients should be provided with ascorbic acid, folate, nicotinic acid, biotin, thiamin, vitamins B_6 and A, and zinc and magnesium adequate to meet increased needs or losses. Fluid loss of burned patients is estimated as

$$ml/h = (25 + \% \text{ burn}) \times \text{surface area (m}^2)$$

Parenteral Nutrition Formulas. Formulas for stressed patients, applicable to those with multiple trauma or burns, are provided in Table 25–5. Altered fuel metabolism in those with severe stress may result in failure to achieve adequate positive nitrogen balance even with provision of adequate calories and a high protein intake. Nitrogen balance may be improved with an amino acid mixture of 45 to 50 percent branched chain amino acids, in amounts of 0.5 g per kg. Preparations of branched chain amino acids (such as

Table 25–5. PARENTERAL NUTRITION FORMULAS FOR THE STRESSED PATIENT

	Level of Stress		
	Low	*High Early*	*High Late*
Amino acid, % (final)	5	5.5	6.5
Dextrose, % (final)	18	15	24.5
Kcal/l (total)	817	735	1099
Nonprotein calorie-to-nitrogen ratio	100:1	90:1	80:1
Fat, ml/%	500/10	500/20	—
		Mixing	
Amino acids, 10%, ml	500	550	650
Dextrose, %/ml	50/360	50/300	70/350
Water, ml	140	150	—

Branch Amin) can be mixed with standard amino acid solutions for injection. Preparations enriched in branched chain amino acids are available for enteral and parenteral administration (see Chapters 11 and 12). It has not yet been shown conclusively that solutions high in branched chain amino acids are more beneficial than balanced amino acid solutions in achieving nitrogen balance.

SEPSIS

Infection is characterized by the presence of fever. With elevated body temperature, energy expenditure increases and the nitrogen-sparing mechanism of starvation may be inhibited (see Chapter 13). Immunologic defense mechanisms are of primary importance in combating infection. The effect of sepsis on nutritional requirements varies with the severity and duration of the infection and whether it is local or generalized. Factors affecting nutritional requirements and metabolism in the septic patient include

- age
- gender
- premorbid nutritional state
- presence of underlying or complicating medical or surgical conditions

Hormonal Changes

A variety of hormones mediate the body's response to fever:

- Increased levels of ACTH are observed, with resultant increased secretion of mineralocorticoids and glucocorticoids.
- Glucocorticoids undergo a short twofold to fivefold rise with loss of the circadian rhythm, and there is a marked rise with septic shock.
- Levels of growth hormone show an exaggerated rise following administration of intravenous glucose.
- Secretion of TSH and TRF is delayed and may be excessive.
- Thyroid hormone levels fluctuate with alteration in thyroxine-binding affinity, increase in reverse T3 and accelerated hepatic removal of T3.
- Secretion of antidiuretic hormone (ADH) may be inappropriate, especially in infections of the central nervous system.
- Insulin is secreted out of proportion to the degree of starvation, is excessive after administration of intravenous glucose, and is cleared slowly.
- Glucagon secretion also is increased.

Nutritional Changes

Infection results in measurable loss of body components, including decreased body weight, muscle mass, and fat. Negative nitrogen balance may be as severe as -20 to -90 g per day, with associated loss of potassium, magnesium, phosphorus, zinc, and sulfur. Presence of diarrhea, vomiting, exudates, wounds, and drainages accentuates loss of electrolytes (sodium, chloride), water, hydrogen ion, bicarbonate, potassium (with acidosis or other abnormalities of acid-base balance), protein, and red blood cells.

Excess Utilization of Nutrients

Loss of nutrients results from their excess utilization caused by the increased metabolic rate averaging 13 percent per °C of fever. Carbohydrate needs are met by increased gluconeogenesis from amino acids, accentuating nitrogen loss. Ureagenesis and use of vitamins increases, and nutrients are diverted into alternate metabolic pathways.

Sequestration of Nutrients

Sequestration of nutrients also results in functional loss. For example, iron and zinc are lost into storage in the liver (hemosiderin, ferritin, metallothioneins).

- Iron sequestration is especially seen in pyogenic infections, resulting in decreased plasma iron and increased total iron-binding capacity or transferrin and ferritin (see Chapter 15). Teleologically this diversion may aid in combating infection by making iron less available to support the infecting microorganism.
- Zinc is bound to cysteine and histidine and lost in the urine of patients with hepatitis.
- Copper is secreted in ceruloplasmin, which undergoes increased hepatic synthesis in the presence of fever.
- Sodium in extracellular fluid decreases and accumulates in cells due to loss of control of membrane transport.

The Gastrointestinal Tract

Effects of infection on the gastrointestinal tract also influence the nutritional state. Anorexia is often present. Infection may affect multiplication of the tract's mucosal cells or induce protein loss. Bacteria, toxins, or parasites may interfere with absorption, consume blood or protein, compete for dietary nutrients, or be affected by antibiotics, laxatives, or enemas (see Chapter 21).

Electrolytes and other Minerals

Severe infection brings abnormalities in electrolytes. Sodium and chloride are retained because of excessive mineralocorticoid secretion. During convalescence from sepsis, dilutional hyponatremia may occur with subsequent diuresis. Infections that cause paralysis also promote loss of calcium and phosphorus, mobilized from bone.

Monitoring mineral status is another principle of management of the septic patient.

- Serum magnesium may fall, while calcium may decrease or increase depending on the type of infection.
- A fall in serum phosphorus results in decrease in leukocyte ATP and in chemotactic, phagocytic, and bactericidal properties of granulocytes.
- When iron and transferrin are low in patients with kwashiorkor, iron alone should not be administered, as it will feed the microorganisms; first protein should be given to improve protein status.

Alkalosis and Acidosis. Tachypnea may result in loss of CO_2, producing respiratory alkalosis. On the other hand, pneumonia or paralysis of the respiratory muscles may lead to CO_2 retention and acidosis. Metabolic acidosis occurs in shock because of the high level of lactic acid production. With high volume diarrhea, there are increased losses of bicarbonate as ileal secretions are not reabsorbed, leading to a fall in pH (see Chapter 21). Metabolic alkalosis can occur with low volume diarrhea and excessive potassium loss.

Vitamins

Circulating vitamin levels may be decreased in sepsis due to various causes:

- There may be increased urinary loss with negative nitrogen balance (e.g., riboflavin).
- Infesting parasites may take up B vitamins (see Chapter 5).
- Vitamin C is utilized in the activation of phagocytosis, which is stimulated by glucocorticoids.
- B vitamins and folate are required in the replication and function of lymphocytes involved in cell-mediated immune function.
- Vitamins A and E also are involved in host defense mechanisms (see Chapters 2 and 14).
- The absorption of fat-soluble vitamins and folate may be impaired in enteric infections or parasitism (see Chapter 21).
- Infection may precipitate acute avitaminosis such as scurvy, beriberi, pellagra, or night blindness and xerophthalmia (see Chapter 14).
- Antibiotics may reduce intestinal bacterial production of vitamins (vitamin K, biotin).

Protein, Energy, and Fat Metabolism

Anabolism and catabolism of protein are both increased in sepsis (Table 25–6). A variety of cellular proteins important to the inflammatory process are produced by cells involved in cell-mediated immunity and the liver.

- Synthesis of albumin is decreased in infection.
- Hepatic gluconeogenesis increases, from amino acids (alanine, glycine) derived from catabolism of muscle and other somatic tissues, lactate, pyruvate, and glycerol. Failure of hepatic gluconeogenesis from unavailability of substrate or from impaired hepatic function, or both, results in hypoglycemia.
- Serum cholesterol may increase or decrease, while circulating free fatty acids fall and triglycerides increase, especially in gram-negative sepsis.
- Hypertriglyceridemia results from increased lipid synthesis and de-

Table 25–6. PROTEIN METABOLISM IN INFECTION

↑ Catabolism muscle, somatic tissue
↑ Hepatic uptake amino acids
↑ Production phagocytes, lymphocytes, plasma cells
? ↑ Synthesis, release cellular proteins:
    Lactoferrin
    Lysozyme
    Endogenous pyrogen
    Interferon
    Lymphokines
    Cold-insoluble globulin
    Peptide hormones
↓ Hepatic synthesis albumin, transferrin
↑ Hepatic synthesis
    Enzymes
    Metallothioneins
    Complement
    Kinin
    Coagulation factors
    Lipoproteins
    Acute-phase reactant plasma proteins:
        Haptoglobin
        α_1-antitrypsin
        C-reactive protein
        α-acid glycoprotein
        Ceruloplasmin

creased activity of lipoprotein lipase under the influence of cachectin produced in response to bacterial endotoxin (see Chapter 19).

Alterations in energy metabolism with sepsis include increased glucose oxidation and increased utilization of branched chain amino acids.

Nutritional Management

The septic patient should be provided with about 1.5 g per kg protein with a balance of essential amino acids, together with an increase in calories to minimize protein loss. Indications for nutrition support of the septic patient include

- protracted infection
- secondary infection in the patient with medical or surgical problems
- severe burns or trauma
- malnutrition
- severe gram-negative sepsis

The plasma amino acid pattern of the septic patient is characterized by increased levels of phenylalanine, tyrosine, taurine, cysteine, and methionine; and a mild increase in alanine, asparagine, glutamine, and proline. Levels of branched chain amino acids usually are within normal limits. Levels of the first group of amino acids are even higher in preterminal patients, while levels of branched chain amino acids, alanine, and arginine are higher in survivors of severe infection than in preterminal patients. There have been reports of decreases in taurine, alanine, asparagine, glutamine, and proline in septic patients. A solution of amino acids containing 50 percent branched chain amino acids provided at 0.5 g per kg per day may be the minimum to sustain optimum nitrogen retention in patients in a highly catabolic state (excreting more than 8 g nitrogen in the urine when not provided with nutrition support).

Ventilatory Failure

Administration of carbohydrate calories to malnourished or severely stressed injured or septic patients results in increased CO_2 production and an increase in the RQ; this requires increased alveolar ventilation. The response in the stressed patient is much greater than that of the malnourished patient (see Fig. 25–2). This increased CO_2 production may induce ventilatory failure in patients with underlying pulmonary disease or may make it difficult to wean the patient from ventilatory support. In patients with pulmonary insufficiency and ventilatory failure, 25 to 50 percent of calories should be provided from fat. The malnourished patient with weakened respiratory muscles must be fed adequate calories and protein in order to maximize ventilation efficiency.

Subacute or Chronic Infection

Serum albumin and transferrin levels decline and serum iron increases in those with subacute or chronic infection. Adrenocortical hormone levels decrease. Nitrogen balance remains negative with slow depletion of adipose tissue stores resulting in a state of protein-energy malnutrition (see Chapter 13). This deficiency in turn impairs host defense mechanisms of both cell-mediated and humoral immunity. Unless refed, the severely malnourished patient may not manifest fever, leukocytosis, or the granulomatous response to infection.

Convalescence

- The patient with high fever should be treated with antipyretic drugs or other fever-controlling methods to minimize hypermetabolism and sweat losses.
- Provision of fluid and electrolytes is vital for the patient with diarrhea.
- Salt and water derangements may require limiting administration of saline and fluid if there is inappropriate secretion of antidiuretic hormone. Such defective balance is likely not only in patients with central nervous system infections, but also in the aged, in children, and in those with Rocky Mountain spotted fever.
- With convalescence from a febrile illness there is rapid reversal of negative nitrogen balance.
- Anorexia disappears, and the patient should be refed with increased calories and protein. The patient is susceptible to secondary infection at this point.
- Foods high in zinc should be provided.
- Vitamin supplements should be provided at levels equal to or double the RDA.

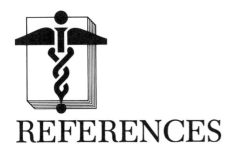

REFERENCES

Alleyne, GAO, Hay, RW, Picou, DI, Stanfield, JP, and Whithead, RG: Protein-energy Malnutrition. Edward Arnold, London, 1977.

Alpers, DH, Clouse, RE, and Stenson, WF: Manual of Nutritional Therapeutics. Little, Brown & Co, Boston, 1983.

Benedict, FG: A Study of Prolonged Fasting. Carnegie Institute Publication No. 203, Washington, DC, 1915.

Cerra, FB: Pocket Manual of Surgical Nutrition. CV Mosby, St. Louis, 1984.

Clark, JW: Nutrition in dental therapy. In Clark, JW (ed): Clinical Dentistry, Vol 1. Harper & Row, Hagerstown, 1983.

Dawber, TR: The Framingham Study. Harvard University Press, Cambridge, MA, 1980.

Diet, Nutrition and Cancer. National Academy Press, Washington, DC, 1982.

Feldman, EB (ed): Contemporary Issues in Clinical Nutrition, Vol 6, Nutrition and Heart Disease. Churchill Livingstone, New York, 1983.

Feldman, EB (ed): Nutrition in the Middle and Later Years. Wright-PSG, Littleton, MA, 1983.

Fischer, JE (ed): Surgical Nutrition. Little, Brown & Co, Boston, 1983.

Floch, MH: Nutrition and Diet Therapy in Gastrointestinal Disease. Plenum Publishing, New York, 1981.

Grand, RJ, Sutphen, JL, and Dietz, WH, Jr (eds): Pediatric Nutrition Theory and Practice. Butterworths, Boston, 1987.

Jeejeebhoy, KN: Total Parenteral Nutrition in the Hospital and at Home. CRC Press, Boca Raton, 1983.

Kerner, JA (ed): Manual of Pediatric Parenteral Nutrition. John Wiley & Sons, New York, 1983.

Keys, A: Seven Countries. Harvard University Press, Cambridge, MA, 1980.

Keys, A, Brozek, J, Hanschel, A, Mickelson, O, and Taylor, A: The Biology of Human Starvation. University of Minnesota Press, Minneapolis, 1950.

Lawrence, RA: Breast Feeding: A Guide for the Medical Profession. CV Mosby, St. Louis, 1980.

Mayo Clinic Diet Manual, ed 5. WB Saunders, Philadelphia, 1981.

Neuman, PA and Halvorson, PA: Anorexia Nervosa and Bulimia: A Guide for Counselors and Therapists. Van Nostrand Reinhold, New York, 1983.

Nutrition Education in U.S. Medical Schools. National Academy Press, Washington, D.C., 1985.

Nutrition Reviews' Present Knowledge in Nutrition, ed 5. The Nutrition Foundation, Inc., Washington, DC, 1984.

Paige, DM (ed): Manual of Clinical Nutrition. Nutrition Publications, Inc., Pleasantville, NJ, 1983.

Passmore, R and Eastwood, MA: Davidson and Passmore Human Nutrition and Dietetics, ed 8. Churchill Livingstone, New York, 1986.

Pediatric Nutrition Handbook, ed 2. American Academy of Pediatrics, Evanston, IL, 1985.

Read, MS, Bodner, J, and Sayadi, H: Guide to materials for use in teaching clinical nutrition in schools of medicine, dentistry and public health II. Am J Clin Nutr 45:643, 1987.

Recommended Dietary Allowances, ed 9. National Academy of Sciences, Washington, DC, 1980.

Roe, DA: Geriatric Nutrition, ed 2. Prentice-Hall, Englewood Cliffs, NJ, 1987.

Rombeau, JL and Caldwell, MD (eds): Clinical Nutrition, Vol 1, Enteral and Tube Feeding. WB Saunders, Philadelphia, 1984. Vol 2, Parenteral Nutrition, 1986.

Schneider, HA, Anderson, CE, and Coursin, DB: Nutritional Support of Medical Practice, ed 2. Harper & Row, Philadelphia, 1983.

Shils, ME and Young, VR (eds): Modern Nutrition in Health and Disease, ed 7. Lea & Febiger, Philadelphia, 1988.

Silberman, H and Eisenberg, D: Parenteral and Enteral Nutrition for the Hospitalized Patient. Appleton-Century-Crofts, East Norwalk, Conn, 1982.

Smith, DK and Feldman, EB: Parenteral Nutrition Handbook, ed 3. Medical College of Georgia, 1988.

Silberman, H and Eisenberg, D: Parenteral and Enteral Nutrition for the Hospitalized Patient. Appleton-Century-Crofts, East Norwalk, Conn, 1982.

Smith, DK, McLeod, NB, and Feldman, EB: Parenteral Nutrition Handbook, ed 2. Medical College of Georgia, 1984.

Suskind, RM (ed): Textbook of Pediatric Nutrition. Raven Press, New York, 1981.

Taylor, KB and Anthony, LE: Clinical Nutrition. McGraw-Hill, New York, 1983.

Weinsier, RL and Butterworth, CE: Handbook of Clinical Nutrition. CV Mosby, St. Louis, 1981.

Winick, M (ed): Nutritional Management of Genetic Disorders. John Wiley & Sons, New York, 1979.

Winters, RW and Greene HL: Bristol-Myers Nutrition Symposia, Vol 1, Nutritional Support of the Seriously Ill Patient. Academic Press, 1983.

Wright, RA and Heymsfield, S (eds): Nutritional Assessment. Blackwell Scientific Publications, Boston, 1984.

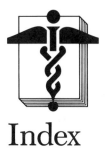

Index

A "t" following a page number indicates a table. An "f" following a page number indicates a figure.

impaired, 384
reduced, 383
zinc and, 52
Dorsolumbar kyphosis, 342
Drinking man's diet, 141
Drug-food interactions, 127–128
in elderly, 247
Drugs. *See also* Medications; specific drugs
absorption and bioavailability of, 128
breast feeding and, 186
influencing nutritional status, 127–128
Dumping syndrome, 489
Duodenal resection, 496
Duodenal ulcer, 488
Duodenostomy, 271
D-xylose malabsorption, 414
D-xylose test, 76
Dyes, organic, 110
Dysbetalipoproteinemia, 444–446
Dysentery, 117
Dyslipoproteinemias, 435
Dystrophic calcification, 483

Eating behaviors. *See also* Anorexia nervosa; Bulimia
cancer effects on, 538–539
motivation to modify, 398
Eating control mechanisms, defects in, 392
Echinococcus, 120
granulosis, 117, 119
Edema, 289
with excess sodium, 290
famine, 326
with liver cirrhosis, 509
management of, 509
Eggs, 95
allergy to, 126
essential amino acids in, 11
Eicosanoids, 21
Elastin degradation, 235
Elderly. *See also* Aging
body composition and metabolism in, 240
chronic illness in, 248
depression in, 246
hospitalized, 248–249
isolation of, 245–246
manifestations of aging in, 235–236
in nursing homes, 249
nutrition of, 234
counseling for, 234, 249
physiology and, 236–240
nutritional deficiencies in, 242–244

nutritional requirements in, 240–244
nutritional risks of, 245–248
overnutrition in, 244–245
scurvy in, 347
Electrocoagulation procedures, 267
Electrolyte(s)
balance of in athlete, 105
filtering of in kidney, 513
imbalance of, 219
with alcoholism, 414
with cardiac arrhythmias, 297
with parenteral nutrition, 299
with renal failure, 515, 519–520
with infection, 557
infusion of, 560
intake of
for dialysis patient, 526–527
in renal failure, 523–524
intravenous, 511
recommendations for infants and children, 211*t*
requirements for, 289–290
in sweat and gastrointestinal fluids, 45*t*
Elimination diet, 127, 227
Emulsifiers, 111
Encephalopathy, 503. *See also* Hepatic encephalopathy
with mercury poisoning, 120
Endocrine function, declining, 235
Endometrial cancer, 393, 534
Endorphins, 389
Endoscopic retrograde cannulation of the pancreas, 512
Energy
deficiency of, 327–328
expenditure of, 7
ideal body weight and, 8
respiratory quotient and, 9
fruits and, 96
intake of
increased, 16–17*f*
nitrogen balance and, 17
recommended, 390*t*
intake-expenditure ratio, with age, 241*f*
metabolism of
during 24-hour fast, 310*f*
with 5 to 6 week-fast, 312*f*
pattern of in trauma, 549*f*
requirements of, 7–8
differences in, 391–392
with infection, 558–559
meeting during starvation, 309
during pregnancy, 149–150